W9-BMG-137

ACADEMIC SKILLS PROBLEMS

The Guilford School Practitioner Series

EDITORS

STEPHEN N. ELLIOTT, PhD
Vanderbilt University

JOSEPH C. WITT, PhD
Louisiana State University, Baton Rouge

Recent Volumes

Academic Skills Problems

DIRECT ASSESSMENT AND INTERVENTION

Third Edition

◆ ◆ ◆

Edward S. Shapiro

◆

THE GUILFORD PRESS
New York   London

© 2004 The Guilford Press
A Division of Guilford Publications, Inc.
72 Spring Street, New York, NY 10012
www.guilford.com

All rights reserved

No part of this book may be reproduced, translated, stored in a retrieval system, or transmitted, in any form or by any means, electronic, mechanical, photocopying, microfilming, recording, or otherwise, without written permission from the Publisher.

Printed in the United States of America

This book is printed on acid-free paper.

Last digit is print number: 9   8   7   6   5   4   3

Library of Congress Cataloging-in-Publication Data

Shapiro, Edward S. (Edward Steven), 1951–
  Academic skills problems: direct assessment and intervention / Edward S. Shapiro.—3rd ed.
    p. cm.—(The Guilford school practitioner series)
  Includes bibliographical references (p.   ) and index.
  ISBN 1-57230-977-6 (hardcover: alk. paper)
  1. Remedial teaching.   2. Basic education.   3. Educational tests and measurements.   I. Title.   II. Series.
  LB1029.R4S5 2004
  372.4′3—dc22

                                           2004010860

To Ace and baseball;
My wife and children certainly understand.

About the Author

♦

Edward S. Shapiro, PhD, is Iacocca Professor of Education, Professor of School Psychology, and Director of the Center for Promoting Research to Practice at Lehigh University, Lehigh, Pennsylvania. He is also Executive Director of Lehigh Transition and Assessment Services, which provides training in the school-to-work transition for secondary school-age students and young adults with disabilities. A recipient of the Lightner Witmer Award from the Division of School Psychology of the American Psychological Association, in recognition of early career contributions to school psychology, he is past Editor of *School Psychology Review,* the official journal of the National Association of School Psychologists. Dr. Shapiro has written numerous books and publications in the areas of curriculum-based assessment, behavioral assessment, behavioral interventions, and self-management strategies for classroom behavior change, including *Conducting School-Based Assessments of Child and Adolescent Behavior* and *Behavioral Assessment in Schools, Second Edition: Theory, Research, and Clinical Foundations* (both coedited with Thomas R. Kratochwill), and *Promoting Children's Health: Integrating School, Family, and Community* (coauthored with Thomas J. Power, George J. DuPaul, and Anne E. Kazak). He is currently codirecting a federal training project focused on developing doctoral school psychologists as pediatric school psychologists, a model of training that attempts to train students to integrate health, psychological, and educational needs for children within school settings.

Preface to the Third Edition

◆

In the 15 years since the first edition of this text was published, significant shifts have been clearly evident in the assessment processes for students with academic skills problems. When the book first emerged, the high level of dissatisfaction with the use of norm-referenced, standardized tests was a driving force in leading many investigators to examine alternative methodologies to these types of measures. One of the alternatives was curriculum-based assessment (CBA). Focused on assessing students from instructional material, CBA began a journey toward increasing acceptance as a valid method for evaluating the academic performance of students. In particular, a striving to link the assessment and intervention processes together was a major element in CBA's attracting the attention of researchers, educational practitioners, psychologists, school administrators, and other key stakeholders concerned with improving the academic performance of students.

Over the past decade, we have witnessed both a shift in thinking and an intensification in the recognition of the importance of the assessment process in the education of students. Policies set at federal and state levels have made high-stakes testing of students a reality for evaluating educational programs. The passage of the No Child Left Behind (NCLB) bill by the U.S. Congress placed a requirement on all schools and states that the academic progress of every child be assessed in every grade, beginning in third grade. The strong emphasis on developing literacy in all children, a fundamental component of NCLB, has left no doubts about very serious efforts to ensure that the reading skills of *all* children in schools in the United States reach acceptable levels that allow them to be productive learners and contributors to society for the rest of their lives. In addition, there is a strong recognition that achieving the literacy goals of NCLB requires a focus on the prevention of the development of reading difficulties and takes aim at working with children long before they reach school age, as well as in the earliest grades of school.

Most recently, the reauthorization of the Individuals with Disabilities Education Act (IDEA) focuses clearly on both prevention of academic skills problems and an assessment methodology for determining eligibility for special education that moves us farther away from the use of published norm-referenced, standardized tests, particularly standardized tests of intellectual functioning. Whereas former models of identification relied primarily on discrepancy formulas examining differences between students' cognitive potential (i.e., intelligence) and their current functioning (i.e., achievement), the developing alternative to the identification of students with disabilities emphasizes a "response to intervention" model of evaluation. In that model, students who are struggling with academics would be provided with empirically based, strong intervention programs. The responsiveness of these students to such strong, research-based interventions would be the key factor in determining whether they are deemed as meeting eligibility criteria for placement in special education. For this model to be a reality, the assessment methodology to evaluate responsiveness to intervention must be capable of assessing a student's sensitivity to intervention over time and reflect the impact of instruction. The system of assessment that is viewed as having one of the strongest research bases is CBA, the methods described in this text.

Readers familiar with previous editions of the text will find that all chapters have been updated, with the incorporation of new references, new tables and figures, and some new thinking on my part. In particular, increased emphasis is provided on a problem-solving process for intervention development. Case studies were selected to reflect more up-to-date issues, such as assessing students whose first language is not English. Substantial reference to available websites on the Internet, as well as commercially available and free products, is made throughout the text. Indeed, the explosion of information available through the Internet since the publication of the second edition presents a tough challenge to an author. I have certainly tried to make sure that links provided in the text are current and accurate, but as we all know, these links change without notice, so apologies ahead of time to any readers who have difficulties finding links that I cite in the text.

As with all previous editions, the text remains useful for all school-based practitioners. Indeed, I have always aimed the text at the practitioner and have tried to write in ways that make the book immediately useful and easy for implementation. Anyone with interest and a need to assess academic skills problems—school psychologists, special education teachers, educational consultants, general educators, reading specialists, and school administrators—should find the book useful. In addition, students in training to enter school-based professions should also find this an excellent resource for understanding this type of assessment methodology.

As do all authors, I need first to thank many people who help to keep this text alive and exciting. Most important, I want to thank my graduate students in school psychology at Lehigh University. Over my 24 years at Lehigh, these bright, articulate, and energetic people have continued to inspire and challenge my own thinking. These students have been willing field-testers of new concepts, and have helped to refine and improve my ideas. These built-in critics have offered me an unparalleled opportunity to make sure that what I recommend has stood the test of the real world. To have watched many of my former students emerge in our field as leaders who continue to teach these same principles has truly been one of the greatest experiences one can have as a professor.

Second, I want to give thanks to the many colleagues in the fields of school psychology and special education around the country whose work I have admired and used as the basis of evolving my own thinking. It is truly exciting to have such a great community of colleagues who can learn from and share with each other. Only as a collective can we really make an impact on improving the lives of children.

Last, but always first in my heart, is thanks to members of my family, who remain incredibly supportive of my career. Over the years since the first edition of this book was published, I have watched my eldest son, Dan, graduate from college and move along in a very successful career path to personal independence from his parents. I have watched my youngest son, Jay, move from playing T-ball to becoming a senior in college, and have seen him travel to Africa to seek dreams of filmmaking and achieve a level of caring for others in his life that is so gratifying to a parent. My wife, Sally, has remained a steady and incredibly supportive partner as I work the long hours that allow me to do my life's passion. Indeed, it is these deep family roots that continue to inspire me to help improve the lives of those children who are less fortunate than my own.

Contents

◆

xiii

CHAPTER 1

◆ ◆ ◆

Introduction

◆

Brian, a second-grade student at Salter Elementary School, was referred to the school psychologist for evaluation. The request for evaluation from the multidisciplinary team noted that he was easily distracted and was having difficulty in most academic subjects. Background information reported on the referral request indicated that he was retained in kindergarten and was on the list this year for possible retention. As a result of his difficulties sitting still during class, his desk has been removed from the area near his peers and placed adjacent to the teacher's desk. Brian currently receives remedial math lessons.

Susan was in the fifth grade at Carnell Elementary School. She had been in a self-contained classroom for students with learning disabilities since second grade and was currently doing very well. Her teacher referred her to determine her current academic status and potential for increased mainstreaming.

Jorgé was in the third grade at Moore Elementary School. He was referred by his teacher because he was struggling in reading and had been in the English as a Second Language (ESL) program for the past year since arriving from Puerto Rico. Jorgé's teacher was concerned that he was not achieving the expected level of progress compared to other students with similar backgrounds.

All of these cases are samples of the many types of referrals for academic problems faced by school personnel. How should the team proceed to conduct the evaluations? The answer to this question clearly lies in how the problems are conceptualized. Most often, the multidisciplinary team

1

will view the problem within a diagnostic framework. In Brian's case, the primary question asked would be whether he is eligible for special education services and if so, in which category. In Susan's case, the question would be whether her skills have improved sufficiently to suggest that she will be successful in a less restrictive setting. Jorgé's case raises questions of whether his difficulties in reading are a function of his status as an ESL learner, or whether he has other difficulties requiring special education services. In all cases, the methodology employed in conducting these types of traditional assessments is similar.

Typically, the school psychologist would administer an individual intelligence test (usually the Wechsler Intelligence Scale for Children—Fourth Edition [WISC-IV; Wechsler, 2003]), an individual achievement test (such as the Peabody Individual Achievement Test—Revised/Normative Update [PIAT-R/NU; Markwardt, 1997], or the Wechsler Individual Achievement Test–II [WIAT–II; Wechsler, 2001]), and a test of visual–motor integration (usually the Bender–Gestalt). Often, the psychologist would add some measure of personality, such as projective drawings. Other professionals, such as educational consultants or educational diagnosticians, might assess the child's specific academic skills by administering norm-referenced achievement tests such as the Woodcock–Johnson Psychoeducational Battery–III (Woodcock, McGrew, & Mather, 2001), the Key Math—Revised/Normative Update (Connoley, 1997), or other diagnostic instruments. Based on these test results, a determination of eligibility (in the cases of Brian and Jorgé) or evaluation of academic performance (in the case of Susan) would be made.

When Brian was evaluated in this traditional way, the results revealed that he was not eligible for special education. Not surprisingly, Brian's teacher requested that the multidisciplinary team make some recommendations for remediating his skills. From this type of assessment, it was very difficult to make specific recommendations. The team suggested that since Brian was not eligible for special education, he was probably doing the best he could in his current classroom. They did note that his phonetic analysis skills appeared weak and recommended that some consideration be given to switching him to a less phonetically oriented approach to reading.

When Susan was assessed, the data showed that she was still substantially below grade levels in all academic areas. Despite having spent the last 3 years in a self-contained classroom for students with learning disabilities, Susan had made minimal progress when compared to peers of similar age and grade. As a result, the team decided to not increase the amount of time that she be mainstreamed for academic subjects.

When Jorgé was assessed, the team also administered measures to assess his overall language development. Specifically, the Woodcock–Muñóz Language Survey (Woodcock & Muñóz-Sandoval, 1996) was given to assess his Cognitive Academic Language Proficiency (CALP), the degree to which students' acquisition of their second language enables them to effectively use the second language in cognitive processing. The data showed that his poor reading skills were a function of less than expected development in English rather than a general underdeveloped ability in his native language. Jorgé, therefore, was not considered eligible for special education services other than programs for second language learners.

In contrast to viewing the referral problems of Brian, Susan, and Jorgé as diagnostic problems, one could also conceptualize their referrals as questions of "which remediation strategies would be likely to improve academic skills." Seen in this way, the assessment process becomes a problem-solving process and involves a very different set of methodologies. First, to identify remediation strategies, one must have a clear understanding of the child's mastery of skills that were taught, the rate at which learning occurs when the child is taught at his/her instructional level, and a thorough understanding of the instructional environment in which learning had occurred. To do this, one must look to the material that was actually instructed, the curriculum, rather than to a set of tasks that may or may not actually have been taught (i.e., standardized tests). The assessment process must be dynamic and evaluate how the child progresses across time when effective instruction is provided. Such assessment needs measures that are sensitive to the impact of instructional interventions. A clear understanding of the instructional ecology is attained only through methods of direct observation, teacher and student interviewing, and examination of student-generated products, such as worksheets. When the assessment is conducted from this perspective, the results are more directly linked to developing intervention strategies and making decisions about which interventions are most effective.

When Brian was assessed in this way, it was found that he was appropriately placed in the curriculum materials in both reading and math. Deficiencies in mastery of basic addition and subtraction facts were identified. In particular, specific problems in spelling and written expression were noted, and specific recommendations for instruction in capitalization and punctuation were made. Moreover, the assessment team members suggested that Brian's seat be moved, because they found that he really was not as distractible as the teacher had indicated. When these interventions were put in place, Brian showed gains in performance in reading and math that equaled those of general education classmates.

Results of Susan's direct assessment were more surprising and in direct contrast to the traditional evaluation. Although it was found that Susan was appropriately placed in the areas of reading, math, and spelling, examination of her skills in the curriculum showed that she probably could be successful in the lowest reading group within a general education classroom. In particular, it was found that she had attained fifth-grade math skills within the curriculum, despite scoring below grade level on the standardized test. When her reading group was changed to the lowest level in fifth grade, Susan's data over a 13-week period showed that she was making the same level of progress as her fifth-grade classmates without disabilities.

Jorgé's assessment was also a surprise. Although his poor language development in English was evident, Jorgé showed that he was successful in learning, comprehending, and reading when the identical material with which he struggled in English was presented in his native language. In fact, it was determined that Jorgé was much more successful in learning to read in English once he was able to read the same material in Spanish. In Jorgé's case, monitoring his reading performance in both English and Spanish showed that he was making slow but consistent progress. Although he was still reading English at a level equal to that of first-grade students, goals were set for Jorgé to achieve a level of reading performance similar to middle second grade by the end of the school year. Data collected over that time showed at the end of the third grade, he was reading at a level similar to students at a beginning second-grade level, making almost 1 year of academic progress over the past 5 months.

The focus of this text is on the direct assessment and intervention methodologies for the evaluation and remediation of academic problems. Specifically, detailed descriptions of conducting a behavioral assessment of academic skills (as developed by Shapiro, 1990, 1996a; Shapiro & Lentz, 1985, 1986) are presented. Direct interventions, those focused on teaching the skills directly assessed, are also presented.

BACKGROUND, HISTORY, AND RATIONALE
FOR ACADEMIC ASSESSMENT AND INTERVENTION

The percentage of children experiencing academic problems consistently has been of concern to school personnel. Over the past 10 years, the percentage nationally of students who have been identified and have received special education services has increased steadily. In 1999–2000, approximately 11.4% of the U.S. population between 6 and 17 years of age were identified as eligible for special education services. According to the *23rd Annual Report to Congress on the Implementation of the Education of the Handicapped Act* (U.S. Department of Education, 2001), there has been a rise of 30.3% in the number of students receiving special education services over this period. Relative to this increase, the group classified as having learning disabilities (LD) has grown the most, making up 50.5% of those classified and receiving special education services in 2000. In comparison, the percentage of students served under most other handicapping conditions has remained stable. Although much of the increase may be due to different ways of defining and assessing students believed to have LD, a significant number of students are having substantial difficulties mastering basic academic skills. These concerns have been extended beyond special education, with the increased effort to develop statewide standards for academic achievement and the establishment of statewide competency-based testing and remediation in regular education (Braden, 2002; Linn, 2000).

Concern about the number of students identified as having LD has challenged the way that assessment for identification of these students has been done. In particular, the use of a discrepancy formula (i.e., making eligibility decisions based on the discrepancies between attained scores on intelligence and achievement tests) has been challenged significantly. Such approaches to determining eligibility have been found to lack empirical support (Fletcher, Morris, & Lyon, 2003; Peterson & Shinn, 2002; Sternberg & Grigorenko, 2002; Stuebing et al., 2002).

Among the alternative approaches to identification, the process known as "responsiveness to intervention" has been proposed. This method requires the identification of the degree to which a student responds to academic interventions that are known to be highly effective. Students who do not respond positively to such interventions would be considered as potentially eligible for services related to LD (Fletcher et al., 2002; Gresham, 2002). Although this procedure still has limited empirical support (e.g., Fuchs, Fuchs, & Speece, 2002) and critics are unconvinced that the responsiveness to intervention approach to assessment will solve the problem of overidentification of LD (Scruggs & Mastropieri, 2002), support for moving away from the use of a discrepancy formula in the assessment of LD appears to be strong. Clearly, data have shown that academic skills problems remain the major focus of referrals for evaluation.

Bramlett, Murphy, Johnson, and Wallingsford (2002) examined the patterns of referrals made for school psychological services. Surveying a national sample of school psychologists, they ranked academic problems as the most frequent reasons for referral, with 57% of total referrals made for reading problems, 43% for written expression, 39% for task completion, and 27% for mathematics. These data were similar to the findings of Ownby, Wallbrown, D'Atri, and Armstrong (1985), who examined the patterns of referrals made for school psychological services within a small school system (school population = 2,800). Across all grade levels except preschool and kindergarten (where few total referrals were made), referrals for academic problems exceeded referrals for behavior problems by almost five to one.

Clearly, there are significant needs for effective assessment and intervention strategies to address academic problems in school-age children.

Indeed, the number of commercially available standardized achievement tests (e.g., Salvia & Ysseldyke, 2001) suggests that evaluation of academic progress has been a long-standing concern among educators. Goh, Teslow, and Fuller (1981), in an examination of testing practices of school psychologists, provided additional evidence regarding the number and range of tests used in assessments conducted by school psychologists. A replication of the Goh et al. study 10 years later found few differences (Hutton, Dubes, & Muir, 1992). Other studies have continued to replicate the original report of Goh et al. (Stinnett, Havey, & Oehler-Stinnett, 1994; Wilson & Reschly, 1996). Shapiro and Heick (2004) found that there has been some shift in the past decade among school psychologists to include behavior rating scales and direct observation when conducting evaluations for students referred for behavior problems.

Despite the historically strong concern about assessing and remediating academic problems, there remains significant controversy about the most effective methods for conducting useful assessments and choosing the most effective intervention strategies. In particular, longtime dissatisfaction with commercially available, norm-referenced tests has been evident among educational professionals (e.g., Donovan & Cross, 2002; Heller, Holtzman, & Messick, 1982; Hively & Reynolds, 1975; Wiggins, 1989). Likewise, strategies that attempt to remediate deficient learning processes identified by these measures have not been found to be useful in effecting change in academic performance (e.g., Arter & Jenkins, 1979; Good, Vollmer, Creek, Katz, & Chowdhri, 1993).

ASSESSMENT AND DECISION MAKING FOR ACADEMIC PROBLEMS

Salvia and Ysseldyke (2001) define assessment as "the process of collecting data for the purpose of (1) specifying and verifying problems, and (2) making decisions about students" (p. 5). They identify five types of decisions that can be made from assessment data: referral, screening, classification, instructional planning, and monitoring pupils' progress. They also add that decisions about the effectiveness of programs (program evaluation) can be made from assessment data.

Not all assessment methodologies for evaluating academic behavior can equally address each of the types of decisions needed. For example, norm-referenced instruments may be useful for classification decisions but are not very valuable for decisions regarding instructional programming. Likewise, criterion-referenced tests that offer intrasubject comparisons may be useful in identifying relative strengths and weaknesses of academic performance but may not be sensitive to monitoring student progress within a curriculum. Methods that use frequent, repeated assessments may be valuable tools for monitoring progress but may not offer sufficient data on diagnosing the nature of a student's academic problem. Clearly, use of a particular assessment strategy should be linked to the type of decision one wishes to make. A methodology that can be used across types of decisions would be extremely valuable.

It seems logical that the various types of decisions described by Salvia and Ysseldyke (2001) should require the collection of different types of data. Unfortunately, an examination of the state of practice in assessment suggests that this is not the case. Goh et al. (1981) reported data suggesting that regardless of the reason for referral, most school psychologists administer an individual intelligence test, a general test of achievement, a test of perceptual–motor performance, and a projective personality measure. A replication of the Goh et al. study 10 years later found that little had changed. Psychologists still spent more than 50% of their time engaged in assessment. Hutton et al. (1992) noted that the emphasis on intelligence tests noted by Goh et al. (1981) had lessened, whereas the use of achievement tests had increased. Hutton et al. (1992) also found that the use of behavior rating scales and adaptive behavior measures had increased somewhat. Stinnett et al. (1994), as well as Wilson and Reschly (1996), again replicated the basic findings of Goh et al. (1981). Shapiro and Heick (2004) in a more recent survey of assessment practices, did find some shifting of assessment practices for students referred for behavior disorders toward the use of measures such as behavior rating scales and systematic direct observation. Shapiro, Angello, and Eckert (2004) also found some self-reported movement of school psychologists over the past decade toward the use of CBA measures when the referral was for academic skills problems. Even so, almost 47% of those surveyed reported that they had not used CBA in their practice.

In this chapter, an overview of the conceptual issues of academic assessment and remediation is provided. The framework upon which behavioral assessment and intervention for academic problems are based is described. First, however, the current state of academic assessment and intervention is examined.

TYPES OF INDIVIDUAL ASSESSMENT METHODS

Norm-Referenced Tests

One of the most common methods of evaluating individual academic skills involves the administration of published norm-referenced, commercial, standardized tests. These measures contain items that sample specific academic skills within a content area. Scores on the test are derived by comparing the results for the child being tested to scores obtained by a large, nonclinical, same-age/same-grade sample of children. Various types of standard scores are used to describe the relative standing of the target child against the normative sample.

The primary purpose of norm-referenced tests is to make comparisons with "expected" responses. Collection of norms gives the assessor a reference point for identifying the degree to which the responses of the identified student differ significantly from those of the average same-age/same-grade peer. This information may be useful when making special education eligibility decisions, since degree of deviation from the norm is an important consideration in meeting requirements for various handicaps.

There are different types of individual norm-referenced tests of academic achievement. Some measures provide broad-based assessments of academic skills, such as the Wide Range Achievement Test—Third Edition (WRAT-III; Wilkenson, 1993); the PIAT-R/NU (Markwardt, 1997); the WIAT-II (Wechsler, 2001); or the Kaufman Test of Educational Achievement—Normative Update (K-TEA/NU; Kaufman & Kaufman, 1997). These tests each contain various subtests that assess reading, math, and spelling, and provide overall scores for each content area. Other norm-referenced tests, such as the Woodcock Reading Mastery Test—Revised/Normative Update (Woodcock, 1998), are designed to be more diagnostic and offer scores on subskills within the content area, such as passage comprehension, word recognition, or phonetic analysis.

Despite the popular and widespread use of norm-referenced tests for assessing individual academic skills, a number of significant problems may severely limit their usefulness. If a test is to evaluate a student's acquisition of knowledge, then the test should assess what was taught within the curriculum of the child. If there is little overlap between the curriculum and the test, a child's failure to show improvement on the measure may not necessarily reflect failure to learn what was taught. Instead, the child's failure may only be related to the test's poor correlation with the curriculum in which the child was instructed. In a replication and extension of the work of Jenkins and Pany (1978), Shapiro and Derr (1987) examined the degree of overlap between five commonly used basal reading series and four commercial, norm-referenced achievement tests. At each grade level (first through fifth), the number of words appearing on each subtest and in the reading series were counted. The resulting score was converted to a standard score ($M = 100$, $SD = 15$), percentile, and grade equivalent, using the standardization data provided for each subtest. Results of this analysis are reported in Table 1.1. Across subtests and reading series, there appeared to be little and inconsistent overlap between the words appearing in the series and on the tests.

Although these results suggest that the overlap between what is taught and what is tested on reading subtests is questionable, the data examined by Shapiro and Derr (1987) and Jenkins and Pany (1978) were hypothetical. It certainly is possible that such poor overlap does not actually exist, since the achievement tests are designed only as samples of skills and not as direct assessments. Good and Salvia (1988) and Bell, Lentz, and Graden (1992) have provided evidence that with actual students evaluated on common achievement measures, there is inconsistent overlap between the basal reading series employed in their studies and the different measures of reading achievement.

In the Good and Salvia (1988) study, a total of 65 third- and fourth-grade students who were all being instructed in the same basal reading series (Allyn & Bacon Pathfinder Program, 1978), were administered four reading subtests: the Reading Vocabulary subtest of the California Achievement Test (CAT; Tiegs & Clarke, 1970), the Word Knowledge subtest of the Metropolitan Achievement Test (MAT; Durost, Bixler, Wrightsone, Prescott, & Balow, 1970), the Reading Recognition subtest of the Peabody Individual Achievement Test (PIAT; Dunn & Markwardt, 1970), and the Reading subtest of the Wide Range Achievement Test (WRAT; Jastak & Jastak, 1978). Results of their analysis showed significant differences in test performance for the same students on different reading tests, predicted by the test's content validity.

Using a similar methodology, Bell et al. (1992) examined the content validity of three popular achievement tests: Reading Decoding subtest of the K-TEA, Reading subtest of the Wide Range Achievement Test—Revised (WRAT-R; Jastak & Wilkinson, 1984), and the Word Identification subtest of the Woodcock Reading Mastery Tests—Revised (WRMT-R; Woodcock, 1987). All students ($n = 181$) in the first and second grades of two school districts were administered these tests. Both districts used the Macmillan-R (Smith & Arnold, 1986) reading series. Results showed dramatic differences across tests when a word-by-word content analysis (Jenkins & Pany, 1978) was conducted. Perhaps more importantly, significant differences were evident across tests for students within each grade level. For example, as seen in Table 1.2, students in one district obtained an average standard score of 117.19 ($M = 100$, $SD = 15$) on the WRMT-R and a score of 102.44 on the WRAT-R, a difference of a full standard deviation.

Problems of overlap between test and text content are not limited to the area of reading alone. For example, Shriner and Salvia (1988) conducted an examination of the curriculum overlap between two elementary mathematics curricula and two commonly used individual norm-referenced standardized tests (Key Math, and Iowa Tests of Basic Skills) across grades 1–3. Hultquist and Metzke (1993) examined the overlap across grades 1–6 between standardized measures of spelling performance (subtests from the K-TEA, Woodcock–Johnson—Revised [WJ-R], PIAT-R, Diagnostic Achievement Battery–2, Test of Written Spelling–2) and three basal spelling

TABLE 1.1. Overlap between Basal Reader Curricula and Tests

	PIAT				WRAT-R				K-TEA				WRM			
	RS	GE	%tile	SS	RS	GE	%tile	SS	RS	GE	%tile	SS	RS	GE	%tile	SS
Ginn-720																
Grade 1	23	1.8	58	103	40	1M	47	99	14	1.6	37	95	38	1.8	38	96
Grade 2	28	2.8	50	100	52	2M	39	96	23	2.6	42	97	69	2.5	33	94
Grade 3	37	4.0	52	101	58	2E	27	91	27	3.2	32	93	83	3.0	24	90
Grade 4	40	4.4	40	96	58	2E	16	85	27	3.2	16	85	83	3.0	10	81
Grade 5	40	4.4	25	90	61	3B	12	82	28	3.4	9	80	83	3.0	4	74
Scott, Foresman																
Grade 1	20	1.4	27	91	39	1M	41	97	12	1.5	27	91	33	1.8	30	92
Grade 2	23	1.8	13	83	44	1E	16	85	17	1.9	18	86	63	2.3	27	91
Grade 3	23	1.8	7	78	46	2B	4	73	17	1.9	5	70	63	2.3	9	80
Grade 4	23	1.8	3	72	46	2B	1	67	17	1.9	2	70	63	2.3	2	70
Grade 5	23	1.8	1	65	46	2B	.7	59	17	1.9	1	66	63	2.3	.4	56
Macmillan-R																
Grade 1	23	1.8	58	103	35	1B	30	92	13	1.6	32	93	42	1.9	44	98
Grade 2	24	2.0	20	87	41	1M	10	81	18	2.0	19	87	58	2.2	22	89
Grade 3	24	2.0	9	80	48	2B	5	76	21	2.3	12	82	66	2.4	10	81

10

Grade 4	24	2.0	4	74	48	2B	2	70	21	2.3	5	75	67	2.5	3	72
Grade 5	24	2.0	2	69	50	2M	1	65	21	2.3	2	70	67	2.5	2	69

Keys to Reading

Grade 1	24	2.0	68	107	41	1M	50	100	15	1.7	42	97	42	1.9	44	98
Grade 2	28	2.8	50	100	51	2M	37	95	20	2.2	27	91	68	2.5	33	94
Grade 3	35	3.8	47	99	59	3B	30	92	24	2.7	19	87	84	3.1	26	91
Grade 4	35	3.8	26	91	59	3B	18	86	24	2.7	9	80	84	3.1	11	82
Grade 5	35	3.8	14	84	59	3B	8	79	25	2.8	5	76	84	3.1	4	74

Scott, Foresman—Focus

Grade 1	23	1.8	58	103	35	1B	30	92	13	1.6	32	93	37	1.8	35	94
Grade 2	25	2.2	28	91	46	2B	21	88	17	1.9	18	86	56	2.1	20	89
Grade 3	27	2.6	21	88	49	2B	6	77	20	2.2	10	81	68	2.5	11	82
Grade 4	28	2.8	11	82	54	2M	8	79	22	2.4	6	77	76	2.8	7	78
Grade 5	28	2.8	6	77	55	2E	4	73	24	2.7	4	64	81	2.9	3	72

Note. The grade-equivalent scores "B, M, E" for the WRAT-R refer to the assignment of the score to the beginning, middle, or end of the grade level. RS, raw scores; GE, grade equivalent; SS, standard score ($M = 100$; $SD = 15$); PIAT, Peabody Individual Achievement Test; WRAT-R, Wide Range Achievement Test; K-TEA, Kaufman Test of Educational Achievement; WRM, Woodcock Reading Mastery Test. From Shapiro and Derr (1987, pp. 60–61). Copyright 1987 by Pro-Ed, Inc. Reprinted by permission.

TABLE 1.2. Student Performance Scores on Standardized
Achievement Tests in Districts 1 and 2

		Test		
Group	n	WRMT-R	K-TEA	WRAT-R
District 1				
Grade 1	52			
M		117.19	110.31	102.44
SD		17.63	15.67	11.55
Grade 2	47			
M		112.61	104.04	103.68
SD		14.98	13.34	11.02
Total	99			
M		115.11	108.76	102.30
SD		15.91	14.74	11.79
District 2				
Grade 1	40			
M		113.08	105.23	100.20
SD		14.57	13.02	12.31
Grade 2	42			
M		108.60	108.86	99.26
SD		14.96	13.04	12.42
Total	82			
M		110.78	106.06	99.73
SD		14.86	12.98	12.29

Note. From Bell, Lentz, and Graden (1992), p. 651). Copyright 1992 by the
National Association of School Psychologists. Reprinted by permission.

series, as well as the presence of high-frequency words. An assessment of
the correspondence for content, as well as the type of learning required,
revealed a lack of content correspondence at all levels in both studies.

One potential difficulty with poor curriculum–test overlap is that test
results from these measures may be interpreted as indicative of a student's
failure to acquire skills taught. This conclusion may contribute to more
dramatic decisions, such as changing an educational placement. Unfortunately, if the overlap between what is tested and what is taught is questionable, then the use of these measures to examine student change across time
is problematic.

Despite potential problems in curriculum–test overlap, individual
norm-referenced tests are still useful for deciding the relative standing of an
individual within a peer group. Although this type of information is valuable in making eligibility decisions, it may have limited use in other types of
assessment decisions. An important consideration in assessing academic

skills is to determine how much progress students have made across time. This requires that periodic assessments be conducted. Because norm-referenced tests are developed as samples of skills and are therefore limited in the numbers of items that sample various skills, the frequent repetition of these measures results in significant bias. Indeed, these measures were never designed to be repeated at frequent intervals without compromising the integrity of the test. Use of norm-referenced tests to assess student progress is not possible.

In addition to the problem of bias from frequent repetition of the tests, the limited skills assessed on these measures may result in very poor sensitivity to small changes in student behavior. Typically, norm-referenced tests contain items that sample across a large array of skills. As students are instructed, gains evident on a day-to-day basis may not appear on the norm-referenced test, since these skills may not be reflected on test items.

Another problem related to individual norm-referenced tests is their inability to contribute effectively to decisions about programmatic interventions. Although norm-referenced tests were never designed to be used to make educational recommendations for remediation, they continue to be employed frequently in this way by school psychologists. In a survey, Thurlow and Ysseldyke (1982) found that the WISC-R, WRAT, and Bender–Gestalt were reported by school psychologists to be most useful in making intervention recommendations, whereas teachers reported the WISC-R, PIAT, and Key Math test to be valuable. With the exception of perhaps the Key Math, all of these tests were being used for a purpose (instructional planning) for which they were never designed.

Overall, individual norm-referenced tests may have the potential to contribute to decisions regarding eligibility for special education. Because these tests provide a standardized comparison across peers of similar age or grade, the relative standing of students can be helpful in identifying the degree to which the assessed student is deviant. Unfortunately, norm-referenced tests cannot be sensitive to small changes in student behavior, were never designed to contribute to the development of intervention procedures, and may not relate closely to what is actually being taught. These limitations may severely limit the usefulness of these measures for academic evaluations.

Criterion-Referenced Tests

Another method for assessing individual academic skills is to examine a student's mastery of specific skills. This procedure requires comparison of student performance against an absolute standard that reflects acquisition of a skill rather than the normative comparison made to same-age/same-grade peers that is employed in norm-referenced testing. Indeed, many of the statewide, high-stakes assessment measures use criterion-referenced scoring procedures, identifying students as scoring in categories such as "below basic," "proficient," or "advanced." Criterion-referenced tests are instruments referenced to domains of behavior and offer intrasubject rather than intersubject comparisons.

Scores on criterion-referenced measures are interpreted by examining the particular skill assessed and then deciding whether the score meets a criterion that reflects student mastery of that skill. By looking across the different skills assessed, one is able to determine the particular components of the content area assessed (e.g., reading, math, social studies) that represent strengths and weaknesses in a student's academic profile. One problem with some criterion-referenced tests is that it is not clear how the criterion representing mastery was derived. Although it seems that the logical method for establishing this criterion may be a normative comparison (i.e., criterion = number of items passed by 80% of same-age/same-grade peers), most criterion-referenced tests establish the acceptable criterion score on the basis of logical rather than empirical analysis.

Excellent examples of individual criterion-referenced instruments are a series of inventories developed by Brigance. Each of these measures is designed for a different age group, with the Brigance Inventory for Early Development–II (Brigance, 2004) containing subtests geared for children from birth through age 7, the Brigance Comprehensive Inventory of Basic Skills—Revised (CIBS-R; Brigance, 1999) providing inventories for skills development between prekindergarten and grade 9, and the Brigance Diagnostic Inventory of Essential Skills (Brigance, 1981) aiming at secondary-age students. Each measure includes skills in academic areas such as readiness, speech, listening, reading, spelling, writing, mathematics, study skills. The inventories cover a wide range of subskills, and each inventory is linked to specific behavioral objectives.

Although individual criterion-referenced tests appear to address some of the problems with norm-referenced instruments, they may only be useful for certain types of assessment decisions. For example, criterion-referenced measures may be excellent tests for screening decisions. Because we are interested in identifying children who may be at risk for academic failure, the use of a criterion-referenced measure should provide a direct comparison of the skills present in our assessed student against the range of skills expected by same-age/same-grade peers. In this way, we can easily identify those students who have substantially fewer or weaker skills and target these students for more in-depth evaluation.

By contrast, criterion-referenced tests usually are not helpful in making decisions about special education classifications. If criterion-referenced measures are to be used to make such decisions, it is critical that skills expected to be present in nonhandicapped students be identified. Because these measures do not typically have a normative base, it becomes difficult to make statements about a student's relative standing to peers. For example, to use a criterion-referenced test in kindergarten screening, it is necessary to know the type and level of subskills that children should possess as they enter kindergarten. If this information were known, the obtained score of a specific student could be compared to the expected score, and a decision regarding probability for success could be derived. Of course, the empirical verification of this score would be necessary, since the identification of subskills needed for kindergarten entrance would most likely be obtained initially through teacher interview. Clearly, although criterion-referenced tests could be used to make classification decisions, they typically are not employed in this way.

Perhaps the decision to which criterion-referenced tests can contribute significantly is the identification of target areas for the development of educational interventions. Given that these measures contain assessments of subskills within a domain, they may be useful in identifying the specific strengths and weaknesses of a student's academic profile. The measures do not, however, offer direct assistance in the identification of intervention strategies that may be successful in remediation. Instead, by suggesting a student's strengths, they may aid in the development of interventions capitalizing on these subskills to remediate weaker areas of academic functioning. It is important to remember that criterion-referenced tests can tell us what a student can and cannot do, but they do not tell us what variables are related to the student's success or failure.

One area in which individual criterion-referenced tests appear problematic is in decisions regarding monitoring of student progress. It would seem logical that since these measures only make intrasubject comparisons, they would be valuable for monitoring student progress across time. Unfortunately, these tests share with norm-referenced measures the problem of curriculum–test overlap. Most criterion-referenced measures have been developed by examining published curricula and pulling a subset of items together to assess a subskill. As such, student gains in a specific curriculum may or may not be related directly to performance on the criterion-referenced test. Tindal, Wesson, Deno, Germann, and Mirkin (1985) found that although criterion-referenced instruments may be useful for assessing some academic skills, not all measures showed strong relationships to student progress in a curriculum. Thus, these measures may be subject to some of the same biases raised in regard to norm-referenced tests (Armbruster, Stevens, & Rosenshine, 1977; Bell et al., 1992; Good & Salvia, 1988; Jenkins & Pany, 1978; Shapiro & Derr, 1987).

Another problem related to monitoring student progress is the limited range of subskills included in a criterion-referenced test. Typically, most criterion-referenced measures contain a limited sample of subskills, as well as a limited number of items assessing any particular subskill. These limitations make the repeated use of the measure over a short period of time questionable. Furthermore, the degree to which these measures may be sensitive to small changes in student growth is unknown. Using criterion-referenced tests to assess student progress may therefore be problematic.

Criterion-referenced tests may be somewhat useful for decisions regarding program evaluation. These types of decisions involve examination of the progress of a large number of students across a relatively long period of time. As such, any problem of limited curriculum–test overlap or sensitivity to short-term growth of students would be unlikely to affect the outcome. For example, one could use the measure to determine the percentage of students in each grade meeting the preset criteria for different subskills. Such a normative comparison may be of use in evaluating the instructional validity of the program. When statewide assessment data are reported, they are often used exactly in this way to identify districts or schools that are meeting or exceeding expected standards.

Strengths and Weaknesses
of Norm- and Criterion-Referenced Tests

In general, criterion-referenced tests appear to have certain advantages over norm-referenced measures. These tests have strong relationships to intra-subject comparison methods and strong ties to behavioral assessment strategies (Cancelli & Kratochwill, 1981; Elliott & Fuchs, 1997). Furthermore, because the measures offer assessments of subskills within broader areas, they may provide useful mechanisms for the identification of remediation targets in the development of intervention strategies. Criterion-referenced tests may also be particularly useful in the screening process.

Despite these advantages, the measures do not appear to be applicable to all types of educational decision making. Questions of educational classification, monitoring student progress, and developing intervention strategies may not be addressed adequately with these measures alone. Problems of curriculum–test overlap, sensitivity to short-term academic growth, and selection of subskills assessed may all act to limit the potential use of these instruments.

Clearly, what is needed in the evaluation of academic skills is a method that more directly assesses student performance within the academic curriculum. Both norm- and criterion-referenced measures provide an indirect evaluation of skills by assessing students on a sample of items taken from expected grade-level performance. Unfortunately, the items selected may not have strong relationships to what students were actually asked to learn. More importantly, because the measures provide samples of behavior, they may not be sensitive to small gains in student performance across time. As such, they cannot directly tell us whether our present intervention methods are succeeding.

Equally important is the failure of these measures to take into account the potential influence the environment may have on student academic performance. Both norm- and criterion-referenced instruments may tell us certain things about a student's individual skills but little about variables that affect academic performance, such as instructional methods for presenting material, feedback mechanisms, classroom structure, competing contingencies, and so forth (Lentz & Shapiro, 1986).

What is needed in the assessment of academic skills is a methodology that can more directly assess both the student's skills and the academic environment. This methodology also needs to be able to address most or all of the types of educational decisions identified by Salvia and Ysseldyke (2001).

Direct Assessment of Academic Skills

A large number of assessment models have been derived for the direct evaluation of academic skills (e.g., Blankenship, 1985; Déno, 1985; Gickling & Havertape, 1981; Howell & Nolet, 1999; Salvia & Hughes, 1990; Shapiro, 1989, 1996a; Shapiro & Lentz, 1986). All of these models have in common the underlying assumption that *one should test what one teaches.* As such, the contents for the assessments employed for each model are based on the instructional curriculum. In contrast to the potential problem of poor overlap between the curriculum and the test in other forms of academic assessment, evaluation methods that are based on the curriculum offer direct evaluations of student performance on material that students are expected to acquire. Thus, the inferences that may have to be made with more indirect assessment methods are avoided.

Despite the underlying commonality of the various models of direct assessment, each model has provided a somewhat different emphasis to the evaluation process. In addition, somewhat different terms have been used by these investigators to describe their respective models. Fuchs and Deno (1991) classified all models of curriculum-based assessment as either general outcome measurement or specific subskill-mastery models. General outcome measurement models use standardized measures that have acceptable levels of reliability and validity. The primary objective of the model is to index long-term growth in the curriculum and across a wide range of skills. Although outcomes derived from this model may suggest when and if instructional modifications are needed, the model is not directly designed to suggest what those specific instructional modifications should be.

Measures used in a general outcome measurement model are presented in a standardized format. Material for assessment is controlled for difficulty by grade levels and may or may not come directly from the curriculum of instruction (Fuchs & Deno, 1994). Typically, measures are presented as brief, timed samples of performance, using rate as the primary metric to determine outcome.

In contrast, specific subskill-mastery models do not use standardized measures. Instead, measures are criterion referenced and usually based on the development of a skills hierarchy. The primary objective of this model is to determine whether students are meeting the short-term instructional objectives of the curriculum. The measures may or may not have any relationship to the long-term goals of mastering the curriculum.

Specific subskill-mastery models require a shift in measurement with the teaching of each new objective. As such, measures are not standardized from one objective to the next. Generally, these measures are teacher made, and the metric used to determine student performance can vary widely from accuracy to rate to analysis of error patterns. The model is designed primarily to provide suggestions for the types of instructional modifications that may be useful in teaching a student.

One specific subskill mastery model is Blankenship's (1985) model of "curriculum-based assessment" (CBA). Student performance is evaluated on individual instructional objectives. CBAs can be developed for any part of the curriculum and can include any number of objectives the teacher wishes to assess. Testing on similar objectives is repeated over several days to provide stable indications of student performance. From these CBAs, instructional objectives are derived. Periodic assessment using a CBA is employed to determine whether the student has mastered the content instructed.

In another subskill mastery model of CBA, Gickling and his colleagues (Gickling & Havertape, 1981; Gickling & Rosenfield, 1995; Gickling & Thompson, 1985; Rosenfield & Kuralt, 1990) concentrate on the selection of instructional objectives and content based on assessment. In particular, this model tries to control the level of instructional delivery carefully, so that student success is maximized. To accomplish this task, academic skills are evaluated in terms of student "knowns" and "unknowns." Adjustments are then made in the curriculum to keep students at an "instructional" level, as compared to "independent" or "frustrational" levels (Betts, 1946).

I (Shapiro, 1992) provide a good illustration of how this model of CBA can be applied to a student with problems in reading fluency. Burns and his colleagues (Burns, 2001; Burns, Tucker, Frame, Foley, & Hauser, 2000; MacQuarrie, Tucker, Burns, & Hartman, 2002) have provided a number of studies offering empirical support for various components of Gickling's model of CBA.

Howell and Nolet (1999) have provided a subskill-mastery model called "curriculum-based evaluation" that is wider in scope and application than either the Blankenship or Gickling models. In the model, Howell and

Nolet (1999) concentrate on the development of intervention strategies using task analysis, skill probes, direct observation, and other evaluation tools. Extensive suggestions for intervention programs that are based on curriculum-based evaluation are offered for various subskills such as reading comprehension, decoding, mathematics, written communication, and social skills. In addition, details are provided for decision making in changing intervention strategies.

Among general outcome models of CBA, the assessment model that has had the most substantial research base is that developed by Deno and his colleagues at the University of Minnesota (e.g., Deno, 1985). Derived from some earlier work on "data-based program modification" (Deno & Mirkin, 1977), Deno's model, called "curriculum-based measurement" (CBM), is primarily designed as a progress-monitoring system rather than as a system designed to develop intervention strategies. The most common use of this model employs repeated and frequent administration of skills probes taken from the curriculum in which the child is being instructed. Some research has shown that the model is equally effective in monitoring student progress when a curriculum not matched to the student's instruction is used as well (Fuchs & Deno, 1994). The skill assessed in giving the probes (e.g., oral reading rates) is not necessarily the skill being instructed but is viewed as a "vital sign" that indexes and reflects improvement and acquisition of curriculum content. Deno and his colleagues have provided a large, extensive, and impressive database that substantiates the value of this system for screening decisions, eligibility decisions, progress monitoring, and program evaluation (e.g., Deno, Fuchs, Marston, & Shin, 2001; Deno, Marston, & Mirkin, 1982; Deno, Marston, & Tindal, 1985–1986; Deno, Mirkin, & Chiang, 1982; Fuchs, Deno, & Mirkin, 1984; Fuchs & Fuchs, 1986a; Fuchs, Fuchs, Hamlett, Phillips, & Bentz, 1994; Shinn, Habedank, Rodden-Nord, & Knutson, 1993; Stecker & Fuchs, 2000).

Although each of these models offers useful and important alternatives to norm- and criterion-referenced testing, they all primarily focus on the evaluation of student academic performance to examine student skills. Certainly, the importance of assessing individual academic skills cannot be denied. However, it seems equally important to examine the instructional environment in which the student is being taught. Lentz and I (Shapiro, 1987a, 1990, 1996a, 1996b; Shapiro & Lentz, 1985, 1986) provided a model for academic assessment that incorporated the evaluation of the academic environment, as well as student performance. Calling our model "behavioral assessment of academic skills," we (Shapiro, 1989, 1996a; Shapiro & Lentz, 1985, 1986) drew on the principles of behavioral assessment employed for assessing social–emotional problems (Mash & Terdal, 1997; Ollendick & Hersen, 1984; Shapiro & Kratochwill, 2002) but applied them to the evaluation of academic problems. Teacher interviews, student interviews, systematic direct observation, and an examination of student-produced academic products played a significant part in the evaluation process. Specific variables examined for the assessment process were selected from the research on effective teaching (e.g., Denham & Lieberman, 1980) and applied behavior analysis (e.g., Sulzer-Azaroff & Mayer, 1986). In addition, the methodology developed by Deno and his associates was used to evaluate individual student performance but was combined with the assessment of the instructional environment in making recommendations for intervention. Indeed, it is this assessment of the instructional ecology that differentiates our model from other models of CBA.

In a refinement of this model, I (Shapiro, 1990) described a four-step process for the assessment of academic skills that integrates several of the existing models of CBA. The model has been slightly refined further with the relabeling of Step 2 from "Assess Curriculum Placement" to "Assess Instructional Placement." As illustrated in Figure 1.1, the process

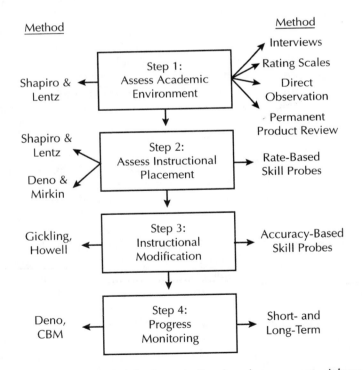

FIGURE 1.1. Integrated model of curriculum-based assessment. Adapted from Shapiro (1990, p. 331). Copyright 1990 by the National Association of School Psychologists. Adapted by permission of the author.

begins with an evaluation of the instructional environment through the use of systematic observation, teacher interviewing, student interviewing, and a review of student-produced academic products. The assessment continues by determining the student's current instructional level in curriculum materials. Next, instructional modifications designed to maximize student success are implemented with ongoing assessment of the acquisition of instructional objectives (short-term goals). The final step of the model involves the monitoring of student progress toward long-term (year-end) curriculum goals. The model integrates several existing models of CBA into a systematic methodology for conducting direct academic assessment. The model is described in more detail in Chapter 3.

One of the important considerations in adopting a new methodology for conducting academic assessment is the degree to which the proposed change is acceptable to consumers who will use the method. Substantial attention in the literature has been given to the importance of the acceptability of intervention strategies recommended for school- and home-based behavior management (e.g., Clark & Elliott, 1988; Miltenberger, 1990; Reimers, Wacker, Cooper, & deRaad, 1992; Reimers, Wacker, Derby, & Cooper, 1995; Witt & Elliott, 1985). Eckert and I (Eckert, Hintze, & Shapiro, 1999; Eckert & Shapiro, 1999; Eckert, Shapiro, & Lutz, 1995; Shapiro & Eckert, 1994) extended the concept of treatment acceptability to assessment acceptability. Using a measure derived from the Intervention Rating Profile (Witt & Martens, 1983), the studies demonstrated that both teachers and school psychologists found CBA, compared to use of standardized norm-referenced tests, to be relatively more acceptable in conducting academic skills assessments. We (Shapiro & Eckert, 1993) also showed in a nationally derived sample that 46% of school psychologists surveyed indicated that they had used some form of CBA in their work. In a replication and extension of our original survey, we found that 10 years later, 53% of those psychologists surveyed indicated that they had used CBA in conducting academic assessments (Shapiro, Angello, & Eckert, 2004). However, our surveys in both 1990 and 2000 also revealed that school psychologists still had limited knowledge of the actual methods used in conducting a CBA. Although there was a statistically significant ($p < .05$) increase in the percentage reporting use of CBA in 2000 compared to 1990, a large proportion of psychologists still reported not using CBA. At the same time, over 90% of those surveyed who had graduated in the past 5 years had been trained in the use of CBA through their graduate programs. Overall, these studies suggest that although CBA is highly acceptable to the consumers (teachers and school psychologists) and is increasingly being taught as part of the curriculum in training school psychologists, it is slow in assuming a prominent role in the assessment methods of practicing psychologists.

Conclusions and Summary

Strategies for the assessment of academic skills range from the more indirect norm- and criterion-referenced methods through direct assessment, which is based on evaluating a student's performance on the skills that have been taught within the curriculum in which the student is being instructed. Clearly, the type of decision to be made must be tied to the particular assessment strategy employed. Although some norm-referenced standardized assessment methods may be useful for making eligibility decisions, these strategies are sorely lacking in their ability to assist evaluators in recommending appropriate remediation procedures or in their sensitivity to improvements in academic skills over short periods of time. Many alternative assessment strategies designed to provide closer links between the assessment data and intervention methods are available. Although these strategies may also be limited for certain types of decision making, their common core of using the curriculum as the basis for assessment allows these methods to be employed more effectively for several different types of decisions.

INTERVENTION METHODS FOR ACADEMIC SKILLS

Remediation procedures developed for academic problems can be conceptualized on a continuum from indirect to direct procedures. Those techniques that attempt to improve academic performance by improving underlying learning processes can be characterized as indirect interventions. In particular, interventions based on "aptitude–treatment interactions" (ATIs) would be considered indirect methods of intervention. In contrast, direct interventions attempt to improve the area of academic skill by directly teaching that particular skill. These types of interventions usually are based on examination of variables that have been found to have direct relationships to academic performance.

Indirect Interventions for Academic Skills

Most indirect interventions for remediating academic skills are based on the assumed existence of ATIs. The basis of the concept of ATI is that different aptitudes require different treatment. If one properly matches the correct treatment to the correct aptitude, then gains will be observed in the child's behavior. Assuming that there are basic cognitive processes that must be intact for certain academic skills to be mastered, it seems logical that identification and remediation of aptitudes would result in improved academic behavior.

In reading, for example, it may be determined from an assessment that a student's failure to acquire mastery of reading is based on poor phonetic analysis skills. Furthermore, the evaluation may show that the student possesses a preference for learning in the visual over auditory modality. Given this information, it may be predicted that the student will succeed if instruction is based more on a visual than on an auditory approach to teaching reading. In this example, the aptitude (strength in visual modality) is matched to a treatment procedure (change to a more visually oriented reading curriculum) in hopes of improving the student's skills.

Probably one of the most extensive uses of the ATI concept for remediating academic problems has been in the area of process remediation. Intervention strategies aimed at process remediation attempt to instruct students in those skills felt to be prerequisites to successful academic performance. For example, if a student having difficulty in reading is assessed to have poor auditory discrimination skills, process remediation strategies would specifically work at teaching the child to make auditory discriminations more effectively. The underlying assumption is that reading skills would show improvement once auditory discrimination is also improved.

Despite the logical appeal of process remediation, studies specifically examining the validity of the method have not been very encouraging. Arter and Jenkins (1979), in a comprehensive, critical, and detailed analysis of both process assessment and remediation programs (called DD-P; Differential Diagnosis–Prescriptive Teaching by Arter and Jenkins), have reported that there is almost no support for the validity of the assessment measures employed to identify specific aptitudes, nor for the remediation programs that are matched to the results of these assessments. Arter and Jenkins furthermore state:

> We believe that until a substantive research base for the DD-PT model has been developed, it is imperative to call for a moratorium on advocacy of DD-PT, on classification and placement of children according to differential ability tests, on the purchase of instructional materials and programs that claim to improve these abilities, and on coursework designed to train DD-PT teachers. (p. 550)

Cronbach and Snow (1977) similarly reported the limited empirical support of ATIs. Although Arter and Jenkins (1979) and Cronbach and Snow (1977) left' room at that time for the possibility that future research would show the value of ATIs, Kavale and Forness (1987), in a meta-analysis from 39 studies searching for aptitude–treatment interactions related to modality assessment and instruction, found no substantial differences between students receiving instruction linked to assessed modality of learning and those receiving no special instruction.

Despite the questionable empirical support for ATI approaches to remediation, their presence continues to be felt in the literature. An excellent example is the publication of the Kaufman Assessment Battery for Children (K-ABC; Kaufman & Kaufman, 1983). The measure was designed based on the hypothesized structure of information processing that divides mental functioning into sequential and simultaneous processing (Das, Kirby, & Jarman, 1975, 1979). Included within the interpretative manual are remedial techniques that describe how to teach skills in reading, spelling, and mathematics differentially, based on whether a child's skills are stronger in sequential or simultaneous processing. Although these remediation strategies are not attempting to train underlying cognitive processes directly (they are not teaching children to be better sequential processors), the specific intervention is clearly linked to a specific aptitude. In fact, Kaufman and Kaufman (1983) specifically recommend this approach.

It is somewhat surprising, given the strong empirical basis upon which the K-ABC was developed, that so little attention was given to empirical evaluation of the recommended ATI approach to remediation. One of the few published studies examining the K-ABC approach to remediation was reported by Ayres and Cooley (1986). Two procedures were developed based directly on Kaufman and Kaufman's (1983) recommended remediation strategies suggested in the K-ABC interpretative manual. One strategy used a sequential processing approach, whereas the other used a simultaneous approach. Students who were differentiated as simultaneous or sequential processors on the K-ABC were divided such that half of each group were trained on tasks matched to processing mechanisms and half on unmatched tasks. The results of the study were startling. Although an aptitude–treatment interaction was found, it was in the opposite direction of that predicted based on the K-ABC!

Good et al. (1993) replicated and extended the previous study, working with first- and second-grade students. Carefully controlling for some of the methodological limitations of the Ayres and Cooley (1986) studies, Good et al. (1993) designed instructional programs that emphasized sequential or simultaneous processing modes. After identifying seven students with strengths in simultaneous processing and 21 with strengths in sequential processing, each student was taught vocabulary words, using each of the two methods of instruction. Results of this carefully conducted study were consistent with previous research (Ayres & Cooley, 1986; Ayres, Cooley, & Severson, 1988), failing to support the K-ABC instructional model.

Despite the consistent findings that indirect interventions based on ATIs are not very effective at remediating academic problems, significant efforts are still being made to use this paradigm to explain academic failure (Gordon, DeStefano, & Shipman, 1985). For example, Naglieri and Das

(1997) developed a measure (the CAS; Cognitive Assessment System) based on the theory of intellectual processing that identifies four components of cognitive processing (PASS; Planning, Attention, Simultaneous, and Sequential). Naglieri and Johnson (2000) found that specific interventions matched to deficits in planning processes resulted in improvements in academic performance, whereas those receiving the intervention but not initially identified as low in planning did not show the same level of improvement. Significant questions about the empirical support for the underlying theory behind the CAS were raised in a series of studies (Keith, Kranzler, & Flanagan, 2001; Kranzler & Keith, 1999; Kranzler, Keith, & Flanagan, 2000).

It appears that the logical appeal of the ATI model may still be outweighing its empirical support. Clearly, for the "moratorium" suggested by Arter and Jenkins (1979) to occur, alternative models for academic remediation that appear to have a significant database must be examined.

Direct Interventions for Academic Problems

Interventions for academic problems are considered direct if responses targeted for change are identical to those observed in the natural environment. For example, in reading, interventions that specifically address reading skills such as comprehension, phonetic analysis, or sight vocabulary are considered direct interventions. This is in contrast to indirect interventions, which may target cognitive processes (e.g., sequencing) that are assumed to underlie and be prerequisite to acquisition of the academic skill.

The types of direct interventions employed for academic skills have been derived from three types of empirical research. One set of intervention strategies has emerged from basic educational research that has explored the relationship of time variables to academic performance (e.g., Denham & Lieberman, 1980; Greenwood, Horton, & Utley, 2002; Rosenshine, 1981). In particular, the time during which students are actively rather than passively engaged in academic responding, or "engaged time," has a long and consistent history of finding significant relationships to academic performance. For example, Berliner (1979), in data reported from the Beginning Teacher Evaluation Study (BTES), found wide variations across classrooms in the amount of time students actually spend in engaged time. Frederick, Walberg, and Rasher (1979), in comparing engaged time and scores on the Iowa Tests of Basic Skills among 175 classrooms, found moderately strong correlations ($r = .54$). Greenwood and his associates at the Juniper Garden Children's Project in Kansas City have examined academic engaged time by focusing on student opportunities to respond. Using the Code for Instructional Structure and Student Academic Response (CISSAR) and its derivatives, the Mainstream Version (MS-CISSAR) and the Ecobehavioral System for Complex Assessments of Preschool Environments (ESCAPE), a number of studies have demonstrated the direct relationships between engagement rates and academic performance (e.g., Berliner, 1988; Fisher & Berliner, 1985; Goodman, 1990; Greenwood, 1991; Greenwood, Horton, & Utley, 2002; Hall, Delquadri, Greenwood, & Thurston, 1982; Myers, 1990; Pickens & McNaughton, 1988; Stanley & Greenwood, 1983; Thurlow, Ysseldyke, Graden, & Algozzine, 1983, 1984; Ysseldyke, Thurlow, Christenson, & McVicar, 1988; Ysseldyke, Thurlow, Mecklenberg, Graden, & Algozzine, 1984).

A number of academic interventions designed specifically to increase opportunities to respond have been developed. In particular, classwide peer tutoring and cooperative learning strategies have been developed for this purpose (e.g., Calhoun & Fuchs, 2003; Delquadri, Greenwood, Stretton, & Hall, 1983; DuPaul, Ervin, Hook, & McGoey, 1998; Fuchs, Fuchs, & Burish, 2000; Greenwood, Arreaga-Mayer, Utley, Gavin, & Terry, 2001; Greenwood, Carta, & Hall, 1988; Greenwood, Terry, Arreaga-Mayer, & Finney, 1992; Johnson & Johnson, 1985; Phillips, Fuchs, & Fuchs, 1994; Sideridis et al., 1997; Slavin, 1983a; Topping & Ehly, 1998).

Another line of research that has resulted in the development of direct interventions for academic problems is derived from performance models of instruction (DiPerna, Volpe, & Elliott, 2002; Greenwood, 1996). These models emphasize that changes in student academic performance are a function of changes in instructional process. In particular, DiPerna and Elliott (2002) identify the influence on academic performance of what they call "academic enablers," those intraindividual behaviors such as motivation, interpersonal skills, academic engagement, and study skills. Others have examined how the processes surrounding instruction, such as teacher instruction, feedback, and reinforcement, have functional relationships to student academic performance (Daly & Murdoch, 2000; Daly, Witt, Martens, & Dool, 1997).

These types of models have resulted in a long and successful history of developing academic remediations by researchers in behavior analysis. Examination of the literature reveals hundreds of studies in which academic skills were the targets for remediation. Contingent reinforcement has been applied to increase accuracy of reading comprehension (e.g., Lahey & Drabman, 1973; Lahey, McNees, & Brown, 1973) and improve oral reading fluency (Daly & Martens, 1994, 1999; Lovitt, Eaton, Kirkwood, & Perlander, 1971), formation of numbers and letters (Hasazi & Hasazi, 1972; McLaughlin, Mabee, Byram, & Reiter, 1987), arithmetic computation (Logan & Skinner, 1998; Lovitt, 1978; Skinner, Turco, Beatty, & Rasavage, 1989), spelling (Lovitt, 1978; Truchlicka, McLaughlin, & Swain, 1998; Winterling, 1990), and creative writing (Campbell & Willis, 1978). Other variables of the instructional environment, such as teacher attention and praise (Hasazi & Hasazi, 1972), free time (Hopkins, Schultz, & Garton, 1971), access to peer tutors (Delquadri, et al., 1983), tokens or points (McLaughlin, 1981), and avoidance of drill (Lovitt & Hansen, 1976a), have all been found to be effective in modifying academic behavior of students. In addition, other procedures, such as group contingencies (Goldberg & Shapiro, 1995; Shapiro & Goldberg, 1986, 1990), monitoring of student progress (Fuchs, Deno, & Mirkin, 1984; McCurdy & Shapiro, 1992; Shimabukuro, Prater, Jenkins, & Edelen-Smith, 1999; Shapiro & Cole, 1994, 1999; Szykula, Saudargas, & Wahler, 1981; Todd, Horner, & Sugai, 1999), public posting of performance (Van Houten, Hill, & Parsons, 1975), peer and self-corrective feedback (Skinner, Shapiro, Turco, Cole, & Brown, 1992), and positive practice (Lenz, Singh, & Hewett, 1991; Ollendick, Matson, Esvelt-Dawson, & Shapiro, 1980), have all been employed as direct interventions for academic problems.

A third line of research from work on effective instructional design (e.g., Kame'enui, Simmons, & Coyne, 2000) has resulted in the development of many direct interventions. In particular, the research using a Direct Instruction approach to intervention has provided extensive efforts to develop strategies that target specific academic skills and metacognitive processes that lead to improved academic performance and conceptual development (e.g., Adams & Carnine, 2003; Kame'enui, Simmons, Chard, & Dickson, 1997). These studies have been effective at teaching explicit skills to students who are struggling. For example, strategies to teach reading to young children have typically focused on teaching skills such as decoding, word identification, fluency building, word attack, and other phonological awareness skills (Lane, O'Shaughnessy, Lambros, Gresham, & Beebe-Frankenberger, 2001; McCandliss, Beck, Sandak, & Perfetti, 2003; O'Connor, 2000; Trout, Epstein, Mickelson, Nelson, & Lewis, 2003). Others have emphasized specific strategy instruction to teach skills to help struggling readers become more fluent by using techniques such as repeated readings, modeling, and previewing (e.g., Chard, Vaughn, & Tyler, 2002; Hasbrouck, Ihnot, & Rogers, 1999; Skinner, Cooper, & Cole, 1997; Stoddard, Valcante, Sindelar, & O'Shea, 1993; Tingstrom, Edwards, & Olmi, 1995).

Similar efforts to develop skills focused interventions have been evident for other academic subjects. For example, in mathematics, strategies have been used to improve both basic computational skills and more complex problem-solving. Among the strategies "cover–copy–compare" (e.g., Skinner, Bamberg, Smith, & Powell, 1993), teaching a conceptual schema (Jitendra & Hoff, 1996; Jitendra, Hoff, & Beck, 1999), self-regulated learning (Fuchs, Fuchs, Prentice, et al., 2003), and peer-assisted learning (Calhoun & Fuchs, 2003) have all been highly effective. Others have shown that basic skills such as written composition and spelling can also be directly targeted by teaching self-regulated strategies, as well as specific skills (Berninger et al., 1998; Graham & Harris, 2003; Graham, Harris, & Troia, 2000).

Clearly, the range of variables that can be modified within the instructional environment is impressive. Included are those strategies that focus more on the events surrounding the academic skills, as well as those that target the skills themselves. More importantly, in most of these studies, changes in academic behaviors were present without concern about supposed prerequisite, underlying skills.

In the chapters that follow, a full description is provided of the four-step model for conducting an assessment of children referred for academic skills problems. Because assessment is considered a dynamic event that requires evaluation of a child's responsiveness to effective intervention, substantial coverage of many of the interventions mentioned previously is provided.

Dir Instruction techn.

Show suces in he'ping std

1.) self-regulated stat.
   cover,
2. copy, compare
3. stegulae to increase opport. to
   respond
4. improve / increase engaged time

CHAPTER 2

♦ ♦ ♦

Choosing Targets for Academic Assessment and Remediation

♦

When a child is referred for academic problems, the most important questions facing the evaluator are "What do I assess?" and "What behavior(s) should be targeted for intervention?" As simple and straightforward as these questions seem to be, the correct responses to these inquiries are not as logical as one might think. For example, if a child is reported to be showing difficulties in sustaining attention to task, it seems logical that one would assess the child's on-task behavior and design interventions to increase attention to task. The literature, however, suggests that this would not be the most effective approach to solving this type of problem. If a child is not doing well in reading skills, one obviously should assess reading skills to determine whether the selected intervention is effective. But reading is an incredibly complex skill consisting of many subskills. What is the most efficient way to determine student progress? Clearly, the selection of behaviors for assessment and intervention is a critical decision in remediating academic problems.

The complexity of target behavior selection for assessment and intervention is reflected in a number of articles published in a special issue of *Behavioral Assessment* (1985, Vol. 7, No. 1). For example, Evans (1985) suggested that identifying targets for clinical assessment requires an understanding of the interactions among behavioral repertoires. He argued for the use of a systems model to plan and conduct appropriate target behavior selection in the assessment process. Kazdin (1985) likewise pointed to the known constellations of behavior, which suggest that focus on single targets for assessment or remediation would be inappropriate. Kratochwill (1985b) has discussed the way in which target behaviors are selected through behavioral consultation. He noted the issues related to using verbal behavior as the source for target behavior selection as problematic.

Nelson (1985) has pointed to several additional concerns in the selection of targets for behavioral assessment. The choice of behaviors may be based on both nonempirical and empirical guidelines, for example, choosing positive behaviors that need to be increased over negative behaviors that need to be decreased. Likewise, when a child presents several disruptive behaviors, the one chosen for intervention may be the one that is the most irritating to the teacher or causes the most significant disruption to other students. *Picking the most irratating behav is not empl*

Target behaviors may also be selected empirically by using normative data. Those behaviors that are evident in peers but not in the targeted child may then become the targets for assessment and intervention (Ager & Shapiro, 1995; Hoier & Cone, 1987; Hoier, McConnell, & Palley, 1987). Other empirical methods for choosing target behaviors have included use of regression equations (McKinney, Mason, Perkerson, & Clifford, 1975), identification of known groups of children who are considered to be demonstrating effective behavior (Nelson, 1985), use of functional analysis that experimentally manipulates different behaviors to determine which result in the best outcomes (e.g., Broussard & Northrup, 1995; Cooper, Wacker, Sasso, Reimers, & Donn, 1990; Cooper et al., 1992; Ervin, DuPaul, Kern, & Friman, 1998; Finkel, Derby, Weber, & McLaughlin, 2003; Lalli, Browder, Mace, & Brown, 1993), and use of the triple-response mode system (Cone, 1978, 1988). Clearly, selection of behaviors for assessment and intervention for nonacademic problems considers both the individual behavior and the environmental context in which it occurs to be equally important. There appears to be a tendency in assessing academic problems, however, not to consider the instructional environment, or to consider it only rarely, when a child is referred for academic problems (but see Christenson & Ysseldyke, 1989; Greenwood, 1996; Greenwood, Carta, & Atwater, 1991; Lentz & Shapiro, 1986). Traditional assessment measures, both norm- and criterion-referenced, and many models of CBA (e.g., Deno, 1985), make decisions about a child's academic skills without adequate consideration of the instructional environment in which these skills have been taught. Unfortunately, a substantial literature has demonstrated that a child's academic failure may reside in the instructional environment rather than in the child's inadequate mastery of skills (Lentz & Shapiro, 1986; Thurlow, Ysseldyke, Wotruba, & Algozzine, 1993; Ysseldyke, Spicuzza, Kosciolek, & Boys, 2003). Indeed, if a child fails to master an academic skill, it directly suggests potential failure in the instructional methodologies.

true and for good reason

SELECTING TARGETS FOR ASSESSMENT

We (Lentz & Shapiro, 1985) have listed several basic assumptions in assessing academic problems. Each assumption is consistent with a behavioral approach to assessment and recognizes the important differences between assessment for academic problems and assessment for behavioral–emotional problems (in which behavioral methods more typically are used).

1. *Assessment must reflect an evaluation of the behavior in the natural environment.* Behavioral assessment emphasizes the need for collecting data under conditions that most closely approximate the natural conditions under which the behavior originally occurred. A child can perform academically in many ways, including individual seatwork, teacher-led small-group activities, teacher-led large-group activities, independent or small peer groups at learning centers, teacher-led testing activities, cooperative groups, peer-tutoring dyads, and so forth. Each of these instructional arrangements may result in differential academic performance under the same task. Whatever method is chosen for the assessment of academic skills, the procedure should be closely related to the way in which the behavior of interest occurs during the regular instructional period.

2. *Assessment should be idiographic rather than nomothetic.* The concerns that often drive the assessment process are the identification and evaluation of potential intervention procedures that may assist the remediation process. In assessing academic skills, it is important to determine how the targeted student is performing against a preintervention baseline rather than normative comparisons. In this way, any changes in performance subsequent to interventions can be observed. Although normative comparisons are important in making eligibility decisions and for setting goals, intraindividual rather than interindividual comparisons remain the primary focus of the direct assessment of academic skills.

3. *What is taught and expected to be learned should be what is tested.* One of the significant problems with traditional norm-referenced testing, as noted in Chapter 1, is the potential lack of overlap between the instructional curriculum and the content of achievement tests (Bell et al., 1992; Good & Salvia, 1988; Jenkins & Pany, 1978; Martens, Steele, Massie, & Diskin, 1995; Shapiro & Derr, 1987). In the behavioral assessment of academic skills, it is important that there be significant overlap between the curriculum and the test. Without such overlap, it is difficult to separate a child's failure on these tests due to inadequate mastery of the curriculum from failure to teach material covered on the test.

4. *The results of the assessment should be strongly related to planning interventions.* A primary purpose of any assessment is to identify those strategies that may be successful in remediating the problem. When assess-

ing academic skills, it is important that the assessment methods provide some indications of potential intervention procedures.

5. *Assessment methods should be appropriate for continuous monitoring of student progress, so that intervention strategies can be altered as indicated.* Because the assessment process is idiographic and designed to evaluate behavior across time, it is critical that the measures employed be sensitive to change. Indeed, whatever methods are chosen to assess academic skills, these procedures must be capable of showing behavioral improvement (or decrements), regardless of the type of intervention selected. If the intervention chosen is effective at improving a child's math computation (e.g., single-digit subtraction), the assessment method must be sensitive to any small fluctuations in the student's performance. It is also important to note that, because of the frequency with which these measures are employed, they must be brief, repeatable, and usable across types of classroom instructors (e.g., teachers, aides, peers, parents).

6. *Measures used need to be based upon empirical research and to have adequate validity.* Like all assessment measures, methods used to conduct direct assessment of academic skills must meet appropriate psychometric standards. From a traditional perspective, this would require that the measures display adequate test–retest reliability and internal consistency, sufficient content validity, and demonstrated concurrent validity. In addition, because these measures are designed to be consistent with behavioral assessment, the measures should also meet standards of behavioral assessment, such as interobserver agreement, treatment validity, and social validity. Although there have been substantial research efforts to provide a traditional psychometric base for direct assessment measures (e.g., Shinn, 1988, 1998) there have been few efforts to substantiate the use of the measures from a behavioral assessment perspective (Lentz, 1988); however, see Derr and Shapiro (1989) and Derr-Minneci and Shapiro (1992).

7. *Measures should be useful in making many types of educational decisions.* Any method used for assessing academic skills should contribute across different types of decisions (Salvia & Ysseldyke, 2001). Specifically, the assessment should be helpful in screening, setting individual educational plan (IEP) goals, designing interventions, determining eligibility for special services, and evaluating special services.

The keys to selecting the appropriate behaviors for assessing academic problems are their sensitivity to small increments of change, their ability to reflect improvement in more molar areas of academic skills (e.g., reading), the curriculum validity of the observed behaviors (match between the assessment measure and the instructional objectives), their ability to assist in the development of intervention strategies, the ability to meet appropriate psychometric standards, and the inclusion of both the academic environment and individual skills in the assessment process. Interestingly, an examination of the literature from somewhat different perspectives (cognitive psychology, educational psychology, applied behavior analysis, and special education) provides significant support for the selection of specific classes of behavior from which one should choose the appropriate targets for evaluation of both the academic environment and the individual's skills.

Assessing the Academic Environment

Academic Engaged Time

Considerable effort has been given to the identification of the critical instructional variables affecting student mastery of basic skills. Much of this research was derived from Carroll's (1963) model of classroom learning, which hypothesized that learning is a function of time engaged in learning relative to the time needed to learn. Although a few researchers have examined issues related to the time needed for learning (e.g., Gettinger, 1985), most efforts have concentrated on the relationship of engaged time to academic performance (Caldwell, Huitt, & Graeber, 1982; Goodman, 1990; Karweit, 1983; Karweit & Slavin, 1981).

One of the most significant projects that examined relationships between time and academic achievement was the Beginning Teacher Evaluation Study (BTES; Denham & Lieberman, 1980). Observations were conducted on the entire instructional day in second- and fifth-grade classrooms across a 6-year period. Data were collected on the amount of time allocated for instruction, how the allocated time was actually spent, and the proportion of time that students spent actively engaged in academic tasks within the allocated time. From the BTES was derived the concept of "academic learning time" (ALT), a variable that incorporates allocated time, engaged time, and success rate.

Berliner (1979), in data reported from the BTES study, compared the amount of allocated time (time assigned for instruction) and engaged time (time actually spent in academic tasks) in second- and fifth-grade classrooms. Although there were wide variations in levels of performance across classes, many were found to have under 100 cumulative hours of engaged time across a 150-day school year. Frederick et al. (1979) examined engaged time and scores on the Iowa Tests of Basic Skills among 175 classrooms in Chicago, and found engagement rates and achievement scores to be moderately correlated ($r = .54$). The importance of engaged time has led to a number of studies examining the levels of student engagement across special education classrooms. Leinhardt, Zigmond, and Cooley (1981) examined engagement rates within reading instruction periods of self-contained classrooms for students with learning disabilities. Results of their investigation noted that reading behavior was significantly predicted by pretest scores, teacher instructional variables, and teacher contact. However, students were found to spend only 10% of their academic day in oral or silent reading activities with teachers, averaging 16 minutes daily of actual direct instruction. Haynes and Jenkins (1986), examining resource rooms for students with learning disabilities (LD), found similar results, with students engaged in silent or oral reading activities only 44% of the time scheduled for reading within the resource room. Similarly, most student time (54%) in these settings was spent in individual seatwork.

In a review of the engaged time literature, Gettinger (1986) noted that there appears to be "a positive association between academic engaged time and learning" (p. 9). She did offer substantial caution, however, that the literature is far from definitive and that other factors that may interact with engaged time (e.g., time needed for learning) need continued investigation. Despite these cautions, it appears that academic engaged time may be a critical variable for the assessment of academic skills. Indeed, Gettinger offers a significant number of excellent recommendations for increasing engaged time that have been supported by research. These suggestions include increasing direct instruction and reducing reliance on independent seatwork, improving teacher monitoring of student performance, reducing student behaviors that compete with engaged time (such as off-task), increasing teacher feedback to students, improving classroom organization, frequent monitoring of student progress, and adhering to the schedule of planned academic activities.

Although there is clear evidence of the importance of engaged time and its relationship to academic achievement, the translation of engaged time to targets for academic assessment is not as direct as it appears. Greenwood, Delquadri, and Hall (1984) at the Juniper Garden's Children's Project have examined engaged time by focusing on opportunities to respond. "Opportunity to respond" is a concept that incorporates the antecedent–behavior relationships surrounding the instructional process. Specifically, the concept includes the academic environment or ecology, along with the student response. Thus, measurement of opportunities to respond must include assessment of the instructional environment, along with the child's responses. Greenwood and his colleagues have developed a series of observational codes matched to different educational settings designed to provide a detailed analysis of these variables. The Code for Instructional Structure and Student Academic Response (CISSAR; Stanley & Greenwood, 1981) is used for the assessment of non-special education students in regular education settings; the Code for Instructional Structure and Student Academic Response—Mainstream Version (MS-CISSAR; Carta, Greenwood, Schulte, Arreaga-Mayer, & Terry, 1987) is used for assessing identified special education students within mainstream settings; and the Ecobehavioral System for Complex Assessments of Preschool Environments (ESCAPE; Carta, Greenwood, & Atwater, 1985) is used for assessing students within kindergarten and preschool settings. These codes have been configured for computerized data collection and analysis using laptop computers into a system called the Ecobehavioral Assessment Systems Software (E-BASS; Greenwood, Carta, Kamps, & Delquadri, 1993). Table 2.1 provides a listing of the CISSAR categories and codes. Similar sets of codes are used for the MS-CISSAR and ESCAPE. As one can see, the code is extremely complex and offers substantially detailed information about teacher and student behavior. Greenwood, Delquadri, and Hall (1984) make clear that the concept of opportunities to respond is not identical to the more typical observational category of on-task behavior common to many direct observational data-collection systems. The key difference is the active responding involved in opportunities to respond, compared to the more passive response of on-task behavior.

A large number of studies have been conducted using CISSAR, MS-CISSAR, and ESCAPE (e.g., Ager & Shapiro, 1995; Carta, Atwater, Schwartz, & Miller, 1990; Friedman, Cancelli, & Yoshida, 1988; Greenwood, Carta, Kamps, Terry, & Delquadri, 1994; Greenwood, Delquadri, & Hall, 1989; Hall et al., 1982; Kamps, Leonard, Dugan, & Boland, 1991; Stanley & Greenwood, 1983; Thurlow, Ysseldyke, Graden, & Algozzine, 1983, 1984; Ysseldyke et al., 1984). Researchers consistently have found results similar to those from the BTES and other studies suggesting that the levels of academic engaged time are surprisingly low. In addition, Thurlow et al. (1983, 1984) and Ysseldyke et al. (1984) also found few differences in engagement rates across types of LD services. Other studies that have used less complex processes for recording engaged time have achieved similar results (e.g., Gettinger, 1984; Greenwood, Horton, et al., 2002; Leach & Dolan, 1985). DiPerna et al. (2002) also included academic engaged time as a critical variable in their model of academic enablers—variables within the academic environment other than a student's skills that contribute to academic performance.

It is clear that any assessment of academic skills must include a measure that either assesses engaged time directly or provides a close approximation of engagement rate. Although observational codes that assess engagement directly do exist (e.g., CISSAR), these codes may be unnecessarily complex for clinical use. What is critical in the behavior or behaviors selected for assessment that represent engaged time is that they clearly should show the level of *active* student responding and not simply be measures of on-task time alone. Two codes that provide such a variable and have been found to be very useful for classroom observation are the Behavioral Observation of Students in Schools (BOSS; Shapiro, 1996b, 2003a) and the State–Event Classroom Observation System (SECOS; Saudargas,

engaged time - important to assess

BOSS we have it already

TABLE 2.1. CISSAR Categories, Descriptions, and Codes

Ecological categories	Number of codes	Description	Codes
Activity	12	Subject of instruction	Reading, mathematics, spelling, handwriting, language, science, social studies, arts/crafts, free time, business management, transition, can't tell
Task	8	Curriculum materials or the stimuli set by the teacher to occasion responding	Readers, workbook, worksheet, paper/pencil, listen to lecture, other media, teacher–student discussion, fetch/put away
Structure	3	Grouping and peer proximity during instruction	Entire group, small group, individual
Teacher position	6	Teacher's position relative to student observed	In front, among students, out of room, at desk, side, behind
Teacher behavior	5	Teacher's behavior relative to student observed	Teaching, no response, approval, disapproval, other talk
Student behavior categories			
Academic response	7	Specific, active response	Writing, reading aloud, reading silent, asking questions, answering questions, academic talk, academic game play
Task management	5	Prerequisite or enabling response	Attention, raise hand, look for materials, move, play appropriate
Competing (inappropriate responses)	7	Responses that compete or are incompatible with academic or task management behavior	Disrupt, look around, inappropriate (locale, task, play), talk nonacademic, self-stimulation
Total codes	53		

Note. From Greenwood, Dinwiddie, et al. (1984, p. 524). Copyright 1984 by the Society for the Experimental Analysis of Behavior, Inc. Reprinted by permission.

1992). Furthermore, it is also possible that approximations of engaged time can be obtained by combining observations on interrelated behaviors that together represent academic engaged time. The observational systems described here take this approach by collecting data about a child's academic behavior from various sources (teacher interview, student interview, direct observation, permanent products) and combining these to determine the student's level of academic responding. Detailed discussion of the use of these codes is provided in Chapter 3.

Classroom Contingencies

Academic responding does not occur in a vacuum. Each response is surrounded by various stimuli within the instructional environment that significantly affect performance. Stimuli immediately preceding the academic responses (e.g., teacher instructions), stimuli preceding the response but removed in time (e.g., studying for a test the night before), consequences immediately following the response (e.g., teacher feedback), delayed consequences (e.g., grades), and contingencies that compete against academic responses (e.g., student–student off-task, disruptive behavior) may all interact in complex ways to affect student academic performance. A significant and substantial research base has developed in applied behavior analysis that demonstrates the relationships of such variables to academic performance.

Antecedent conditions that occur immediately prior to academic responding have been investigated in a number of studies. For example, instructional pacing and teacher presentation during instruction have also been found to be potentially important antecedents to academic performance. Carnine (1976) demonstrated that students answered correctly about 80% of the time when in a fast-paced condition (12 questions per minute) as compared to answering correctly 30% of the time in a slow-rate condition (5 questions per minute). Indeed, recommendations made by those advocating direct methods of instruction (e.g., Becker & Carnine, 1981; Rosenshine, 1979) suggest that students will be more attentive to a fast-paced instructional strategy.

Another form of immediate antecedent that appears to influence academic responding involves the use of self-talk. An emerging literature demonstrates that a child's academic responses can be altered by teaching the child to perform self-instructions. Although first applied and developed for impulsive children (Meichenbaum & Goodman, 1971), self-instruction training has been applied across populations such as preschoolers (e.g., Bornstein & Quevillon, 1976; Duarte & Baer, 1994), children with mental retardation (e.g., Johnston, Whitman, & Johnson, 1980), and elementary-age children with LD (e.g., Lloyd, 1980; Wood, Rosenberg, & Carran,

1993). In addition, the procedure has been successfully applied to academic problems (Fox & Kendall, 1983; Graham & Wong, 1993; Lloyd, Kneedler, & Cameron, 1982; Wood et al., 1993).

Although there has been substantial support for the effects of immediate antecedent stimuli on academic responding, little research has examined the impact of antecedent conditions that are removed in time from the academic responses but may equally affect performance. Obviously, there is a substantial problem in trying to establish causal inferences when antecedents and responses are not contiguous. This probably accounts for the lack of research conducted on such events. Still, it is common to encounter teachers who attribute a child's failure to perform in school to events that occurred some time ago. Furthermore, it seems logical that a child who arrives at school without breakfast, and who has been awake most of the night listening to parents fight, may not perform as well as expected, despite past evidence of skill mastery in the area being assessed. Given that these types of antecedents that are removed temporally from the response may affect academic performance, they clearly provide important variables for assessment.

In general, the types of antecedent stimuli that need to be assessed are primarily found in observation of teacher behavior and the way the instructional environment is arranged. Evaluation of the academic ecology must include some provision for the collection of data around teaching procedures. These variables include methods of presenting instructional stimuli, teacher instructions, student use of self-instructional and other metacognitive strategies, and details about any possible temporally removed antecedents to the observed student's academic responding.

Significant effort has been devoted in the literature on applied behavior analysis to the application of consequences contingent upon academic responding. One of the simplest yet effective procedures to alter academic responding has been the use of feedback about performance. Van Houten and Lai Fatt (1981) examined the impact of public posting of weekly grades on biology tests with 12th-grade high school students. In two experiments, they demonstrated that public posting alone increased accuracy from 55.7% to 73.2% correct responses. These results are consistent with those of earlier studies examining the use of explicit timing and public posting in increasing mathematics and composition skills in regular elementary school students (Van Houten et al., 1975; Van Houten & Thompson, 1976).

Whinnery and Fuchs (1993) examined the impact of a goal-setting and test-taking feedback strategy on the performance of 40 students with LD. In both conditions, students set CBM performance goals after a 20-week intervention period. In one condition, students engaged in weekly CBM test taking, whereas no test taking was done in the other. Results showed that the group engaged in the CBM test-taking strategy had higher performance at the completion of the 20 weeks.

In another example of the impact of feedback on student academic performance, Fuchs, Fuchs, Hamlett, and Whinnery (1991) examined the effect of providing goal lines superimposed on graphs on the math performance of 40 students with LD. Results showed that providing goal-line feedback to students produced greater performance stability among students than providing graphs without goal-line feedback.

We (Skinner et al., 1992) compared corrective feedback for completion of math problems given under either peer- or self-delivered conditions across six second-grade students. In the self-delivered condition, students were instructed to first look at the problem with its answer, cover the problem with a cardboard marker, copy the problem as they recalled it, and then compare the copied and correct responses. This procedure, called "cover–copy–compare" was contrasted against a procedure in which peers examined student responses and provided feedback. Results showed that self-determined feedback resulted in greater performance for four of the six students. Similar results were found by Skinner, Ford, and Yunker (1991) in working with students with behavior disorders.

Other forms of contingent consequences have been examined extensively in the literature. For example, Trice, Parker, and Furrow (1981) found that feedback and contingent reinforcement, using a written format for responses to reading materials, significantly improved the number of words written in replies to questions and the spelling accuracy of a 17-year-old boy with LD. Allen, Howard, Sweeney, and McLaughlin (1993) found that contingency contracting was effective at improving the academic and social behavior of 3 second- or third-grade elementary school students. McLaughlin and Helm (1993) used contingent access to music for 2 middle school students to increase the number of correct problems completed in mathematics. Several studies (Daly & Martens, 1994; Freeman & McLaughlin, 1984; Shapiro & McCurdy, 1989; Skinner & Shapiro, 1987) explored the effectiveness of reading words contiguously with a tape recording. Lovitt and Hansen (1976a) examined the use of a skipping and drilling activity contingent upon improved reading. Skinner and his colleagues (e.g., Skinner, 2002; Skinner, Hurst, Teeple, & Meadows, 2002) used an interspersal technique in which students are given easier problems embedded within more difficult material to increase performance and productivity in mathematics. Gettinger (1985) investigated the use of imitation to correct spelling errors. Many, many other studies have been completed in which some form of contingent consequence has been employed to improve academic responding.

The extensive literature on consequences to academic responding suggests strongly that assessment of academic skills must include an evaluation of events following the academic responses. Included among those events are frequency and type of teacher responses to academic performance (both immediate and delayed). It is also important to assess the instructional environment to determine whether the classroom management system provides opportunities for consequences to be appropriately applied to academic responses.

Other important variables that clearly affect academic performance and are derived from applied behavior analysis are competing contingencies. These are classroom events that compete with the potential affects of antecedent–consequence relationships of academic responses. For example, if a student is frequently drawn off-task by peers asking for help, the observed student may be making fewer academic responses than are desirable. Likewise, if a target student engages in high rates of contact with other students, out-of-seat or out-of-area responses, disruptiveness, or other behaviors that prevent student academic performance, it is likely that the student's academic achievement will be limited. Although Hoge and Andrews (1987) raise some questions about the actual relationship between modifications of disruptive behavior and improvements in academic responding, it remains important in the assessment process to examine the student behaviors that may be affecting the student's academic responding. The assessment of competing contingencies, therefore, requires careful examination of student behaviors that typically occur in classrooms and are considered disruptive or related to poor academic performance. These would include such behaviors as being out of seat, student–student contacts, talking out, physical and/or verbally aggressive behavior, and general inattentiveness.

One final set of instructional environmental variables that should be assessed includes teacher expectations for students, goal setting, and progress monitoring. There is some evidence that students make greater gains in academic performance when teachers formally monitor progress across time (L. S. Fuchs, 1986; L. S. Fuchs, Deno, & Mirkin, 1984). Also, goal setting, whether performed by the teacher or by the student, appears to be critical in improving academic performance (Kelley & Stokes, 1982, 1984; Lee & Tindal, 1994; Lenz, Ehren, & Smiley, 1991; Schunk & Schwartz, 1993).

Summary and Conclusions

The assessment of the academic environment requires an evaluation of those variables that have an impact upon academic performance. These academic enablers (DiPerna & Elliott, 2002; DiPerna et al., 2002) include areas related to motivation, interpersonal skills, study skills, and time. In particular, variables that need to be assessed would include behaviors that are related to academic engaged time (e.g., opportunities to respond), teacher instructional procedures (e.g., presentation style, antecedents and consequences of academic responding), competing contingencies (e.g., disruptiveness, student–student contacts), and teacher–student monitoring procedures and expectations. Although it is impossible to conclude that any one of these variables alone is critical for academic responding, the thorough examination of the academic ecology becomes a crucial portion of the evaluation of a student's academic skills.

Assessing Individual Academic Skills

There has been historical dissatisfaction with the use of traditional methods of assessing academic performance (e.g., Carver, 1974; Hively & Reynolds, 1975; Neill & Medina, 1989; Tindal, Fuchs, et al., 1985). Typically, these procedures involve the administration of published, standardized, norm-referenced achievement tests before and after the implementation of an intervention. Significant questions have been raised about the value of these methods for assessing student progress (Fuchs, Fuchs, Benowitz, & Barringer, 1987), the poor overlap with instructional curricula (Bell et al., 1992; Good & Salvia, 1988; Jenkins & Pany, 1978; Martens et al., 1995; Shapiro & Derr, 1987), and the relevance of these measures for assessing students with disabilities (D. Fuchs et al., 1987; L. S. Fuchs, Fuchs, & Bishop, 1992). In addition, the measures were never designed to be repeated frequently or to assist in deriving appropriate intervention strategies.

A number of alternative measurement systems have been developed for assessing academic skills. They are designed to be reliable and to provide direct assessment of skills based on the curricula, are repeatable, are sensitive to student growth, and can assist in deriving appropriate strategies for academic performance (e.g., Deno & Mirkin, 1977; Gickling & Rosenfield, 1995; Gickling & Havertape, 1981; Howell & Nolet, 1999; Idol, Nevin, & Paolucci-Whitcomb, 1996; Lindsley, 1971; Salvia & Hughes, 1990; Shapiro, 1990; Shapiro & Lentz, 1985, 1986; White & Haring, 1980). Each of these systems is based on principles of CBA. Data are obtained using material taken directly or indirectly from the curriculum in which a student is being taught. Measures collected are brief and repeatable, and generally consist of timed or untimed skill probes. Critical to each system are the graphing and use of the data in educational decision making. The measures are also employed in the development of goals for IEPs and, in some cases, are used to help plan remediation strategies.

L. S. Fuchs and Deno (1991) classified approaches to CBA into two groups. Subskill mastery models assess distinct skills in the learning process. Each of these skills is assessed, and instruction is focused on the teaching of the specific skill. Once competency in that skill is attained, a new measure is developed for assessing the subsequent skill, and teaching of that skill occurs. This process continues through a skills hierarchy that leads to mastery of the required curriculum materials. In particular, the model serves as a mechanism for teachers to identify specific skills in need of remediation and to design effective interventions to remediate those skills. Models such as those identified by Idol et al. (1996), Gickling and Havertape (1981), or Howell and Nolet (1999) typify this model.

General outcome measurement (GOM) models provide a standardized assessment tool across curricular objectives. The measures are designed to be sensitive to instructional gains across time. Measurement systems are consistent across skills taught and serve as indices of whether the instruction is effective, regardless of the specific curriculum being taught. The model serves best as a means to monitor a student's progress across the instructional process. When student performance deviates from the identified goal or expected level of performance, the teacher is signaled that a change in the instructional process is needed. Although GOM models are able to suggest potential skills in need of remediation, the model was designed primarily to let teachers know that "something is not right about the instructional process," then to specifically identify remediation strategies to solve the identified problem. CBM is perhaps the most well-known and well-researched GOM model (Deno, 1985).

Despite the underlying similarity of the two measurement systems in assessing ongoing student progress throughout the instructional process, specific strategies for the two models are quite distinct. For example, Idol et al. (1996) use measures of the acquisition of students skills within grades. In their model, student skills within grades are assessed by teacher-made tests. These measures offer remediation recommendations for skill development, and students are reassessed on these criterion-referenced tests following the implementation of an instructional technique designed to improve the identified skill deficit.

Gickling and Havertape (1981), Gickling and Rosenfield (1995), and Gickling and Thompson (1985) describe a subskill mastery model based on principles of controlling the difficulty level of material presented to students during the instructional process. This is accomplished by examining the content of curriculum material and making instructional decisions based on the ratio of curricular material known by the student (immediate and correct responses) to material unknown by the student. Gickling notes that student learning is maximized when material that is unknown by the student is always between 15 and 30% of known material. In order to determine what students know and do not know, specific skill probes tied to instructional objectives are administered. Remediation strategies are then developed and implemented, with repeated assessment of that specific skill used to determine when the skill has been acquired by the student.

Another example of a subskill mastery model is that described by Howell, Fox, and Morehead (1993) and further elaborated by Howell and Nolet (1999). In this model, a broad-based survey assessment, similar to a GOM model, is initially conducted. Based on the outcomes of that assessment process, more specific-level assessment of problematic skills is conducted. Based on the specific-level assessment measure, potential strategies for intervention are identified. Once these interventions are implemented, specific-level assessment continues until the student demonstrates acquisition of the identified skill.

Although the empirical research base for subskill mastery models is somewhat limited, there have been some efforts to offer support for the model described by Gickling. For example, Burns and his colleagues (2000) have reported that the reliability properties (interscorer, alternate-form, internal consistency, and test–retest) of the model exceeded levels expected for purposes of screening. Furthermore, Burns (2001) examined the concept of using rates of acquisition and retention as a means to determine student learning. Using material unknown to the students across grades 1, 3, and 5, students were taught the material employing a technique labeled "incremental rehearsal" (Tucker, 1989). The technique, also known as "folding in" (Shapiro, 1996b), carefully controls for the ratio of known and unknown material during the teaching process. Burns (2001) showed that student performance between acquisition and retention of the material over a 14-day period were highly correlated for grades 3 and 5 ($r > .90$). Other studies have also shown validation of Gickling's suggested ratio for instructional material (Roberts & Shapiro, 1996; Roberts, Turco, & Shapiro, 1991) as well as support for the instructional process based on the Gickling model (Shapiro, 1992).

The most substantial research base documenting psychometric properties of CBA has been the efforts of Deno and his colleagues. The reliability and validity of their GOM system, called "curriculum-based measurement" (CBM), has been thoroughly investigated. In particular, concurrent validity of CBM with standardized, norm-referenced tests in reading, spelling, and written language has been examined. In addition, the correspondence between CBM and traditional assessment methods for making decisions about student eligibility for special education has been examined. Shinn (1989a, 1998) provides an excellent review of the research in CBM.

The development of CBM began with an earlier effort entitled "data-based program modification" (Deno & Mirkin, 1977). This program described a methodology for special education consultants that used skill probes taken directly from the curriculum as the assessment strategy for determining student progress in academic subjects. Oral reading rates were used to assess reading; performance on timed sheets of math problems encompassing specific computational objectives was used to assess skills in math; words spelled correctly during a timed and dictated word list assessed spelling; and words written correctly in writing a story during 3 minutes were used to assess written language. Results from these assessments were graphed and analyzed to assess students' progress through a curriculum, as well as their performance on specific objectives.

The psychometric properties of these measures in reading, spelling, and written expression were investigated in a series of studies (Deno, Marston, & Mirkin, 1982; Deno, Mirkin, Lowry, & Kuehnle, 1980; Deno, Mirkin, & Chiang, 1982). Shinn, Tindal, and Stein (1988) noted that for each measure, reliability (test–retest, internal consistency, and interscorer) and concurrent validity had to be demonstrated.

In reading, Deno, Mirkin, and Chiang (1982) compared various types of reading probe measures: the number of words read aloud from a list of words randomly taken from the basal reader; the number of words read aloud from basal reader passages; the number of correctly defined words from the basal reader; the number of correct words provided in a cloze procedure taken from the basal reader; and the number of correct words underlined in a passage. All of these measures had been used as methods of informal assessment in the evaluation of reading. Measures were examined for their correlation with numerous subtests from norm-referenced, commercially available standardized tests such as the Stanford Diagnostic Reading Test (Karlsen, Madden, & Gardner, 1975), the Peabody Individual Achievement Test (PIAT; Dunn & Markwardt, 1970), and the Woodcock Reading Mastery Test (Woodcock, 1987). These data showed that the number of words read aloud correctly in 1 minute from either word lists or passages taken from the basal readers had the highest correlations with the various reading subtests, ranging from .73 to .91. Similarly, internal consistency and test–retest reliability, as well as interscorer agreement, ranged from .89 to .99.

L. S. Fuchs, Deno, and Marston (1983) examined the effects of aggregating scores on reliability of oral reading probes. Results showed that measures of correct reading rates were extremely stable across observations and that aggregation of scores had little effect in increasing reliability. For error rates, aggregation substantially improved reliability. Correlations with the Reading Recognition subtest of the Woodcock Reading Mastery Test showed that CBM was just as precise using only a single measure assessed on one occasion.

In a series of studies, L. S. Fuchs, Tindal, and Deno (1984) examined the use of 30- versus 60-second reading samples, as well as a comprehension measure. They also investigated the stability of CBM for reading in two second-grade girls. Results showed that the 30- and 60-second samples had high correlations with each other and substantially high correlations with the comprehension measure (cloze procedure). The second study, however, showed that the degree of instability in performance across time was much higher when 30-second rather than 60-second samples were used.

In spelling, Deno et al. (1980) found that the number of words spelled correctly or the number of correct letter sequences, a measurement procedure used in precision teaching (White & Haring, 1980), during a 2-minute period, had correlations between .80 and .96 with the Test of Written Spelling (Larsen & Hammill, 1976), the PIAT Spelling subtest (Dunn & Markwardt, 1970), and the Stanford Achievement Test—Primary III (Madden, Gardener, Rudman, Karlsen, & Marwin, 1973). Reliability estimates of internal consistency, test–retest, and interscorer agreement ranged from .86 to .99. Further research by Deno et al. (1980) found that 1-, 2-, or 3-minute dictation samples all had equally strong correlations with the criterion spelling measures.

The same research strategy for written expression found that the number of words written during a writing sample was highly correlated (> .70) with various criterion measures, such as the Test of Written Language (Hammill & Larsen, 1978), the Word Usage subtest of the Stanford Achievement Test (Madden et al., 1973), and the Developmental Sentence Scoring System (Lee & Canter, 1971). Additional research related to stimuli used to generate writing samples (e.g., pictures, story starters, or topic sentences) and to time limits found no significant relationships between the criterion measures and CBM. As a result, Deno, Marston, and Mirkin (1982) recommended that a 3-minute response time be used with story starters. Although researchers have continued to find that the words written metric is a good discriminator of students across grades (Malecki & Jewell, 2003), others have suggested that supplemental metrics, such as correct punctuation marks, may be valuable in assessing written language (Gansle, Noell, Van Der Heyden, Naquin, & Slider, 2002).

Surprisingly, there has been very little systematic investigation into CBM measures for mathematics, although it has been used as an outcome measure in numerous studies (e.g., L. S. Fuchs, Fuchs, Phillips, Hamlett, & Karns, 1995; L. S. Fuchs, Fuchs, Hamlett, et al., 1991; Stoner, Carey, Ikeda, & Shinn, 1994). Although Deno and Mirkin (1977) offer some very specific recommendations for assessing computational skills, there have been only a few published attempts to demonstrate reliability and validity of the measures. Typically, CBM measures for mathematics use the original Deno and Mirkin procedures of giving timed skill probes taken from across grade-based objectives and counting the number of correct digits per minute (Germann & Tindal, 1985; Marston & Magnusson, 1985). In some subskill mastery models of CBA, computational probes for single operations have been used. In GOM models such as CBM, mixed operations have been employed. Additionally, L. S. Fuchs, Fuchs, Phillips, et al. (1995) in their effort to combine classwide peer tutoring and CBM, have used measures of mathematics concepts and applications.

Although these measures appear to be useful and valid for assessing math performance, their technical adequacy still remains largely unknown.

Efforts to demonstrate the technical adequacy of CBM measures in mathematics have demonstrated that assessments need to include both computation and application measures (Thurber, Shinn, & Smolkowski, 2002). Hintze, Christ, and Keller (2002) also showed that single- and multiple-skill probe assessments measure somewhat different constructs (i.e., a specific skill vs. skills across the curriculum). Some studies have shown moderate to strong correlations between CBM computational measures and student performance on published, standardized, norm-referenced tests (L. S. Fuchs, Hamlett, & Fuchs, 1999c). In addition, some efforts to find CBM measures of mathematics performance able to be used for students at secondary levels have also been reported (Calhoun & Fuchs, 2003; Foegen & Deno, 2001).

Although the data showing the technical adequacy of CBMs in mathematics is thin, L. S. Fuchs, Hamlett, and Fuchs (1990a) have developed a computerized program for conducting CBM monitoring of students in math. In addition, L. S. Fuchs, Fuchs, Hamlett, Walz, and Germann (1993) have provided data on the expected rate of progress in math among students in general education when CBM is conducted across an entire year. Indeed, the computer program has been an integral part of an effort to use classwide peer-tutoring procedures and CBM measures in improving the math performance of students (L. S. Fuchs, Fuchs, & Karns, 2001; L. S. Fuchs, Fuchs, Prentice, et al., 2003; L. S. Fuchs, Fuchs, Yazdian, & Powell, 2002). We (Shapiro et al., in press) showed that CBM measures in computation and concepts/applications to be sensitive to changes in performance among students with learning disabilities. Together, the research and outcomes reported here allow evaluators to use CBM in math with some degree of confidence.

In a review of CBM research, Shinn (1989a, 1998) describes the extensive efforts to replicate the technical adequacy findings of Deno and colleagues (Deno, Mirkin, & Chiang, 1982; Deno et al., 1980). Test–retest and alternate-form reliabilities over a 5-week period remained high for reading and spelling measures (.80–.90) and moderate for written expression (.60). Marston and Magnusson (1985), in a replication of the Deno, Mirkin, and Chiang (1982) findings, found that correlations between subtests of the Stanford Achievement Test, the Science Research Associates (SRA) Achievement series (Naslund, Thorpe, & Lefever, 1978), and the Ginn Reading 720 Series (Clymer & Fenn, 1979), with oral reading rates taken from basal readers, showed coefficients between .80 and .90. In addition, Marston and Magnusson (1985) found correlations between teacher judgments of student achievement levels in reading to be strongest for CBM measures compared to standardized test scores.

Over the past decade substantial attention has been devoted to the development of curricular standards that drive the instructional process.

Considering the increasing national emphasis on using statewide assessments to judge student academic performance (e.g., Garcia & Rothman, 2002), some studies have examined relationships between CBM measures and statewide, high-stakes tests. Good, Simmons, and Kame'enui (2001) reported correlations between measures of oral reading fluency for students in third grade and scores on the reading subtest of the Oregon State Assessment to be .67. Crawford, Tindal, and Stieber (2001) found similar correlations between reading and math both in the same year and 1 year earlier for the Oregon State Assessment. In other states (Pennsylvania, Washington, Illinois, Florida, Michigan), studies seem to be finding the same outcomes (McGlinchey & Hixson, in press; Powell-Smith, 2004; Shapiro, Edwards, Lutz, & Keller, 2004; Stage & Jacobsen, 2001). These studies offer preliminary evidence that CBM, especially in reading, can be a valuable and powerful predictor of student performance on high-stakes, statewide assessments.

One of the concerns that emerged in the development of CBM measures of reading was the significant shift in the type of materials used for reading instruction. Schools have shifted to using literature-based materials and whole-language instructional methods rather than basal texts and skills-oriented approaches to teaching reading. Although there has been a significant return to approaches to teach phonemic awareness to young children over the past few years, making popular curriculum materials that focus on the development of phonics and the building blocks of early literacy, most schools still use literature-based reading series in the instructional process beyond early grades. Questions have been raised as to whether the measures typical of CBM derived from grade-based reading material are equally applicable when working with nongraded material typical of a literature-based reading series. L. S. Fuchs and Deno (1994) examined the necessity of deriving the assessment material directly from the curriculum of instruction. Their analysis suggests that it may not be critical that the measures developed for purposes of assessment come directly from the material being instructed. Indeed, L. S. Fuchs and Deno (1992), in a study of 91 elementary-age students, found that the oral reading rate metric was a developmentally sensitive measure regardless of the series in which the students were being instructed. However, Hintze, Shapiro, and Lutz (1994), Hintze and Shapiro (1997), and Bradley-Klug, Shapiro, Lutz, and DuPaul (1998) have found that there may be some differences in the sensitivity of CBM passages derived from literature-based and basal reading series when the measures are used to monitor progress across time. Others studies (Powell-Smith & Bradley-Klug, 2001) found no differences in sensitivity of the two types of CBM passages to monitoring growth of student performance, only that students may perform somewhat higher in generic passages derived from basal reading series.

Results from these studies suggest that it is important to use passages that are carefully controlled for grade-level readability when working from a literature-based reading series. It was found, however, that generic CBM measures derived from basal reading material can be used to monitor student progress regardless of which type of curriculum series a student is being taught. Given the ease and availability of generic passages, recommendations have been made that such measures be used over those that may be developed directly from literature-based series in which students are being instructed.

Strong evidence that CBM reading measures are valid and effective predictors of student performance has led some researchers to suggest that CBM may be an effective metric for an alternative approach to the classification of students with learning disabilities in the area of reading. L. S. Fuchs and Fuchs (1998) and L. S. Fuchs et al. (2002) recommended a model for identifying students with learning disabilities based on treatment validity. Their model requires assessments of two discrepancies—student performance against a set of local peers at a specific point in time and the rate of student performance across time against the expected rate of local peers. This dual set of discrepancies requires that students are identified as having a learning disability only after they are provided with intervention strategies that are known to be effective in remediation reading problems. The model, known as "responsiveness to intervention" (Gresham 2002), requires that a measure sensitive to instructional change over time must be used to evaluate student performance. At present, CBM in reading is one of the only metrics with the needed levels of empirical support. Indeed, the Oral Reading Fluency metric was one of the recommended scientifically based measures for assessing reading noted in the National Report of Reading Assessment (Kame'enui, 2002). Preliminary evidence supporting the model using the CBM Oral Reading Fluency measure was reported by Speece and Case (2001).

Beyond the data suggesting that CBM can be used reliably to discriminate categories of learning-disabled and non-learning-disabled students, an important aspect of CBM is its ability to be sensitive to student progress across time. Clearly, one of the key advantages of CBM is its repeatability over time. Indeed, Jenkins, Deno, and Mirkin (1979) have offered strong and persuasive arguments for the use of these measures in writing and setting IEP goals (see Deno et al. 1985).

Shinn et al. (1993) demonstrated how CBM can be used potentially to impact decisions to reintegrate students from special education to general education settings. In two studies involving children in grades 3–5, CBM was used to identify special education students who performed in reading at or above the level of those students in the low-reading groups from general education classes. Results showed that approximately 40% of the special education students could be candidates for potential reintegration using this approach.

In a similar study, Shinn, Powell-Smith, and Good (1996) showed how CBM was effective in measuring the reading progress of 18 students receiving special education services in pull-out settings, when they were placed into the general education setting for reading instruction. Of the 18 students, 9 were judged as being successfully reintegrated, with only 3 viewed by experts as having received no benefits. Powell-Smith and Stewart (1998) further described how CBM can play an important role in decisions regarding when students with special education needs are ready and capable of moving to less restrictive settings.

L. S. Fuchs, Deno, and Mirkin (1984) reported what is perhaps historically one of the most important and significant studies investigating the relationship between teacher monitoring of progress and student achievement. Special education teachers in the New York City public schools were assigned randomly to either a repeated-measurement or a conventional-measurement group. Those in the repeated-measurement group were trained to assess reading using 1-minute probes taken from the goal level of the basal reading series. Data from these probes were graphed and implemented using a data-utilization rule that required teachers to introduce program changes whenever a student's improvement across 7 to 10 measurement points appeared inadequate for reaching their goal. Teachers in the conventional measurement group set IEP goals and monitored student performance as they wished, relying predominantly on teacher-made tests, nonsystematic observation, and scores on workbook exercises. Data were obtained on a CBM of reading (using third-grade reading material), the Structural Analysis and Reading Comprehension subtests of the Stanford Diagnostic Reading Test (Karlsen et al., 1975), the Structure of Instruction Rating Scale (Deno, King, Skiba, Sevcik, & Wesson, 1983), a teacher questionnaire designed to assess progress toward reading goals and describe student functioning, and a student interview.

Results of the study showed that children whose teachers used repeated measurement made significantly better academic progress. These improvements were noted not only on the passage-reading tests, which were similar to the repeated-measurement procedure, but also on decoding and comprehension measures. In addition, teachers using repeated-measurement procedures were able to write precise and specific goals for students, and students whose behavior was measured repeatedly showed significantly more knowledge about the progress they were making. In a similar study, Marston, Fuchs, and Deno (1986) directly compared the sensitivity of standardized achievement tests and CBM of reading and written language across 10- and 16-week periods. Results of their investigation showed that

CBM consistently reflected student progress and was related to teacher judgments of pupil growth across time.

L. S. Fuchs and Fuchs (1986b), in a meta-analysis of formative evaluation procedures on student achievement, examined 21 studies in which evaluation procedures employed systematic examination of ongoing student progress and continual modification of instructional procedures. The analysis showed an average weighted effect size of .70. Fuchs and Fuchs suggested that from their data, one can expect students with handicaps whose programs are monitored to average 0.7 standard deviation units higher than nonmonitored students on evaluation measures. Results of their analysis were consistent across students' age, treatment duration, frequency of measurement, and handicap status. In particular, the strongest effect sizes were related to use of behavior modification procedures as intervention strategies, data-utilization rules by teachers, and a graphic method for displaying data. Overall, the study by Fuchs and Fuchs provides significant evidence for the importance of monitoring student progress and using data in decision making.

L. S. Fuchs and Fuchs (1986a) also conducted a meta-analysis of studies that used different methods of measuring outcomes on IEPs. Comparisons were made between CBA methods, employing subskill mastery methods that assess directly attainment of curriculum objectives (e.g., Blankenship, 1985; Idol-Maestas, 1983) and general outcome measurement CBM-type methods, which assess performance on identical measures across time (e.g., L. S. Fuchs, Deno, & Mirkin, 1984). Analysis of these data showed that the largest effect size was associated with the type of measure employed, but not with the goal on which monitoring occurred. In other words, when progress toward long-term goals was measured, the use of general outcome methods was more likely to show progress than the use of subskill mastery methods assessing attainment of curriculum objectives. Likewise, when progress toward short-term goals was measured, methods assessing mastery of objectives were more likely to reflect progress than those measuring global performance. These findings together suggest that subskill mastery and general outcome measurement may be useful for planning and assessing interventions for remediation of specific academic deficiencies.

In general, there is a substantial research base justifying the use of CBA methods, particularly CBM-type, in the evaluation of academic problems. These measures appear to possess acceptable psychometric characteristics (reliability and criterion-related validity) and are sensitive to student growth. The measures appear to be important in affecting academic performance and can be useful in differentiating students with and without handicaps.

Although the research validating CBA measures has provided strong evidence of psychometric properties, another set of studies has examined the validity of CBA methods based on parameters of behavioral assessment methods such as accuracy, generalizability, and treatment validity (Cone, 1981, 1988; Cone & Hoier, 1986; Lentz, 1988). For example, to what degree does a student's oral reading rate vary when he or she reads aloud in a small group to the teacher, individually to the teacher, individually to a stranger, in a small testing room, and so forth? How closely related are a child's spelling scores when the words are taken from the basal reader versus the spelling curriculum? Do we have to make assessments from the same basal reader that the student is reading, or can we use any basal reader? If a teacher does not employ a basal reading series, can we still demonstrate student growth over time by assessing across a basal reading series? These latter questions are particularly important for students with disabilities, who may be changing reading series when they return from a self-contained to a mainstreamed setting.

In an attempt to examine the accuracy of CBM, Derr and Shapiro (1989) and Derr-Minneci and Shapiro (1992) investigated the relationship between differential arrangements of how a CBA in reading is conducted. In our studies, 126 third- and fourth-grade students in general education classes were administered sets of reading passages under conditions that varied the location of the assessment, who conducted the evaluation, and whether students knew they were being timed or not. Results showed that oral reading rates were significantly different depending on the conditions of the assessment. These effects were present regardless of whether students were low-, average-, or high-ability readers. The outcome of these studies suggested that the results of a CBA in reading may be affected significantly by the methodology for data collection.

We (McCurdy & Shapiro, 1992) conducted another study to examine the impact of the way CBM data are collected on student performance in reading. Using 48 elementary-age students with LD, progress monitoring in reading was conducted for 9 weeks. Students were randomly assigned to either teacher-monitoring, peer-monitoring, or self-monitoring conditions. Analysis of the group data showed that students in all conditions made equal levels of progress across time. However, when the data were examined at an idiographic level, students in the teacher-monitoring condition showed the most progress. The study did demonstrate that students with LD were able to reliably collect CBM data on themselves and their peers, thus demonstrating the potential reduction in teacher time devoted to the data-collection process.

Hintze, Owen, Shapiro, and Daly (2000) examined the use of generalizability (G) theory as an alternative to validating direct behavioral measures. Whereas most studies validating CBM have used classical reliability theory, where the amount of error evident in repeated measurement is determined, G theory examines multiple sources of variance simultaneously. Using G theory, one can partition the sources of variance to estimate proportions of contribution by components such as different rates, different forms, or occasions. In addition, G theory can allow one to determine the precision of decisions made with various measurement techniques. Results showed that CBM oral reading fluency measures can be used to compare student performance against one's peers as well as against one's own past performance. Hintze and Pelle Pettite (2001), using G theory, have similarly found that CBM in reading is a valid and reliable predictor of student performance across both general and special education students.

The use of CBM appears quite promising. Indeed, as noted by Shapiro and Eckert (1993) and Shapiro, Angello, and Eckert (2004), CBA appears to have made a substantial impact on the practice of school psychologists. For example, Shapiro, Angello, and Eckert (2004) noted that among school psychologists entering the field in the past 6 years, over 90% indicated that they had received training in CBA through their graduate education. Roberts and Rust (1994) found that school psychologists in Iowa spent a significant amount of time in CBA activities. CBA measures seem to be able to overcome many of the problems of the traditional standardized assessment instruments and have been shown in many field settings to be highly acceptable. In a series of studies, Shapiro, Eckert, and colleagues have found that CBA methods are more acceptable to teachers and school psychologists than standardized, norm-referenced tests for assessing academic achievement (Eckert & Shapiro, 1999; Eckert et al., 1995; Shapiro & Eckert, 1994). Despite the overwhelming support for CBA methods in the research literature, Shapiro, Angello, and Eckert (2004), in a national survey of knowledge, use, and attitudes toward CBA, reported that over the past decade, the percentage of school psychologists who use CBA in their typical practice increased only from 47% to 53%. Clearly, the data supporting the impact that CBA can have on assessing academic performance in students suggest a need for school psychologists to make CBA a much more important part of their day-to-day assessment process.

SELECTING TARGETS FOR REMEDIATION: LINKING ASSESSMENT TO INTERVENTION

Choosing target behaviors for remediation of academic problems is not always as simple as it seems. When behavioral assessments are conducted for nonacademic problems, the behaviors chosen for assessment are usually the direct targets for remediation. If a child is referred because of excessive talking out during group instruction, the number times the child talks out is recorded, and remediation strategies are developed specifically to reduce the talking-out behavior. If a student is referred because of low rates of peer interaction, the number of peer interactions is assessed, and interventions are implemented to increase the frequency of positive peer interactions. When the problem is academic, however, the link between what is assessed and what is targeted for remediation is not as straightforward. Although a student may have significant problems in reading, the complexity of reading behavior makes selection of the specific skill to be assessed quite difficult. For example, a student who is a poor reader may have a deficiency in the component skill of sequencing—a problem that is viewed by some as a prerequisite skill to developing effective reading skill. If one follows the same logical linkage between the assessment and intervention strategies as in a behavioral assessment for nonacademic problems, one should probably design an intervention to remediate sequencing skills, readministering the assessment measures used to identify the deficient component skill. Despite the logical appeal of this approach, a substantial literature suggests that such an approach may improve sequencing but not reading.

Arter and Jenkins (1979), in an extensive and comprehensive review of the literature examining the assessment and remediation in diagnostic-prescriptive teaching, found very few studies in which the remediation of an underlying perceptual process led to improvements in the overall academic skill of interest. Consistently, the literature showed that even when specific component skills underlying basic academic skills (such as auditory memory or perceptual–motor integration) could be adequately identified and remediated, changes would only be observed for the component skill trained (i.e., auditory memory or perceptual–motor integration). Any transfer from improvements in these skills to increases in academic performance in reading or math were negligible. The evidence against the use of this approach was so overwhelming that, as noted previously, Arter and Jenkins called for a moratorium on the classification and placement of children according to differential ability tests, and on the use of instructional materials and programs that claim to improve these abilities.

The critical issue in selecting the appropriate behaviors for assessment is the functional relationship between the assessed behavior and remediation strategies designed to improve the skill. Daly, Witt, Martens, and Dool (1997) provided a conceptual framework for a functional assessment of academic skills. Based on the literature, Daly et al. identified five potential hypotheses as to why students have academic difficulties. Specifically, they noted that students fail because they lack motivation, have had insufficient practice, have had insufficient instruction, have not been expected to perform the academic task in the way they are being asked to perform, and/

or the expected academic performance contains skills that have prerequisites that are far above the students' instructional level. Intervention development is linked to which of these hypothesized areas is problematic. Of course, many academic skills problems are a function of the combination of these variables, but the linking of the assessment to intervention development is the critical component of the approach.

Hoge and Andrews (1987) have provided an extensive review of the literature on selecting targets for remediation of academic problems. Typically, studies that have aimed at improving academic skills have focused either on enhancing classroom behavior or on improving academic performance. Those looking at classroom performance have argued that academic survival skills, such as attention to task, compliance, and nondisruptive behavior, have direct and functional links to improvements in academic responding (e.g., Cobbs & Hopps, 1973; DiPerna & Elliott, 2002; DiPerna et al., 2002; Friedling & O'Leary, 1979; Greenwood, Hops, & Walker, 1977; Greenwood et al., 1979; Hallahan, Lloyd, Kneedler, & Marshall, 1982). Others have examined the relationship of direct remediation of academic skills to both academic performance and classroom behavior (e.g., Harris, Graham, Reid, McElroy, & Hamby, 1994; Maag, Reid, & DiGangi, 1993; Reid & Harris, 1993; Speltz, Shimamura, & McReynolds, 1982; Stevenson & Fantuzzo, 1984). Still other researchers have made direct comparisons between interventions designed to improve academic performance and interventions aimed directly at classroom behavior (e.g., Lam, Cole, Shapiro, & Bambara, 1994; Skinner, Wallace, & Neddenriep, 2002). According to Hoge and Andrews (1987), all of these studies clearly showed that the most direct effects upon academic performance are evident when academic performance rather than classroom behavior is the target for remediation.

What becomes clear in the selection of behaviors for assessing academic problems is the necessity for these behaviors to reflect change in the academic skill, should the selected remediation strategy be effective. Indeed, the methods developed by Deno and his colleagues for CBA and CBM in particular have been shown to be sensitive to remediation of the skills. An important question that must be raised is the process by which the intervention strategy would be selected. Fuchs and colleagues (e.g., L. S. Fuchs, Fuchs, Hamlett, & Allinder, 1991a; L. S. Fuchs, Fuchs, Hamlett, & Ferguson, 1992; L. S. Fuchs, Fuchs, Hamlett, & Stecker, 1991; Phillips, Hamlett, Fuchs, & Fuchs, 1993) have increasingly demonstrated that CBM can be used to identify a student's strengths and weaknesses in skills development and assist the teacher in selecting an intervention method that may improve a student's skills. However, although the use of CBM data as described by Deno and colleagues offers an excellent method for monitoring the effectiveness of academic interventions (e.g., L. S. Fuchs, Deno, &

Mirkin, 1984; L. S. Fuchs & Fuchs, 1986a, 1986b), the method was not designed primarily to suggest which remediation strategies may be effective. How does one choose the intervention procedure likely to remediate the academic problem?

SELECTING INTERVENTION PROCEDURES

Choosing an appropriate remediation strategy should be based on a linkage between assessment and intervention. In choosing interventions for non-academic problems, Nelson and Hayes (1986) describe three procedures: functional analysis, the keystone behavior strategy, and the diagnostic strategy. A fourth procedure, the template-matching strategy, is also described here.

Functional Analysis

The purpose of functional analysis is to determine empirically the relationships between the variables controlling the target behavior and, subsequently, to modify these behaviors. In terms of selecting a treatment strategy, the identification of specific environmental variables related to behavior change should differentially lead to the selection of various treatment procedures. Hypothetically, choosing the strategy with a functional relationship to the target behavior should result in improvement, whereas choosing strategies without a functional relationship should not result in any change in the targeted response. Functional analysis has long been suggested as a viable strategy for linking assessment and intervention in behavior analysis (e.g., Ferster, 1965), and many empirical investigations demonstrating the utility of this methodology have appeared in the literature. Based on the work of Iwata, Dorsey, Slifer, Bauman, and Richman (1982), Mace and his colleagues, in a series of studies, have provided several examples of the potential use of the functional analysis methodology.

Mace, Yankanich, and West (1988), McComas and Mace (2000), and McComas, Hoch, and Mace (2000) have provided both descriptions and examples of the application of this methodology to individuals with developmental disabilities. The method begins with a problem identification interview with the referral source (teachers, parents, or caretakers), followed by data collection to generate a series of potential hypotheses regarding variables that may be functioning to maintain the aberrant response. These hypotheses are then evaluated through the development of analogue conditions, typically employed in an alternating treatments design. Data are graphed and examined to determine which variables are functionally related to the response, and a relevant treatment procedure based on this knowledge is then generated, implemented, and evaluated. If the analysis is accurate, the aberrant behavior should be significantly altered once the appropriate treatment procedure is implemented.

In an example of this methodology, Mace and Knight (1986) described the analysis and treatment of pica behavior in a 19-year-old individual with mental retardation. Data collected through direct observation and interviews with staff members suggested the possibility that levels of staff interaction may have been related to the pica behavior. As shown in Figure 2.1, the lowest levels of pica were evident during the condition of frequent staff interaction. Throughout this phase, the client continually wore a protective helmet with a face shield, prescribed by a physician as a mechanism for reducing pica. An additional phase was conducted to examine the relationship of pica to wearing the helmet, with and without the face shield. From this analysis, it was determined that frequent interaction without the helmet was likely to result in the most significant reductions of pica behavior. Staff feedback suggested that frequent interaction would be difficult to maintain, so a treatment consisting of limited interaction plus no helmet was implemented. As evident in Figure 2.1, this treatment was successful in substantially reducing the frequency of pica behavior.

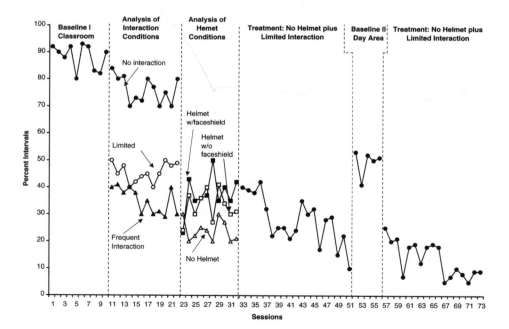

FIGURE 2.1. Pica behavior across baseline, analysis, and treatment conditions. From Mace and Knight (1986, p. 415). Copyright 1986 by the Society for the Experimental Analysis of Behavior, Inc. Reprinted by permission.

This same methodology has been applied by Mace, Browder, and Lin (1987) in reducing stereotypical mouthing, and Carr, Newsom, and Binkoff (1980) in analyzing escape behavior in maintaining the aggressive responses of two children with mental retardation. In all cases, the use of functional analysis provided direct links between the process of assessment and the development of intervention strategies.

Although few studies have directly applied this methodology to the selection of effective treatment strategies for academic problems, the procedures described by Mace et al. (1987) seem to have direct applicability to such problems. For example, hypotheses could be generated based on direct observation and interview data collected during the initial analysis phase. These hypotheses could be tested through analogue conditions, and differential treatment procedures could be generated. From these data, one could determine the effective treatment and the functional variables related to academic performance. Thus, one student who is performing poorly in math may be found to be having problems related to competing contingencies (being drawn off-task by peers), whereas another student may need to have the level of difficulty reduced. Each of these cases would require differential interventions, which could be systematically evaluated and implemented within the classroom setting.

Broussard and Northrup (1995) demonstrated the use of functional analysis in the evaluation of 3 elementary-age students who were referred for extreme disruptive behavior. Based upon the descriptive assessment phase, one of three hypotheses was chosen for functional analysis: Disruptive behavior was related primarily to teacher attention, peer attention, or escape from an academic task. For each student, two conditions were constructed that represented occurrences or nonoccurrences of the consequences associated with each hypothesis. For example, for the contingent teacher-attention hypothesis, the evaluator made a disapproving statement (e.g., "Pay attention to your work") each time the targeted student engaged in a disruptive behavior. For nonoccurrence of this condition, the evaluator had the teacher provide noncontingent attention ("Good job") every 60 seconds, independent of the student's behavior. Similar conditions were constructed for the contingent peer-attention and escape-from-academic-task hypotheses. Using a reversal design, the effects of the differing conditions were compared. Results of the functional analysis demonstrated that the same disruptive behaviors were controlled by differing contingencies for different students.

In another extension of functional analysis methodology, Cooper et al. (1990) conducted an analysis of variables that were maintaining behavior among children with conduct disorders. Completed in an outpatient clinic setting, the children's parents were instructed to present one of four conditions following a no-demand baseline phase, to present the children with difficult or easy tasks, and to attend to or ignore appropriate behavior.

Two replications of the conditions were then conducted. Results again showed that the same behavioral responses were maintained by differing sets of consequences.

In working with a 12-year-old girl with a long history of severely disruptive behavior, Dunlap, Kern-Dunlap, Clarke, and Robbins (1991) demonstrated the relationships between the student's school curriculum and her disruptive behavior. Following a descriptive analysis and data-collection process, four hypotheses were generated: (1) The student is better behaved when engaged in large-motor as opposed to fine-motor activities; (2) the student is better behaved when fine-motor and academic requirements are brief as opposed to lengthy; (3) the student is better behaved when engaged in functional activities with concrete and preferred outcomes; and (4) the student is better behaved when she has some choice regarding her activities. In the initial phase of the study, each of these hypotheses was evaluated systematically during 15-minute sessions using materials taken directly from the classroom curriculum.

Results of the analysis of the first hypothesis showed that the student had zero level of disruptive behavior and consistently high levels of on-task behavior under gross-motor conditions compared to fine-motor activities. Data from the second hypothesis showed substantially better performance under short versus long tasks. The third hypothesis test revealed that she did much better when the task was functional. The results of the final hypothesis showed superior performance when choice was provided in activities. Thus, the analysis of the student's performance revealed that her best performance would occur using functional, gross-motor activities of a short duration when she had a choice of tasks.

Following the assessment phase, the student's curriculum was revised to incorporate the variables associated with high rates of on-task behavior and low rates of disruptive behavior. Based on the analysis, a set of guidelines was constructed to assist the teacher in developing lesson plans for the student. Specifically, it was suggested that sessions involving fine-motor activities be of short duration (e.g., 5 minutes or less). These activities should be interspersed with gross-motor activities, since these were found to result in low levels of disruption. Whenever possible, the activities should lead to functional and concrete outcomes. In addition, the student should be offered choices regarding activities. Through the help of classroom consultants, these changes were implemented throughout the student's day.

The results were dramatic and immediate. Once the intervention was begun, classroom disruption occurred only once across 30 days of observation. Follow-up data collected up to 10 weeks later showed maintenance of this zero rate of disruption. The student also showed substantial increases in appropriate social behavior and decreases in inappropriate vocalizations.

Roberts, Marshall, Nelson, and Albers (2001) examined how CBA and functional assessment procedures can be combined to identify antecedents to off-task behavior of students in a general education setting. The initial academic assessment using CBA procedures pointed to a hypothesis that difficulty level of material may have been related to levels of off-task behavior. In the functional analysis phase of the study, the hypothesis was evaluated by specifically manipulating task difficulty. Outcomes of the study confirmed the hypothesis and demonstrated that functional analysis procedures can be used within general education settings.

Conducting a functional analysis in a regular classroom setting requires a high degree of expertise in behavior analysis. Clearly, such a procedure necessitates the use of a classroom consultant who could effectively direct the classroom teacher and arrange for the analysis to be properly conducted. The outcomes of the analysis are especially useful when the teacher is faced with a difficult and challenging set of behaviors that may have not responded to more common methods of analysis. Functional analysis does offer an opportunity to provide a strong idiographic analysis of student behavior.

Keystone Behavior Strategy

A second method described by Nelson and Hayes (1986) for selecting intervention strategies is the "keystone behavior strategy." This procedure recognizes that multiple behaviors are usually linked to a particular behavior problem. Within the set of behaviors, a particular response is identified, which, if changed, would result in significant and substantial change in the overall group of behaviors. Thus, one attempts to identify a key response that is functionally related to all others. Nelson and Hayes noted that the primary difference between functional analysis and the keystone behavior strategy is that functional analysis is based on stimulus–response relationships, whereas the keystone strategy is based on response–response interactions.

McKnight, Nelson, Hayes, and Jarrett (1984) provided some evidence for this procedure in a study of depressed women with social skills problems, who showed improved social skills and reduced depression when treated with social skills training as compared to cognitive therapy. Similarly, those with depression and assessed cognitive distortion improved more when treated with cognitive therapy then with social skills training. Thus, assessing and treating the correct behavior was a keystone in reducing depression.

Another example of a keystone behavior is the development of language in nonverbal children with autism. Lovaas (1977) and Lovaas, Koegel, Simmons, and Long (1973) reasoned that the development of language would be a keystone behavior in the amelioration of other aberrant responses in children with autism. Thus, much of Lovaas's effort in treating these children was aimed at teaching and establishing functional language.

Despite these hypotheses, there have been few cases described in which establishing language in children with autism resulted in substantial improvement in other behaviors.

Although the keystone behavior strategy certainly has applicability to the selection of interventions for academic problems, no studies reported to date have specifically examined this procedure. However, Jenkins, Larson, and Fleisher (1983) and Roberts and Smith (1980) conducted studies that would be analogous to a keystone strategy in the remediation of reading problems. In the Jenkins et al. (1983) study, the relationships between reading comprehension and two instructional strategies for correcting reading errors, word supply and word drill, were examined. Results showed that drill had substantially more impact on word recognition and comprehension than word supply. Similarly, Roberts and Smith (1980) examined the effects on comprehension of interventions aimed at either increasing oral reading rate or decreasing error rate. Results suggested that improvements in rates (correct or error) did not affect comprehension. When comprehension was targeted, collateral changes did occur in both reading rates. Shapiro (1987a) showed the interrelationships between comprehension and correct oral reading rates when a contingent reinforcement procedure was applied differentially to these behaviors. Results of this analysis are shown in Figure 2.2.

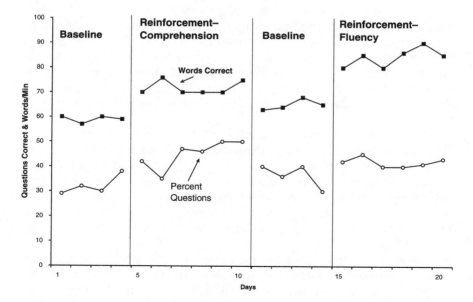

FIGURE 2.2. Collateral effects on oral reading rates and comprehension on a student in a reading program using contingent reinforcement. From Shapiro (1987c, p. 377). Copyright 1987 by John Wiley & Sons, Inc. Reprinted by permission.

Diagnostic Strategy

The diagnostic strategy for choosing interventions is one that is based on the traditional medical model, that is, the notion that effective diagnosis leads to effective treatment. In this model, the diagnosis is determined from the assessment information and is based on a particularly nosology, for example, the fourth edition of the *Diagnosis and Statistical Manual of Mental Disorders* (DSM-IV; American Psychiatric Association, 1994). The specific intervention plan is determined on the basis of this diagnosis. For example, an individual diagnosed as phobic might receive exposure treatment (Barlow & Wolfe, 1981), and a depressive might receive cognitive therapy (Beck, Rush, Shaw, & Emery, 1979). Treatment selection is based on known relationships between treatment effectiveness and specific disorders (Nelson, 1988).

Applications of this approach to academic problems are somewhat vague, since educators do not use the same type of nosological classifications as clinicians (Power & Eiraldi, 2000). However, a child diagnosed as having attention-deficit/hyperactivity disorder may be viewed as a good candidate for pharmacological therapy to indirectly affect academic performance. Likewise, a child with a conduct disorder, who is having academic problems, may be viewed as more likely to respond to contingency management aimed at the disruptive behavior rather than at the academic performance problem (Hoge & Andrews, 1987).

In educational settings, children with academic problems are often considered for placement into special education. In a sense, the decision as to a child's eligibility for special education is a diagnostic decision, since eligibility determination is based on meeting the criteria for a specific classification (e.g., learning-disabled, behavior-disordered, educationally handicapped). Yet these diagnostic labels have little to do with educational treatment. Indeed, substantial data suggest that the instructional processes in classes for children with mild handicaps are more similar than they are different (e.g., Fletcher, et al., 1998; Fletcher, Morris, & Lyon, 2003; Reynolds, 1984; Rich & Ross, 1989; Thurlow, Graden, Greener, & Ysseldyke, 1983; Thurlow, Ysseldyke, et al., 1983, 1984; Vellutino, Scanlon, & Lyon, 2000; Ysseldyke et al., 1984). Thus, the diagnostic–treatment link is equally weak for academic problems.

Template-Matching Strategy

Hoier and Cone (1987), Cone and Hoier (1986), and Hoier et al. (1987) describe a procedure called "template matching" that may have implications for selection of intervention strategies. Data are obtained on individuals deemed to possess effective levels of the desired behaviors. These profiles, or "templates," are compared to those individuals who are targeted for remediation in order to identify the specific behaviors that need to be remediated. Hoier (1984; cited in Hoier & Cone, 1987) compared the social skills of third- and fourth-grade students against those of classmates considered exemplary in their behavior, using primarily peer-assessment data. Discrepancies between the exemplary students' and the other students' behavior became targets for intervention. In a validation of the process, it was found that as a child's template approached the exemplary template, increases in peer interaction were evident.

Although designed primarily to identify behaviors for remediation, the procedure may have implications for choosing intervention strategies. For example, once specific behaviors are identified, one may decide on alternative treatments for differential templates. By matching the template to the treatment procedure, one may be able to make effective recommendations for interventions. Still, the applicability of these procedures to academic interventions may be somewhat questionable.

For example, we (Ager & Shapiro, 1995) used template matching to develop strategies to facilitate the transition between preschool and kindergarten for students with disabilities. Using the ESCAPE and the Assessment Code/Checklist for Evaluating Survival Skills (ACCESS), templates of the expected behaviors in kindergarten classes of students without disabilities were constructed. These templates were constructed in the classrooms in which the target group of students with disabilities would be placed during the following school year. Data were then collected on the same behaviors in the preschoolers' classrooms. Using the discrepancies between the preschool and kindergarten environments, a series of interventions were implemented to align more closely the expectations of the kindergarten classroom with those of the preschool. At follow-up, those students for whom the interventions based on template matching were implemented exhibited fewer disruptive behaviors and showed high levels of independent work.

SUMMARY OF PROCEDURES
FOR CHOOSING INTERVENTIONS

Despite the potential of functional analysis, the keystone behavior strategy, or template matching in applications for remediating academic problems, the current methods for choosing an intervention strategy for academic skills problems remain largely based on clinical judgment. Typically, teachers are interviewed about the child's problem; the data are examined regarding potentially important variables that may affect academic performance; the literature is consulted for studies that have previously shown the variables critical to achievement; and recommendations are made for interventions. These recommendations often are based on the teacher's experiences with other students with similar problems, past successes and failures, the range of expertise of the teacher and consultant, the structure of the classroom, the time available for remediation, the resources offered by the setting, and other variables that may or may not have direct relationships to the problem at hand. Clearly, a more empirical analysis of these effects would be worthwhile. At present, the methodology suggested by Mace et al. (1987) and Roberts et al. (2001) may have the most applicability. Still, significant work must be done to demonstrate that the procedures described for assessing and treating aberrant behavior are also applicable for assessing and treating problems in academic skills acquisition. It is important to remember that the variables surrounding an academic ecology may be significantly more complex than those surrounding behaviors such as pica or stereotypical head weaving (Lentz, 1988; Lentz & Shapiro, 1986). Furthermore, moving functional analysis methodology into school-based applications may require additional modifications of the procedure. Despite these cautions, this method appears to offer significant promise for making the assessment–intervention link an empirically based decision.

An equally important consideration is the level of analysis at which each of the procedures is aimed. With the exception of the functional analysis, empirical support for the procedures described is based on the aggregation of data across cases. These methods rely on the ability to make effective generalizations based on assessment data. Unfortunately, almost all concerns of the practitioner are at the level of the individual. What is important is the ability to effect change in a specific student's problem. Whether the individual student is like other students with similar problems is of interest in general, but not necessarily of concern to the person conducting the assessment at that time. This makes a methodology such as functional analysis, which examines the problem at the individual-student level, rather attractive.

Substantial work needs to be done to bring the decision-making process for choosing intervention strategies into line with the assessment methodology employed. Conceptually, behavioral assessment is designed to offer this link. Although the empirical link is somewhat questionable at this time, behavioral assessment continues to offer the best opportunity for using the assessment data to make one's "best guess" as to the critical elements needed for an effective intervention.

CHAPTER 3

◆ ◆ ◆

Step 1: Assessing the Academic Environment

◆

The process of conducting an assessment of academic behavior incorporates several different methods, each designed to contribute to the overall understanding of the problem. It is important to remember that because academic responses occur in the context of an instructional environment, an effective evaluation of academic problems must contain more than just an assessment of academic skills. Procedures employed in the assessment process are those typical of behavioral assessment for nonacademic problems (interviews, direct observation, examination of permanent products, rating scales) and those developed by Deno and others for CBA. Specifically, interviews, direct observation, examination of permanent products, and completion of rating scales provide the assessment of the academic environment, whereas the CBA procedures provide assessment of individual academic skills. Interpretation of the data, conclusions, and recommendations from the assessment requires careful examination and integration of the data collected from each part of the assessment process.

Several objectives guide an assessment of academic problems. First, it is important to determine the degree to which the academic ecology is contributing to the observed academic problem (Lentz & Shapiro, 1986). Understanding how events such as instructional presentation, feedback, and class structure relate to academic responding may provide significant clues regarding potential intervention strategies for remediating the academic problems. Second, the assessment is designed to separate the degree to which the child's problem is a skills versus performance deficit. In many cases, students exhibit a "won't do" rather than "can't do" problem. These students possess the necessary skills for performance but do not exhibit these skills when the situation for performance arises in the classroom. Other students may show similar deficits in performance; however, careful assessment reveals that their failure is due primarily to inadequate mastery of needed skills. Clearly, the remediation recommendations in each case would be different (Daly et al., 1997).

A third objective of the assessment for academic problems is to determine where in the curriculum the child has achieved mastery, where he or she should be instructed, and where he or she is frustrated. It is surprising to find how many times students are moved on in curricular materials despite their failure to achieve mastery of prerequisite skills. Considering that most curricula are based on principles of both repetition (spiraling) and scaffolding (interrelated skill development), failure to master certain skills will almost always lead to difficulty in subsequent parts of the curricula.

Fourth, the academic assessment should serve to assist several types of educational decisions. Salvia and Ysseldyke (2001) noted that educational assessments are used to make decisions about referral, screening, classification, instructional planning, and pupil progress. Among these, we (Lentz & Shapiro, 1985) strongly suggest that the most important purpose of an evaluation is to provide suggestions for the development of interventions aimed to remediate the problem areas.

A critical and underlying assumption of assessing academic skills is a function of environmental *and* individual variables. As such, one cannot simply focus upon the child's academic skills as the source of academic failure. It is equally important to examine events within the instructional environment that may be contributing significantly to the child's problems. In addition, careful examination of the teaching procedures, contingencies for performance, classroom structure, and other such instructional events may often suggest appropriate remediation strategies.

When academic skills are assessed, the child's academic behavior that represents the closest duplication of responses made during typical classroom instruction should be the target for evaluation. This requires that the assessment procedures be derived directly from the outcomes of what is expected of students within curriculum materials in which the child is being instructed. In this way, one is able to determine the degree to which a child has mastered what he or she has been expected to learn. In other words, if the expected outcome of instruction in reading is that a student read better, then one should assess how well a student reads. Furthermore, examination of permanent products (e.g., worksheets, homework assignments, etc.) may offer significant information about the child's academic problems.

Many different terms have been used to describe the type of academic assessment under discussion. Deno and his colleagues refer to the procedure as curriculum-based measurement (CBM). Howell et al. (1993) called it "curriculum-based evaluation." Others (Gickling & Havertape, 1981; Idol et al., 1986; Shapiro & Lentz, 1986; Tucker, 1985) have labeled the procedure "curriculum-based assessment" (CBA). Although each of these emphasizes somewhat different aspects of the evaluation process, they all have in common assessing a child's academic problems on the basis of the curriculum in which the child is instructed. One important difference, however, is that most models other than the one Lentz and I described (Shapiro, 1987a, 1989, 1990, 1996a; Shapiro & Lentz, 1985, 1986) do *not* incorporate significant efforts at evaluating the academic environment, along with the child's skills. Efforts to add this component to CBM have been offered by Ysseldyke and Christenson (1987, 1993). The model we have suggested is most consistent with the assumptions and methods of behavioral assessment. As such, our model of CBA is conceptualized as the behavioral assessment of academic skills. For the simplicity of communication, however, future mention of CBA in this text will refer to the model we have described (Shapiro & Lentz, 1985, 1986) as "behavioral assessment of academic skills."

WHAT CURRICULUM-BASED ASSESSMENT IS

CBA is designed to assess individuals who have deficits in *basic academic skills*. This means that the procedures are relevant for those pupils having difficulty reading, writing, spelling, or doing math. Students of all ages, *including secondary-age students*, with deficiencies in these areas can be assessed using CBA. Students with these types of problems are found typically in the elementary grades, however. After all, once students reach the middle and high school levels, their academic skills should have progressed to the point at which they can be instructed effectively in content areas (i.e., social studies, science, history, etc.). However, we have all come across students who are failing history because they cannot read the text, or those who fail math because they cannot read the word problems. CBA is a relevant method of assessment for these students.

Attempts to bring CBA methods to content-area instruction have not been widely reported in the literature. Tindal and Parker (1989) examined the development of several possible metrics to conduct progress monitoring for students in 6th-, 8th-, and 11th-grade subject matter. Espin, Scierka,

Scare, and Halverson (1999) reported on the use of curriculum-based measures in the assessment of writing proficiency among high school students. Espin and Tindal (1998) also proposed a conceptual model for developing curriculum-based measures for assessing secondary students with learning disabilities (LD). Despite these initial attempts, continuous performance measures analogous to those developed for assessing basic skills at the elementary level have not been successful.

Efforts to establish measures for purposes of development of early reading skills have been successful, resulting in the Dynamic Indicators of Basic Early Literacy (DIBELS; Good & Kaminski, 1996; Kaminski & Good, 1996). In addition, efforts are under way to establish continuous performance measures that extend downward to early language development (Greenwood, Luze, Cline, Kuntz, & Leitschuh, 2002; Priest et al., 2001). At present, it is recommended that CBA, as described in this text, be limited to working with students who have basic skills deficiencies and are primarily in elementary level grades. Extension of one aspect of CBA, measurement of the development of early reading skills, also has strong empirical support and is covered somewhat in Chapter 4 of this volume.

CBA can contribute to a number of decisions regarding a student with an academic problem. Specifically, it can do the following:

1. Serve as an effective means for providing evaluation prior to placement in special education programs.
2. Determine whether a student is accurately placed in curriculum materials.
3. Assist in developing strategies for remediation of academic problems.
4. Suggest changes in the instructional environment that may improve the student's performance.
5. Provide a means for setting IEP short- and long-term goals for students in special education programs.
6. Provide a method for monitoring progress and performance of students across time.
7. Provide an empirical method for determining when an intervention is effective or not.
8. Make the assessment relevant to what the child has been expected to learn in the curriculum.
9. Provide a potential strategy for screening students.
10. Offer an empirical method for deciding whether a student needs to move to a more restrictive setting.
11. Provide accountability for teachers and psychologists when making eligibility decisions.

WHAT CURRICULUM-BASED ASSESSMENT IS NOT

CBA is a set of new skills for purposes other than psychodiagnostic assessments. Specifically, CBA is designed to assist in assessment and intervention prior to making a decision regarding eligibility of a student for special education services. The data derived from CBA are intended to help make decisions regarding the variables contributing to academic performance. A significant assumption of CBA is that these variables lie *both* within the individual skills of the student *and* within the academic environment.

CBA is not designed to replace current service delivery systems completely. The legal requirements for most eligibility decisions still include the administration of norm-referenced instruments, such as individual intelligence and achievement tests. Although substantial questions have been raised about the ability of these measures to effectively diagnose LD (Fletcher et al., 1998, 2002; Stuebing et al., 2002) and there are efforts to examine models of making eligibility decisions based on a student's responsiveness to intervention that uses CBA and CBM in particular as the outcome measure for determining success of interventions (Fuchs & Fuchs, 1998; Fuchs, Fuchs, & Speece, 2002; Gresham, 2002), the data substantiating these models are still questionable (Scruggs & Mastropieri, 2002). CBA can certainly contribute to the decision-making process for eligibility; however, questions of whether it can meet legal mandates for making eligibility decisions are yet to be administered. Some school settings, however, have experimented with the use of CBA data alone for making eligibility decisions (Marston & Magnusson, 1985; Tindal, Wesson, et al., 1985), and at least one study has found support for the responsiveness to intervention model in young children (Speece & Case, 2001).

CBA, at least the model presented here, is also not designed to evaluate problems in content areas such as American history or chemistry. Although there are CBA models that can address these areas (see Idol et al., 1996; Howell & Nolet, 1999), students having difficulty in these areas more often seem to have trouble in study skills, memory, and cognitive tasks that require different types of assessment strategies.

Finally, it is important to remember that although the data on academic skills collected during a CBA can on their own be extremely useful, CBA, in combination with a general behavioral consultation approach, can work effectively as a method for service delivery. The integration of CBA with behavioral consultation is described elsewhere (Gravois, Knotek, & Babinski, 2002; Lentz & Shapiro, 1985; Reschly & Grimes, 1991; Rosenfield, 1987, 1995; Rosenfield & Gravois, 1995; Shapiro, 1987a, 1996a).

ASSESSING THE ACADEMIC ENVIRONMENT: OVERVIEW

The assessment of the academic environment incorporates examination of variables that have been found to affect academic performance significantly. These variables include academic engaged time (scheduled time, allotted time, time on-task, opportunities to respond, response rates), events that are concurrent with engagement (instructional presentation, contingencies for performance, and classroom structure), events that are temporally removed from academic responding but may significantly influence performance (instructions, contingencies for completion, and accuracy), and teacher methods of planning and evaluation. Although all of these variables can be directly assessed through observation, it would become impractical to try consistently to observe each of these for each assessment method. As such, the use of teacher interviews, combined with direct observation of related variables such as on-task behavior, teacher attention to academic performance, teacher-completed rating scales, and the examination of actual student products can permit the observer to examine (at least indirectly) each of the variables of concern.

Beyond these data, it is also important to determine the student's perspective on the instructional process. For example, does the student know how to access help when he or she runs into difficulty? Does the student know the objectives of the instructional lesson? What is the student's self-perception of his or her ability to successfully meet the requirements of the task? Does the student understand the instructions of the task? Answers to these types of questions may add substantially to the analysis of the instructional ecology. To obtain this information, a student interview needs to be conducted. Table 3.1 provides a list of both relevant variables for assessing the academic environment and which method (teacher interview, student interview, observation, or permanent products) offers data on that variable.

The model we have described (Shapiro & Lentz, 1985, 1986) was modified by Shapiro (1990) and is displayed in Figure 1.1 (see Chapter 1). This approach combines components from several other models of CBA and involves a four-step process: (1) assessment of the instructional environment, (2) assessment of instructional placement, (3) instructional modification, and (4) progress monitoring. The process begins with the teacher interview. Data obtained from the interview will often suggest relevant and critical settings in which direct observation will need to be made, as well as the important areas of academic skills in need of assessment. A student interview is also conducted in conjunction with the direct observation. Finally, permanent products obtained during these observations will again help in interpreting and confirming the interview and observational data. Figure 3.1 includes a flowchart of the sequence of methods used to conduct the assessment of the academic environment.

TABLE 3.1. Assessment Procedures for Achievement-Related Variables

Variable	Procedures
Actual placement of student in curriculum according to skill	Direct assessment using skill probes, curriculum tests, criterion-references tests
Expected placement	Teacher interview
Actual placement procedures used by teacher	Teacher interview, permanent product review
Allotted time	Teacher interview, direct observation
Student motivation	Teacher interview, rating scale
Teacher perceptions of skills	Teacher interview, rating scale
Opportunities to respond	Direct observation, permanent products
Active and passive engaged time	Direct observation
Student perceptions of teacher expectations	Student interview
Student academic self-efficacy	Student interview
Immediate contingencies	Direct observation
Competing contingencies	Direct observation, teacher interview, student interview
Orientation to materials	Direct observation
Teacher feedback	Direct observation, teacher interview, student interview
Teacher planning	Teacher interview

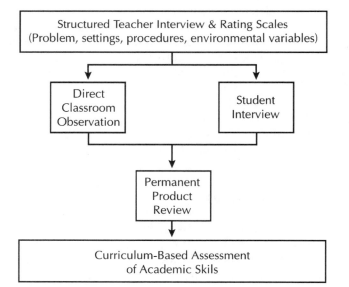

FIGURE 3.1. Flowchart or procedures for assessing academic skills.

TEACHER INTERVIEWS

The first step in conducting the CBA is to interview the teacher. During the interview, information is obtained about each area of basic skills (reading, math, spelling, written language). Specifically, questions are asked about the curriculum, instructional procedures, and the child's performance. Data are sought regarding the current level and instructional level of the child in the curriculum, the specific materials used for instruction, the expected levels of performance of "typical" students in the classroom, the types of instructional settings used by the teacher (large group, small group, learning centers, cooperative learning), monitoring procedures employed to assess student progress, specific contingencies for performance, details of specific interventions that have already been tried, and global indications of the child's behavior during the instructional process. Questions are asked regarding on-task levels, homework completion, class participation, and other events that might affect academic performance.

The format for the interview process is based on the behavioral consultation process described by Bergan (1977), Bergan and Kratochwill (1990) and Kratochwill and Bergan (1990). The model incorporates the use of a series of interviews designed to identify the problem, analyze the critical variables contributing to the problem, design and implement intervention strategies, and evaluate the effectiveness of the intervention. The interview process described by the model offers a comprehensive analysis of verbal behavior and a methodology for training consultants to conduct these interviews. Bergan's interview procedures can be used reliably (Bergan, 1977; Erchul, Covington, Hughes, & Meyers, 1995; Gresham, 1984; Kratochwill, Elliott, & Busse, 1995), and the types of consultant verbalizations needed for a problem analysis interview have been validated (Gresham, 1984; Witt, 1990; Witt, Erchul, McKee, Pardue, & Wickstrom, 1991). In addition, outcome data reported by Bergan and Tombari (1975) and Miltenberger and Fuqua (1985) show the importance of effective problem identification for the problem-solving process.

Although there have been other behavioral interviewing formats for school consultation (e.g., Alessi & Kaye, 1983; Lentz & Wehmann, 1995; Witt & Elliott, 1983), the format described by Bergan appears to be most often cited in the behavioral consultation literature. For example, Graden, Casey, and Bonstrom (1985) and Graden, Casey, and Christensen (1985) used Bergan's behavioral consultation model in an investigation of a prereferral intervention program across six schools. Noll, Kamps, and Seaborn (1993) reported that a prereferral intervention program using a behavioral consultation model over a 3-year period resulted in between 43% and 64% of students referred remaining in general education classrooms.

Appendix 3A provides a convenient form that has been developed to facilitate the teacher interview process. The section on reading is straightforward. After identifying the specific name and type of reading series (i.e., basal, literature-based, trade books), as well as the target student's current level within the series, the teacher is also asked to identify the point in the reading series that the average student in the class has reached at this time. If the teacher is having some difficulty in defining the "average student," the interviewer may want to suggest that he or she think about the students in the average or middle reading group. It is helpful to get information as specific as possible regarding the targeted student's and his/her peers' placement in the reading series, including the particular page or story on which the students are working currently. However, this may not be useful information if the teacher is using a literature-based series, since the difficulty level of material varies greatly within levels of a typical literature-based reading series. How the student was placed into the text, however, may be an important indication of the duration of the student's problem.

The interviewer also asks for information about how the instructional time is allotted and divided. In reading, one needs to determine whether students are instructed in small or large groups, the size of the target student's group, what the expectations are for students when they are not engaged in direct teacher instruction, and other structural aspects of the teaching process. Furthermore, any specific contingencies, such as stickers, points, or rewards for completion and/or accuracy, need to be recorded.

Another important question in the interview concerns how changes are made in the instructional program. In some schools, any changes in the reading program must be cleared through the district reading specialist. This information may be influential in a teacher's decision not to alter instruction, despite a student's failure to master the given material. Equally important is information on how student performance is monitored.

The next part of the form asks questions designed to focus on intervention methods already attempted. Given that students for whom this type of interview is being conducted are likely to have been referred for ongoing problems in reading, teachers will likely have tried different interventions to solve the problem. These interventions could range from simple strategies linked to improving motivation, instructions, or the way feedback is given, to more complex interventions, such as altering the curriculum materials, the modalities of instruction, or peer tutoring. Questions need to be asked that determine the nature of the interventions, the frequency of these specific strategies, the intensity with which they were implemented, and the integrity with which they were used.

The interview form also asks teachers to provide some indication of the target student's skills in certain basic components of reading, such as oral reading, word attack, word knowledge and sight vocabulary, and comprehension. In each of these areas, the teacher is asked to compare the target student to peers in the same reading group, as well as to those in the entire class. Additionally, specific questions about the nature of a student's comprehension skills are asked to determine whether for this student, oral reading fluency will be an accurate index of comprehension. Although students known as "word callers," those who are fluent readers but cannot understand what they read, make up a small percentage of students referred for reading problems (Hamilton & Shinn, 2003), comprehension is certainly a key component of the reading process for all children, and evidence that oral reading fluency accurately reflects levels of comprehension is often a question that must be addressed when making recommendations for intervention.

Finally, the teacher is asked to complete a brief rating form describing different types of behavior problems that commonly interfere with successful academic performance. These include participation in the reading group, knowing the appropriate place in the book when called on, staying on-task and in-seat during independent seatwork, and handing in homework on time that is complete and accurate. Each of these behaviors is rated on a 5-point scale.

Content for the interview in mathematics is similar but contains a few critical differences. The CBA interview in mathematics examines a student's skills in both computation and concepts–application. The primary concern in the CBA begins by assessing computational skills. Typically, students who cannot master basic computational skills are unable to effectively master applications of mathematics, such as measurement, time, money, or geometry. However, given that research has shown that mathematics does divide into two areas of skills development, consisting of computation and concepts especially for older elementary students (Thurber et al., 2002), assessment of problem-solving and application areas is needed. Indeed, many math curricula have deemphasized the development of computational mastery and enhanced efforts to teach students to be mathematical problem solvers.

Despite the emphasis in many curricula on problem solving, students are taught and develop computational skills in a consistent sequence regardless of the type of curricula used for instruction. Skills are generally hierarchical and are taught in such a way that acquisition of one skill will provide a basis for learning later skills. For example, students are taught single-digit addition facts with sums less than 10 before sums greater than 10 are taught. Students are taught addition and subtraction without regrouping before regrouping is instructed. Typically, all students are placed within the same level of the math curriculum. Asking a teacher where a student is currently placed in the curriculum may be somewhat helpful, but it may not specifically define the computational objectives that have or have not been mastered. To determine the computational skills of the student from the teacher interview, one needs to examine the list of computational objectives for that particular district and curriculum. This can be obtained from the scope and sequence charts of the curriculum, if it is not available from the district curriculum officer.

Although using the district-based list of computational objectives is ideal, the order in which these skills are instructed does not usually vary significantly. It is therefore possible to use an already existing set of objectives taken from any curriculum or district. Provided in Appendix 3B is the list of computational objectives taken from a small urban school district in the northeastern United States. When such a list is used during the interview, the teacher is asked to mark the approximate objective the target student has mastered, the objective at which the student is being instructed, the objective at which the student is frustrated, the objective the average student in the class has mastered, and the objective at which the average student in the class is being instructed.

At times, teachers may not have clear knowledge of a student's performance on specific instructional objectives. Because one can divide math computational objectives into broad categories, interviewers can use general questions in each of these areas when teachers are unable to identify a student's skills from a list of computational objectives. Figure 3.2 provides a list of these broad categories.

Computation operations	Computational skills to be assessed
Addition	• Single-digit facts to 9 • Single-digit facts to 18 • No regrouping • Regrouping
Subtraction	• Single-digit facts to 9 • Single-digit facts to 18 • No regrouping • Regrouping
Multiplication	• Facts: 1, 2, 5 • Other facts • 1 × 2 digits • Multiple digits
Division	• Facts: 1, 2, 5 • Other facts • 1 ÷ 2 digits • Long division without remainders • Long division with remainders

FIGURE 3.2. Order of assessing computation skills across operations.

Similar questions are included to assess a student's concepts and applications of mathematical principles in areas such as numeration, estimation, time, money, geometry, measurement, graphic representation, and interpretation of data. These data will play an important role in the subsequent direct assessment of math skills.

Other questions on the interview for math are identical to those on the interview for reading. Questions are asked about the instructional process (large group, small groups, independent seatwork, learning centers, cooperative learning), how progress is monitored and changes are made in instruction, what contingencies are in place for completion or accurate performance, how much time is allotted for instruction, and what interventions have been attempted to solve the student's difficulties in math. In addition, a similar behavior checklist is completed.

The interview for spelling is straightforward and asks questions very similar to those in the reading interview. However, given that spelling is often taught as an integrated part of language arts that includes writing and reading, less attention is given to this area of assessment. Items related to intervention are asked as well, including questions about types of interventions used to remediate any problems in spelling.

Finally, the teacher is asked to describe the types of writing assignments used in the classroom. The specific difficulties of the target student are then described in the areas of expression of thought, mechanics, grammatical usage, handwriting, and spelling. An additional opportunity is included for the teacher to express any concern about potential social–emotional adjustment problems that may be interfering with academic performance.

Figure 3.3 illustrates a completed teacher interview form for a fourth-grade boy, Sunny. His primary academic problems were reported to be in mathematics, writing, and spelling. The interview conducted with Sunny's teacher touched on all areas of academic skills development, to support reports in areas not considered problematic, such as reading.

In reading, the teacher indicated that Sunny is currently placed in the fourth-grade-level P book of the Houghton Mifflin reading series, having moved from level O to P earlier this year. Of the four reading groups in her class, Sunny is in the lowest group. Approximately 75 minutes each day are allotted for reading; this time is divided into teacher-led large-group instruction, followed by small-group instruction mixed with individual seatwork assignments when the teacher is not working with the group. During large-group instruction, the teacher uses modeling, direct instruction, and teaching strategies for comprehension. Students are expected to practice these skills in small groups and during independent work assignments. Sunny's teacher has characterized his oral reading, sight-word, vocabulary, and word attack skills as the same or somewhat better than

[text continues on p. 86]

TEACHER INTERVIEW FORM FOR ACADEMIC PROBLEMS

Student: _Sunny_   Teacher: _Mrs. W_

Birth date: _1/20/93_   Date: _3/4/03_

Grade: _4_   School: _Reiger_

          Interviewer: _T. D._

GENERAL

Why was this student referred? _Academic difficulties_

What type of academic problem(s) does this student have?

Math, writing, and spelling

READING

Primary type of reading series used
- ☒ Basal reader
- ☐ Literature-based
- ☐ Trade books

Secondary type of reading materials used
- ☐ Basal reader
- ☒ Literature-based
- ☐ Trade books
- ☐ None

Reading series title (if applicable) _Houghton Mifflin: Traditions (large group)_

     Grade level of series currently placed _4 (P)_

     Title of book in series currently placed _I'm New Here_

How many groups do you teach? _4_

Which group is this student assigned to? _Lowest_

At this point in the school year, where is the average student in your class reading?

     Level and book _Level 5, 4th grade_

     Place in book (beg., mid., end, specific page) _Middle_

     Time allotted/day for reading _75 minutes, 9–10:15 A.M._

How is time divided? (Independent seatwork? Small group? Cooperative groups? Large groups?)

Teacher-led small group, 30 min. whole class, 5–10 min. sharing/summarizing

FIGURE 3.3. Teacher interview for Sunny.

How is placement in reading program determined? _Diagnostic test decides placement,_
teacher determines placement

How are changes made in the program? _Periodic testing, teacher judgment_

Does this student participate in remedial reading programs? How much?
No, current school does not offer, participated in previous school

Typical daily instructional procedures _Large-group instruction (direct instruction, modeling,_
practice strategies for comprehension) followed by small-group work emphasizing vocabulary building,
silent reading, with discussion. Independent work and silent reading when teacher is not with group.

Contingencies for accuracy? _Verbal feedback, praise_

Contingencies for completion? _Stickers for completing activities, students keep reading logs_

Types of interventions already attempted:

Simple (e.g., reminders, cues, self-monitoring, motivation, feedback, instructions):
Praise, feedback, and reminders to use strategies

Moderate (e.g., increasing time of existing instruction, extra tutoring sessions):
Extra peer-tutoring beyond regular instructional time

Intensive (e.g., changed curriculum, changed instructional modality,
changed instructional grouping, added intensive one-to-one):

Frequency and duration of interventions used:
Daily basis, peer-tutoring 3 times per week.

Extent to which interventions were successful:
Responds to interventions, improved performance during the year

FIGURE 3.3. *(continued)*

Daily scores (if available) for past 2 weeks <u>None available</u>

Group standardized test results (if available) <u>None available</u>

ORAL READING

How does he/she read orally compared to others in his/her reading group?

___ Much worse   ___ Somewhat worse   _X_ About the same
___ Somewhat better   ___ Much better

In the class?

___ Much worse   ___ Somewhat worse   _X_ About the same
___ Somewhat better   ___ Much better

WORD ATTACK

Does he/she attempt unknown words? <u>Yes</u>

WORD KNOWLEDGE/SIGHT VOCABULARY

How does the student's word knowledge (vocabulary) compare to others in his/her reading group?

___ Much worse   ___ Somewhat worse   ___ About the same
_X_ Somewhat better   ___ Much better

In the class?

___ Much worse   ___ Somewhat worse   _X_ About the same
___ Somewhat better   ___ Much better

How does the student's sight-word vocabulary compare to others in his/her reading group?

___ Much worse   ___ Somewhat worse   _X_ About the same
___ Somewhat better   ___ Much better

In the class?

___ Much worse   ___ Somewhat worse   _X_ About the same
___ Somewhat better   ___ Much better

FIGURE 3.3. *(continued)*

COMPREHENSION

How well does the student seem to understand what he/she reads compared to others in his/her reading group?

_____ Much worse   _____ Somewhat worse   _X_ About the same

_____ Somewhat better   _____ Much better

In the class?

_____ Much worse   _X_ Somewhat worse   _____ About the same

_____ Somewhat better   _____ Much better

Areas of comprehension where student has success (+)/difficulty (−):

_+_ Main ideas

_−_ Prediction

_+_ Recollection of facts

_−_ Identifying plot

_+_ Identifying main characters

_−_ Synthesizing the story

_____ Other (describe):

_____

_____

BEHAVIOR DURING READING

Rate the following areas from 1 to 5 (1 = very unsatisfactory, 3 = satisfactory, 5 = superior).

Reading Group

a. Oral reading ability (as evidenced in reading group)   3
b. Volunteers answers   3
c. When called upon, gives correct answer   4
d. Attends to other students when they read aloud   4
e. Knows the appropriate place in book   3

Independent Seatwork

a. Stays on task   4
b. Completes assigned work in required time   3
c. Work is accurate   3
d. Works quietly   5
e. Remains in seat when required   5

FIGURE 3.3. *(continued)*

79

Homework (if any)

a. Handed in on time   2

b. Is complete   2

c. Is accurate   2

MATHEMATICS

Curriculum series _Chicago Everyday Math_

What are the specific problems in math? _Multiplication facts, word problems, time, money_

Time allotted/day for math _60 minutes, 1–2 P.M._

How is time divided? (Independent seatwork? Small group? Large group?

Cooperative groups?) _Large-group instruction, independent seatwork in partner pairs_

Are your students grouped in math? _No_

If so, how many groups do you have, and in which group is this student placed? _N/A_

For an **average** performing student in your class, at what point in the planned course format would you consider this student at mastery?

(See computational mastery form.) _#34—Addition w/regrouping, all columns; #37—_
Subtraction w/regrouping all columns; #41—Multiply 3-digit x 1-digit w/regrouping

For an **average** performing student in your class, at what point in the planned course format would you consider this student instructional?

(See computational mastery form.) _#46—Divide 4-digit by 1-digit number w/remainder_

For an **average** performing student in your class, at what point in the planned course format would you consider this student frustrational?

(See computational mastery form.) _Divide multiple numbers w/remainders_

For the **targeted** student in your class, at what point in the planned course format would you consider this student at mastery?

(See computational mastery form.) _#23—Addition w/regrouping 1–3 columns; #32—_
Subtraction w/regrouping 10's to 100's columns

FIGURE 3.3. *(continued)*

For the **targeted** student in your class, at what point in the planned course format would you consider this student instructional?

(See computational mastery form.) _#34—Addition w/regrouping all columns; #37—_ _Subtraction w/regrouping in all columns_

For the **targeted** student in your class, at what point in the planned course format would you consider this student frustrational?

(See computational mastery form.) _#33—Multiplication facts 3–9; #42—Division_ _facts 0–9_

How is mastery assessed? _Pre- and posttest every chapter_

Describe any difficulties this student has in applying math skills in these areas:

Numeration _____

Estimation _____

Time _Struggles with nondigital time telling_____

Money _Inaccuracies in making change_____

Measurement _____

Geometry _____

Graphic display _____

Interpretation of graph _____

Word problems _Does not use context cues within word problems; poor at using strategies_

Other _____

How are changes made in the student's math program? _Consultant with learning support_ _teacher_

Does this student participate in remedial math programs? _No_

Typical daily instructional procedures _Review assigned work from previous day in whole group_ _and with partners; work with partner on applications and homework assignments; teach entire_ _group new material._

Contingencies for accuracy? _Verbal praise, acknowledge 100% on homework, praise and_ _stickers for accuracy on tests and quizzes._

Contingencies for completion? _Praise and stickers for homework accuracy; if homework is_ _not done, students remain indoors during breaks to complete._

FIGURE 3.3. *(continued)*

Types of interventions already attempted:

Simple (e.g., reminders, cues, self-monitoring, motivation, feedback, instructions):

Reminders and cue cards

Moderate (e.g., increasing time of existing instruction, extra tutoring sessions):

Increased partner tutoring time

Intensive (e.g., changed curriculum, changed instructional modality, changed instructional grouping, added intensive one-to-one):

Frequency and duration of interventions used:

Partner time 2 extra per week

Extent to which interventions were successful:

Not successful, still struggling

Daily scores (if available) for past 2 weeks _90% correct on multiplication test;_
Unsatisfactory on last 2 tests, < 60%.

Group standardized test results (if available) _Not available_

BEHAVIOR DURING MATH

Rate the following areas from 1 to 5 (1 = very unsatisfactory, 3 = satisfactory, 5 = superior)

Math Group (large)

a. Volunteers answers   _2_
b. When called upon, gives correct answer   _2_
c. Attends to other students when they give answers   _2_
d. Knows the appropriate place in math book   _3_

FIGURE 3.3. *(continued)*

Math Group (small)

a. Volunteers answers   2
b. When called upon, gives correct answer   2
c. Attends to other students when they give answers   2–3
d. Knows the appropriate place in math book   3

Math Group (cooperative)

a. Volunteers answers   2
b. Contributes to group objectives   3
c. Attends to other students when they give answers   3
d. Facilitates others in group to participate   —
e. Shows appropriate social skills in group   3–4

Independent Seatwork

a. Stays on task   3–4
b. Completes assigned work in required time   3
c. Work is accurate   2
d. Works from initial directions   2
e. Works quietly   5
f. Remains in seat when required   5

Homework (if any)

a. Handed in on time   5
b. Is complete   5
c. Is accurate   2

SPELLING

Type of material used for spelling instruction:

☒ Published spelling series

    Title of series _Rebecca Sitton_

☐ Basal reading series

    Title of series _____

☒ Teacher-made materials _Teacher made spelling list from frequently misspelled words_

☐ Other _____

Level of instruction (if applicable) _4th grade_

At this point in the school year, where is the average student in your class spelling?

    Level, place in book _4th grade_

Time allotted/day for spelling _10 minutes; 10:55–11:05 A.M._

FIGURE 3.3. *(continued)*

How is time divided? (Independent seatwork? Small group? Cooperative groups?)
Whole group review of spelling homework, no groups

How is placement in the spelling program determined? _Test at beginning of year_

How are changes made in the program? _Quarterly review by teacher_

Typical daily instructional procedures _Words introduced Monday, review word families,_
endings, other skills during week, Friday spelling test

Types of interventions already attempted:

Simple (e.g., reminders, cues, self-monitoring, motivation, feedback, instructions):
None

Moderate (e.g., increasing time of existing instruction, extra tutoring sessions):
None

Intensive (e.g., changed curriculum, changed instructional modality,
changed instructional grouping, added intensive one-to-one):
None

Frequency and duration of interventions used:
_N/A_

Extent to which interventions were successful:
_N/A_

Contingencies for accuracy? _Verbal praise, share responses with class_

Contingencies for completion? _Letter home to parent, reports homework completion_

FIGURE 3.3. *(continued)*

WRITING

Please describe the type of writing assignments you give? _Research reports, writer's_
journals, essays, narratives, poetry

Compared to others in your class, does he/she have difficulty with (please provide brief descriptions):

- ☒ Expressing thoughts _Simple sentences, no development_
- ☒ Story length _Too short_
- ☒ Story depth _Poor because of lack of sentence development_
- ☒ Creativity _Not confident, does not attempt own ideas_

Mechanics:

- ☒ Capitalization
- ☒ Punctuation
- ☐ Grammar
- ☒ Handwriting
- ☒ Spelling

Comments: _Needs lots of reminders; knows rules, does not apply them_

BEHAVIOR

Are there social–behavioral adjustment problems interfering with this student's academic progress? (be specific)

None

Check any item that describes this student's behavior:

_____ Distracted, short attention span, unable to concentrate

_____ Hyperactive, constant, aimless movement

_____ Impulsive aggressive behaviors, lacks self-control

__X__ Fluctuating levels of performance

_____ Frequent negative self-statements

_____ Unconsciously repeating verbal or motor acts

_____ Lethargic, sluggish, too quiet

_____ Difficulty sharing or working with others

FIGURE 3.3. *(continued)*

those of his classmates. Comprehension is reported as somewhat worse, but with difficulties related to inferential comprehension skills, such as prediction and synthesis. Few specific interventions in reading beyond regular instruction have been needed, although some additional peer tutoring has been provided to Sunny. Mrs. W reports that Sunny's behavior is excellent during instruction. He sometimes does not complete all his homework, however.

Examination of the entire interview reveals that the areas of most concern are mathematics and written language. In mathematics, Sunny was reported to have particular problems with mathematics concepts and applications, although he is also struggling with basic computational skills in multiplication and division. Interventions that have been tried by Mrs. W include peer tutoring, reminder cards, and requiring completion of homework during free time if its was not done at home. Sunny also was noted as struggling in aspects of writing, both in production of written material and mechanics.

The entire interview, once an interviewer is skilled in its administration, should take no more than 15–20 minutes. It is important to become thoroughly familiar with the questions, since teachers will often provide responses in many categories when asked a single question. Although the process of interviewing teachers is common in assessment, the types of questions being asked here are not typical of most interview processes. Clearly, asking teachers to describe and think about the instructional process, to describe how they monitor student progress, to detail the nature and integrity of intervention, and to discuss how they make decisions about moving students through the curriculum may result in unexpected defensiveness on the part of the teachers. It is essential that the purpose of this type of interview be explained to teachers prior to beginning the interview. Although asking these types of questions may appear to be potentially dangerous to maintaining effective rapport with teachers, it has been found over hundreds of cases that the common response to being asked these questions is very positive. Often, teachers will remark that they had not asked themselves these questions, which they recognize are important for understanding the students' problems.

Despite the positive testimonials regarding the method, there have not yet been any systematic investigations examining the acceptability of these types of interviews. Until such time, the user of this interview process for CBA is cautioned to be sensitive to a teacher's responses to these questions and to reassure the teacher that his or her answers to these questions are being used to help the evaluator understand the child's academic problem.

An additional adjunct to the teacher interview may be the completion of a more formal teacher-rating scale related to academic skills problems. DuPaul, Rapport, and Perriello (1991) developed the Academic Performance Rating Scale (APRS) to have teachers report their perceptions of student academic behavior. Similar measures can be found as part of the Social Skills Rating Scales—Teacher (Gresham & Elliott, 1990). A copy of the APRS, along with normative data to interpret the measure, can be found in the workbook accompanying this text.

Another rating-scale measure that may be found useful in understanding teacher perceptions of student academic performance is the Academic Competence Evaluation Scales (ACES; DiPerna & Elliott, 2002). Based on research (DiPerna & Elliott, 1999), the ACES asks specific questions about the academic enablers (total of 40 items) of a student's motivation, engagement, study skills, and interpersonal behavior across academic areas. Specific questions are asked about skills (total of 33 items) in reading, mathematics, and critical thinking. Versions of the ACES for teachers, parents, and students have been developed, allowing for a full understanding of academic performance from different perspectives. In addition, the measure covers the entire K–12 grade period, along with versions that have been developed for preschool- and college-age students as well. ACES has strong psychometric properties of reliability and validity, and has been normed on a national sample of 1,000 students, with careful attention given to representation across groups differing in cultural and linguistic backgrounds.

From the interview and rating-scale data, one is able to discern the specific areas of academic problems, the types of settings (small groups, independent seatwork, etc.) that may differentially affect student performance, the types of instructional methods employed by the teacher, and the environmental conditions for reinforcing appropriate academic behavior. Types and nature of academic enablers such as a student's motivation, perceived level of on-task behavior, and skills development, are also assessed if one uses a measure such as the ACES. In addition, one obtains vital information regarding teacher expectations and actual student performance, along with indications about specific types of skills deficiencies.

Questions sometimes arise as to whether information obtained from interviews and rating scales is redundant. Research has supported the strong relationship between the use of these two methods (e.g., McConaughy & Achenbach, 1989, 1996). At the same time, others have noted the complementary rather than redundant nature of interviews and rating scales (DuPaul, Guevremont, & Barkley, 1991; Elliott, Busse, & Gresham, 1993). In the context of assessing academic skills, no studies have specifically examined the question of whether information obtained from teachers through rating-scale methods is redundant to teacher interviews. From a clinical perspective, however, it would seem that these methods nicely complement each other, and together can provide a fuller picture of a student's academic performance. At the same time, interviewing may offer the assessor an opportunity to delve into details in areas not specifically covered by a rating scale. Given practical realities of schools and time available for assessment, it is more often the case that either rating scales or interviews are done.

Although data from the interview and rating scales are extremely valuable and useful in the assessment process, they still represent a teacher report (verbal or written) and are subject to potential biases inherent in such methods of data collection. These types of data collection processes are considered indirect methods of assessment (Shapiro & Kratochwill, 2000), and are examining the teacher's perception of the student's performance. Assessing the academic environment requires the confirmation of some of these variables through direct observation. In addition, important data about the child's actual performance during the instructional period are needed.

DIRECT OBSERVATION

One objective of collecting data through direct observation is to provide data that may (or may not) verify the information obtained through teacher report. In particular, the direct observation data give quantitative indications about the student's reported behavior during the instructional process. For example, data collected on the levels of on-task and disruptive behavior during different formats of reading instruction (small groups vs. independent seatwork) may confirm the teacher's report that a student is substantially more disruptive when working alone then when with his or her reading group.

A second objective of direct observation is to provide data on student–teacher interactions under naturalistic conditions of instruction. It is especially important that the assessment involve evaluation of not only individual student behaviors that may be related to effective development of academic skills but also those types of student–student and student–teacher interactions that may be related significantly to academic performance.

Finally, given the extensive literature on the role of academic engaged time and academic performance (e.g., Greenwood, 1991), the direct observation of academic skills should include data collection on variables that can approximate engaged time. This would include data obtained on on-task behavior or opportunities to respond (e.g., Greenwood, Delquadri, & Hall, 1984; Greenwood, 1996).

In combination with direct observation, it is also important to examine the products of the student's academic performance while the direct observations were being conducted. The worksheets or academic activities that the student produces can be valuable pieces of information that allow a more accurate interpretation of the observational data. For example, although the data collected through direct observation may show that a student has a high level of on-task behavior, examination of the worksheet produced during the observation may show that the student only completed a small number of items correctly. Thus, this may be a student who has learned to appear to be working well and paying attention in class but is really struggling academically.

Getting Reading to Observe

Before one begins the observation process, it is important to determine the classroom rules operating while the observations are being conducted. These rules may affect how certain behaviors are defined and can easily be obtained by either asking the teacher or looking to see whether they are posted somewhere in the room. It will also be important to find out the teacher's planned schedule of activities during the observation period. Knowing what is supposed to occur should help the observer determine the exact periods when the targeted student should be observed. Finally, it may also be useful to sketch out a seating chart depicting where the target student is sitting in relation to peers. In addition, important components of the physical classroom structure can be noted, such as the use of learning centers, boy–girl ratios, location of teacher and aides' desks, and places where educational materials are stored. All of these data may be useful in interpreting the quantitative data to be collected.

The observer should find a place in the classroom that is unobtrusive but provides a clear view of the referred child and is close enough that the child can be overheard. However, the observer should be careful not to be disruptive or so prominent that he or she ends up distracting the target child. All materials should be ready before the observation process begins. The observer should ask the teacher before beginning the observation what can be expected to happen during the instructional period. This will be important in the examination of student work products, which usually follows the direct observation.

During the teacher interview, the observer should have identified information to be verified while observing. Specifically, this includes the actual time allotted for instruction, contingencies for accuracy and/or work completion, instructional arrangements described by the teacher, and so forth. The observer may want to jot these items down at the bottom of the observation form to serve as reminders of things to check while conducting the observations.

When Should Observations Be Conducted?

Observations should be planned during activities related to the child's referred problems. This is why it is particularly important to conduct the teacher interview prior to the direct observations. During the interview, the observer should be able to determine the most important instructional periods for observation. For example, if reading is the referred problem, and the teacher expresses dissatisfaction during the interview with the child's performance during large-group and independent seatwork activities in reading, it is important to observe the child during both of these activities. If the activities occur consecutively (as they often do in many classrooms), then observation should be planned to cover both instructional settings. Likewise, if the teacher reports the student to be having difficulties in more than one academic area, observations may be needed in both instructional periods.

It is particularly important to be sensitive to teacher-reported discrepancies with regard to the student's behaviors during different instructional arrangements. For example, if a teacher states in the interview that the referred student is disruptive and fails to complete work accurately during all independent seatwork activities (regardless of academic subject area), but is usually compliant and attentive during teacher-led group activities, then the observation should be planned to sample the student's behavior during independent work across academic subjects, as well as at least one occasion of teacher-led group activity. The purpose of these observations would be to confirm or disconfirm the teacher's report during the interview.

How Often Should Observations Be Conducted?

The question of how often observations should be conducted is difficult to answer. One aspect to consider is that of time constraints on the observer. The number of observations that can be conducted is going to be partially related to the amount of time available to whomever is conducting the observation. Ideally, enough observation needs to be scheduled to give an accurate picture of the referred child's behavior and the instructional environment. The teacher interview may provide some guidance for deciding observational frequency, if the interviewer asks questions concerning the variability of student behavior. Students who are reported as different from day to day may need more observations than those reported to behave consistently. A "best-guess" recommendation is to observe for at least one full period in which problems exist, and then portions of that period on 1 or 2 other days. Spreading the observations across 2 or 3 days may be very helpful if a student's behavior is atypical on the first day of observation.

It is important to recognize that the process of conducting observations itself may alter a student's behavior in a classroom. Anyone who has conducted direct observations has had teachers tell him or her when an observation is finished: "I can't believe how good Kevin was today. He's never like this." These types of reports are critical in determining whether the observational data collected can be adequately interpreted. Following each observation, one should ask the teacher whether the student's behavior during the observation session was typical. If the teacher suggests that the student's behavior was atypical, additional observation under the same conditions will be necessary.

The primary objective of direct observation is to obtain data that are stable, conform to teacher reports, and offer an "accurate" picture of the student's typical behavior when the observer is not in the classroom. It should be kept in mind that reactivity to observation is often a transient phenomenon. Students usually habituate to observers in classrooms and act in ways that are consistent with other periods of the instructional process. The observer is cautioned, however, to try not to make it known to the target student that the object of the classroom visit is specifically to observe him/her.

Observation of Comparison Children

Very often, an observer may desire to compare the behavior of the referred child to peers within his or her classroom. These data can be very useful in interpreting the results of observing the target student and can provide a type of minilocal norm. In addition, collection of data on peers may offer information about the degree of discrepancy between the target student's behavior and expected levels of behavior for other students in the classroom.

The first step is to identify the set of children to use as a comparison. One way this can be done is by asking the teacher prior to beginning the observation to identify some children who are "typical," or who meet his or her expectations during the instructional setting to be observed. The observer should be sure that the teacher identifies students who are average, not those who represent exceptionally good behavior. The advantage of this approach is that the observer can arrange his or her data sheet to specify which children will be observed. A disadvantage, however, is that only a limited number of students will be observed, rather than a sampling across the classroom. As a result, teacher judgment plays a significant role in the selection of peers who are perceived to be typical.

A second procedure for selecting peers is for the observer to select students randomly from the class in which the referred child is being observed. One can choose a specific subset of children (perhaps those sitting in the referred student's proximity), or select students in a random pattern from all parts of the room. The advantage of this method is that any error due to teacher judgment is eliminated. A disadvantage, however, is that the observer is unaware of the behavioral characteristics of those observed and could, without knowing, select a group of students that are not considered as typical responders by the teacher.

Whichever method of choosing comparison students is used, the observer can systematically include these students in the observation process in different ways. One method is to mark off a subset of intervals (approximately five in every 20) during which only the peer comparison student(s) are observed. For example, if interval 5 is selected as a comparison interval, the observer completes the observation of the referred student during intervals 1 through 4, and then switches to the comparison child for interval 5. If the observer is using the random selection method, then a different student, selected randomly, is observed during the next comparison interval (e.g., interval 9).

Another way to observe peers is to alternate between the referred child in one interval and the peer-comparison child(ren) in the next. Still another way is to observe simultaneously both the referred child and a peer during each interval. This procedure obviously requires a modification of the observation form that allows recording of both referred and comparison children at the same time. Although this last method can result in excellent comparison data, it may also result in less than accurate data collection.

Regardless of the method used to collect the peer comparison data, the intervals in which these data are collected are treated as if a single individual were being observed. By aggregating these intervals, a peer norm is provided for comparison against the behavior of the referred student.

Using Existing Observational Codes

Procedures for collecting data systematically through direct observation have been well articulated in the literature (see Daly & Murdoch, 2000; Hintze & Shapiro, 1995; Hintze, Volpe, & Shapiro, 2002; Shapiro 1987a; Skinner, Dittmer, & Howell, 2000). After the target behaviors are identified and operationally defined, a procedure appropriate for the data-collection process is chosen. The method may involve collection of simple frequency counts of behavioral acts or may be a more complex system based on a time-sampling procedure. Although systematic observation systems can be individually tailored to each specific observational situation, this obviously can become a time-consuming and inefficient procedure. Given that the behaviors of interest within instructional settings do not deviate significantly, it may be more logical and cost-efficient to use an existing observation system rather than to try to individualize the observational procedure each time a new student or behavior is observed.

Not surprisingly, a large number of observational systems have been developed and reported in the literature. Some of these systems appear to have been used in many investigations and have been found to be particularly valuable for use in school settings. Table 3.2 provides a list of codes found in the literature that have been used for purposes of assessing school-based behaviors.

Alessi and Kaye (1983) described a code designed primarily to assess types of on- and off-task behavior, as well as teacher and peer response to these behaviors. Although not described in any specific research studies, the code does have an excellent training manual, including a videotape, and appears potentially useful for in-class observation of student behavior.

Saudargas and Creed (1980) developed a code (SECOS, State–Event Classroom Observation System) designed specifically by school psychologists for school psychologists, which appears to have potential usefulness in classroom observation. Unlike the Alessi and Kaye (1983) code, the SECOS offers the opportunity to assess at least 15 different student, and 6 teacher behaviors. Behaviors on the SECOS are divided into States (those behaviors that are continuous and recorded as present or absent) and Events (those behaviors that are discrete and are counted on an occurrence basis). It also allows for behavioral categories to be added that previously were not defined by the code. Furthermore, the system has been used in at least two studies in which certain behavioral categories appear to be significant discriminators of students with and without handicaps (e.g., Saudargas & Lentz, 1986; Slate & Saudargas, 1986).

Normative data have been collected on the code. The use of normative data to interpret observational codes presents a dilemma. On the one hand, the observer may want to know how the level of performance observed for the targeted student compares against performance levels that may be expected for same-age peers observed elsewhere under similar conditions. On the other hand, such information may be irrelevant, since a local context is needed to accurately interpret the data. Given this dilemma, the collection of data on peers from the same classroom as the target student is important. However, establishing whether the target student's behavior is within the level expected against similar-age peers on a larger scale can offer helpful feedback to teachers and evaluators. Haile-Griffey, Saudargas, Hulse-Trotter, and Zanolli (1993) completed SECOS observations on 486 children across grades 1–5 in general education classrooms from one school district in eastern Tennessee. Children were all engaged in independent seatwork, while their teacher worked at his or her desk or conducted a small-group activity in which the targeted student did not partake. Data for six State and six Event behaviors are reported in Tables 3.3 and 3.4. (For a complete set of normative data, contact Richard A. Saudargas, Department of Psychology, University of Tennessee, Knoxville, TN 37996.) These data allow an evaluator to compare the obtained rates of behavior on the SECOS for the particular targeted student against a large, normative database suggesting typical levels of performance. It is important to remember,

TABLE 3.2. Some Available Systematic Observation Codes

Measure/developer/availability	Purpose	Computerized?	Norms available?	Advantages	Disadvantages
BOSS (Behavioral Observation of Students in Schools) Edward S. Shapiro Available from: The Guilford Press (hard copy) and The Psychological Corporation (PDA software)	Classroom observations of independent seatwork, small-group, or other instructional events	Yes, for PDA	No, built-in feature for collecting peer comparison data	Simple to learn and provides data on different types of academic engaged time	Minimal information on teacher behavior and ecological instructional variables
E-BASS (Ecological Behavioral Assessment System) Available from: Juniper Gardens Children's Project 650 Minnesota Ave., Suite 2 Kansas City, KS 66101	Observation of preschool, regular ed, and mainstream settings	Yes, for laptop	No, built-in feature for collecting peer comparison data	Code provides computerized data collection system and detailed analysis of academic ecology	Complex, requires extensive training; analysis may be difficult given the large number of codes
!OBSERVE Sander Martin Available from: Sopris-West (*http://www.soprisuwest.com*)	Observation of academic and nonacademic settings	Yes, for PDA and laptop	No	User-defined codes, built-in behavior, templates; very flexible	Not tied to specific behavioral code
POC (Preschool Observation Code) Ron Bramlett and Dave Barnett	Observation of preschool settings, both instructional and noninstructional	No	No	Code was designed specifically for use in preschool environments	Complex, based on SECOS and requires similar training expertise

	Setting			Advantages	Disadvantages
Available from: Ron Bramlett University of Central Arkansas Psychology and Counseling Department Conway, AR 72035					
PSB (Peer Social Behavior) Hill Walker and Herb Severson Available from: Sopris-West (*http://www.sopriswest.com*)	Observation of nonacademic settings, grades 1–6	Instructional settings	Yes	Code is simple to learn and provides data on play periods and other nonacademic settings, especially playground behavior	Only relevant for nonacademic settings
POP (Portable Observation System, part of Behavior Assessment System for Children) Randy Kamphaus and Cecil Reynolds Available from: American Guidance Services (*http://www.agsnet.com*)	Classroom observations, mostly of independent seatwork	Yes, for PDA	No	Fairly simple code to learn	Questionable whether information obtained will be judged useful; yet to be determined
SECOS (State–Event Classroom Observation Code) Richard Saudargas Available from: Richard Saudargas University of Tennessee Department of Psychology Austin Peay Building Knoxville, TN 37996	Classroom observations of independent-seatwork, small-group, large-group, or other instructional events; elementary and middle school grades	No	Yes, in code manual	Provides detailed information on student, teacher, and student–teacher interaction	Complex and requires some time to master

TABLE 3.3. Normative Results for Six State Behaviors from the SECOS

	SW	LK	OACT	SIC	SIT	OS
Grade 1						
M (SD)	58.4 (17.4)	18.5 (11.7)	10.7 (10.1)	8.3 (10.5)	1.3 (2.8)	8.1 (11.6)
Grade 2						
M (SD)	67.9 (17.4)	13.6 (10.1)	9.1 (9.7)	5.2 (7.2)	0.8 (1.9)	8.5 (10.8)
Grade 3						
M (SD)	69.0 (15.1)	12.2 (9.0)	9.7 (8.7)	4.6 (5.7)	1.4 (3.3)	7.1 (8.9)
Grade 4						
M (SD)	73.9 (15.7)	11.1 (7.7)	6.4 (6.4)	5.7 (8.2)	0.8 (1.8)	5.2 (8.5)
Grade 5						
M (SD)	70.4 (15.1)	10.8 (7.2)	8.1 (8.2)	6.5 (8.0)	1.3 (4.2)	6.8 (1.0)

Note. SW, schoolwork; LK, looking around; OACT, other activity; SIC, social interactions with child; SIT, social interactions with teacher; OS, out of seat. From Haile-Griffey, Saudargas, Hulse-Trotter, and Zanolli (1993). Reprinted by permission of the authors.

however, that these normative data can only be interpreted correctly when observed under conditions of independent seatwork.

Greenwood and colleagues (Carta et al., 1985, 1987; Greenwood, Delquadri, Stanley, Terry, & Hall, 1985; Greenwood, Carta, & Atwater, 1991; Greenwood, Carta, et al., 1993, 1994; Greenwood et al., 1985) developed a series of computer-based observational measures designed to assess the nature of the academic environment that surrounds student class-

TABLE 3.4. Normative Results for Six Event Behaviors from the SECOS

	AC	OCA	TA/SW	TA/OTH	RH	CAL
Grade 1						
M (SD)	.28 (.31)	.25 (.26)	.02 (.04)	.02 (.04)	.03 (.08)	.03 (.06)
Grade 2						
M (SD)	.20 (.25)	.19 (.21)	.01 (.03)	.01 (.04)	.02 (.05)	.02 (.05)
Grade 3						
M (SD)	.18 (.23)	.16 (.21)	.01 (.05)	.01 (.03)	.01 (.02)	.03 (.05)
Grade 4						
M (SD)	.20 (.27)	.16 (.17)	.01 (.03)	.01 (.02)	.02 (.05)	.02 (.04)
Grade 5						
M (SD)	.23 (.35)	.21 (.26)	.03 (.06)	.01 (.03)	.02 (.04)	.02 (.04)

Note. AC, approach child; OCA, other child approach; TA/SW, teacher approach to child engaged in schoolwork; TA/OTH, teacher approach to child not engaged in schoolwork; RH, raise hand; CAL, call out. From Haile-Griffey, Saudargas, Hulse-Trotter, and Zanolli (1993). Reprinted by permission of the authors.

room performance. Their measures, the Ecobehavioral Assessment Systems Software (E-BASS), contain codes that are used for assessing general education student environments (CISSAR; Code for Instructional Structure and Student Academic Response), students with disabilities in mainstreamed settings (MS-CISSAR), and students in preschool settings (ESCAPE; Ecobehavioral System for Complex Assessments of Preschool Environments). Each of the codes includes measures that examine the domains of teachers, students, and the classroom ecology. Each of the very complex codes includes over 50 individual categories grouped into the three domains. The measure uses 20-second momentary time sampling for each of the categories, but its complexity requires extensive training. The entire measure uses software that resides on a laptop, which offers quick analysis and feedback once data are collected. Substantial use of the measure in research has been found (e.g., Carta et al., 1990; Greenwood et al., 1985; Kamps et al., 1991); however, the code's complexity makes it less useful for everyday use by practitioners.

In trying to develop a code which is practitioner friendly but targets those behaviors known to be strongly related to outcomes for student academic performance, I (Shapiro, 1996a, 2003a) developed a code based in part on aspects identified in the codes of Alessi and Kaye (1983) and Saudargas and Creed (1980). As noted in E-BASS developed by Greenwood, Carta, et al. (1993, see Chapter 2), it is important to observe exactly how on-task students are spending their time. Thus, observation systems designed for periods of academic work need to determine more carefully whether students are actively or passively interacting with their academic tasks, something not clearly present in the SECOS or many other codes used to assess students as they perform academic skills. The Behavioral Observation of Students in Schools (BOSS) offers practitioners a simple observational code designed to assess key components of student academic performance. The code necessarily makes some compromises in limiting the range of behavioral categories that are included. However, the code is designed to provide detail about the nature of a student's on- and off-task behavior. In addition, the code can be used in a paper-and-pencil version or using Personal Digital Assistant (PDA) software developed exclusively for this code (Shapiro, 2003a). A description of the code is provided here, with a full and detailed description for its use in the workbook accompanying this text.

Behavioral Observation of Students in Schools (BOSS)

The BOSS divides on-task behavior into two components: active and passive engaged time (see Appendix 3C). Three subtypes of off-task behavior are observed: verbal, motor, and passive. In addition, data are collected on the teacher's directed instruction toward the targeted student. The code is also arranged to collect data on peer-comparison students.

The top of the data sheet asks for a variety of identifying information. In addition to the student's name, grade, name of school, teacher's name, and observer's name, the sheet asks for a record of the academic subject. The observer should write in the exact activity observed. For example, during reading, students may be working in a workbook, engaged in silent reading, or working on assigned worksheets. Simply indicating that the subject observed was "reading" is not sufficient.

To the right of this line is a series of numbers with abbreviated codes. These represent the four most common instructional situations:

1. *ISW:TPsnt—Individual seatwork, teacher present.* The student being observed is engaged in an individual-seatwork activity, while the teacher is circulating around the room checking work or working with individual students. The teacher may also be seated at his/her desk.
2. *ISW:TSmGp—Individual seatwork, teacher working with a small group of students.* The student being observed is working on individual seatwork, while the teacher is working with a small group of students that does not include the target student.
3. *SmGp:Tled—Small group led by the teacher.* The student being observed in this setting is part of the group of students being taught by the teacher.
4. *LgGp:Tled—Large group led by the teacher.* The student being observed in this setting is part of a large group of students, defined as at least half the class.

Occasionally, the observer will encounter a situation that is not covered by any of these four options. One common setting might be when learning centers or cooperative learning are being used. This different situation should simply be noted on the form. If the instructional arrangement changes during the observation, this change should be noted by circling the appropriate interval number where the setting changed and marking on the sheet the nature of the changed instructional environment.

Before beginning the observation, the observer will need some type of timing device to keep track of the intervals. It is strongly recommended that a stopwatch *not* be used. Conducting these types of observations requires extreme vigilance to the occurrence of behavior. Using a stopwatch will require the observer to look frequently down at the watch and back up at the students. Instead of a stopwatch, the observer should use some kind of cuing device. This can be an audiocassette that is cued for the appropriate intervals, a device that makes an audible sound at the set number of seconds, or a device that vibrates at specified intervals. In any case, one should try to use a device, such as wearing an earplug, that avoids any possible distraction that sound would create for the students in the classroom.

Typically, observations are conducted for a period of not less than 15 minutes at any one time. Some observations may last up to 30 minutes. If 15-second intervals are used, at least two sheets (60 intervals) will be needed to conduct the observation. It is suggested that the observer develop sets of recording sheets with intervals numbered 1–120, to permit the collection of data for up to 30 minutes at a time.

The next part of the form lists the behaviors to be observed down the left-hand column. Intervals are listed across the top row, with every fifth interval depicted in a shade of gray, indicating that these are peer comparison intervals. Active and passive engaged time are collected as momentary time samples. Off-task behaviors are collected using a partial-interval recording system. Teacher-directed instruction is sampled once every five intervals, also using a partial-interval recording system.

Each behavioral category is carefully defined through examples of occurrence and nonoccurrence in the BOSS manual (Shapiro, 2003a). For example, both active engaged time (AET) and passive engaged time (PET) require that the student first be "on-task," defined as attending to his/her work or assigned task/activity. If the on-task student is actively writing, raising his/her hand, reading aloud, answering questions, talking to others (peers or teacher) concerning academics, or flipping through a book (e.g., a dictionary), an occurrence of AET would be scored. Similarly, if the student is on-task but his/her behavior is passive, such as reading silently, listening to the teacher or a peer, looking at the blackboard during instruction, or looking at academic materials, an occurrence of PET is scored.

As each 15-second interval begins, the student is scored for the presence or absence of AET or PET at the instant the interval is cued (momentary time sampling). During the remainder of the interval, off-task behaviors (motor, verbal, or passive) are scored as soon as they occur. The BOSS requires only that the behavior has occurred, not a count of its frequency (partial-interval time sampling). In other words, if during an interval a student gets out of his/her seat and talks to a peer, a mark would be placed in the Off-Task Motor (OFT-M) and Off-Task Verbal (OFT-V) categories. However, if the student in the same interval then talked to a second peer, only a single mark, indicating that the behavior had occurred, would be scored.

Every fifth interval, the observer using the BOSS is instructed to randomly select a different nontarget student in the class to observe. Also in that interval, any teacher-directed instruction (TDI) to the class is marked. Thus, when the observation is completed, the BOSS provides data on the targeted student, a peer-comparison score, and a score on the estimated time the teacher spent instructing the class.

Interpreting Data from the BOSS

Data from the BOSS offer information about the nature of a student's on-task and off-task behavior. Although less detailed than the SECOS or E-BASS, the measure provides important insight into the level of engagement that a student is showing in his or her classroom. Not provided in the BOSS is extensive information on either the student–student or student–teacher contact patterns or the academic ecology, as would be captured on measures such as the E-BASS. Although this information is certainly important, obtaining such data does make the observation code extremely complex to learn. It has been my clinical experience over many years that the BOSS offers the essential data needed to more clearly understand the aspects of the educational environment that may be impacting on student performance.

Data from the BOSS can also be very useful in achieving a fuller understanding of the nature of academic engagement among students commonly known to be at-risk for academic failure. For example, in a study of academic skills problems of children with attention-deficit/hyperactivity disorder (ADHD), Gruber, DuPaul, Jitendra, Volpe, and Lorah (2004) used the BOSS to examine differences in the nature of academic engagement and off-task behavior. Her study compared 92 students between first and fourth grade who had confirmed diagnoses of ADHD along with 52 control students matched to the students with ADHD based on gender and grade. Each student was observed using the BOSS for 15 minutes during a period of independent seatwork across both reading and math instruction. Results of the study showed that students with ADHD had significantly lower rates of passive academic engagement and higher rates of off-task behavior than normal controls. In addition, higher rates of active engagement were found during math than during reading, while higher rates of passive engagement were evident during reading.

Data collected from direct observations need to be organized in particular ways if the results are to be effectively interpreted. Typically, observations are made during one academic period, although a single observation may contain several data sheets (three sheets for a 15-minute period, 20 intervals per sheet). It is important, however, to separate observations that occur on different days, even if the same instructional activity is observed. Thus, if independent seatwork is observed during reading on Monday for 15 minutes and on Tuesday for 20 minutes, each of these sets of observations is scored independently. If observations are conducted of the same academic subject in the same day, but during different instructional settings (e.g., large group led by the teacher [LgGp:Tled] versus individual seatwork, teacher present [ISW:TPsnt]), these sets of observations should also be scored separately. The observer must be careful to check whether the instructional setting changes during an observation. For example, if during a 30-minute observation the observer finds during interval 45 that the setting goes from ISW:TPsnt to SmGp:Tled, the data scored during intervals 1–45 should be treated separately from those scored on intervals 45–120.

When performing calculations on the BOSS, the observer must be sure to separate the intervals marked for the referred student and those marked for the comparison student. Once the protocol is scored for the referred child, similar data should be calculated for the peer-comparison observations. As noted previously, data for all comparison-child intervals are combined, even if different students are observed across intervals.

The most significant behaviors observed in the BOSS are AET and PET. Together, these behaviors represent the time on-task. Assessors can indeed add these two categories together if they want to report the level of on-task behavior found for the student. These data do represent an estimate of the percentage of time that the student was attentive to task. More important, however, the relative distribution between active and passive engagement is a more meaningful way of discussing the data. Given that there are known links between a student's level of active engagement and academic outcome (e.g., Greenwood, 1991; Greenwood, Dinwiddie, et al., 1984; Greenwood, Horton, & Utley, 2002), the degree to which a student shows levels of active engagement that approach or exceed passive engagement would be viewed as evidence of a strong academic instructional program. Of course, such interpretations must be tied to the nature of the activity that is observed during the instruction. For example, if a teacher is teaching a large group and using a group question-and-answer format, the level of active engagement is likely to be far lower than if a more cooperative grouping method were being used. At the same time, if during a cooperative grouping lesson a referred student has a very low level of active engagement but a high passive-engagement level, one views that contrast as suggesting the possibility that the student is not significantly contributing to the group responses. This would be a clear point of potential intervention.

An important component to interpreting the level of AET and PET is related to the products that result during the individual work period. It is critical to examine the work products (e.g., worksheets, workbook pages, writing assignments, math sheets, etc.) that the student produced during the observation. For example, if during the work session the student is found to have a 40% level of engagement (AET + PET), but completes all the work with 80% accuracy, then the problem may lie more with the assignment than with the student. On the other hand, if the student is found to complete 50% of the work with low levels of accuracy, then this may imply that the student lacks sufficient skills to complete the assignment accurately. Furthermore, examination of work products may show that the student only completes 50% of the assignment, but with 100% accuracy. This may suggest either that the student has a problem with rate of performance (accurate but too slow), or that the student lacks sufficient motivation to try and move faster (in which case the contingencies for reinforcement need to be examined).

Understanding why a student may have lower than expected levels of AET and PET is also facilitated by examining what the student is doing instead of working. For example, if the student is found to have high levels of Passive Off-Task (OFT-P), it suggests that the child is not paying attention to the assignment. Alternatively, if the student has high levels of OFT-M, it suggests that the student is actively moving around, but not in ways required by the teacher. Finally, if the student shows high levels of OFT-V, it suggests that the student's interactions with peers, as well as potential calling out, may be interfering with assignment completion. By anecdotally noting the quality of these interactions (aggressive or passive?) and the content (are they discussing the assignment?), the observer can determine the possible reasons for the high levels of peer interaction.

Another important comparison is between the level of behaviors in different types of instructional settings. Differences between group and individual seatwork assignments may suggest that a student has the most difficulty under only certain types of instructional conditions. Table 3.5 shows the outcomes of BOSS observations conducted with Sunny (the child described in Figure 3.3) during two different types of writing assignments. The data show that his behavior was much more disruptive (much higher motor and OFT-V behavior) relative to peers when asked to write in an independent versus a whole-class instructional period. Sunny's level of engagement, both active and passive, was also much below his peers. It was

TABLE 3.5. Comparison of BOSS Observations in Whole-Class and Independent Writing Assignments for Sunny

	Whole-class instruction		Independent writing	
	Sunny (48 intervals)	Peers (12 intervals)	Sunny (48 intervals)	Peers (12 intervals)
Active Engaged Time	04.17%	16.67%	14.58%	41.67%
Passive Engaged Time	87.50%	75.00%	08.33%	33.33%
Off-Task Motor	00.00%	04.17%	60.42%	25.00%
Off-Task Verbal	02.08%	00.00%	16.83%	04.17%
Off-Task Passive	02.08%	00.00%	02.08%	04.17%
Teacher-directed Instruction (12 intervals)		83.33%		58.33%

also important to note that even under whole-class instruction, when Sunny showed overall engagement equal to that of his peers (i.e., the combination of active and passive engagement), Sunny's level of active engagement was only one-fourth that of his peers. Given the importance of active engagement for students who struggle academically, interventions targeted at increasing Sunny's level of active engagement appear to be warranted.

Examination of the level of TDI in the classroom offers some indication of the degree to which the teacher is actively engaged in teaching the students during the observation. These data play an important role in determining that the frequency of teacher to student interaction is sufficient to expect students to maintain effective levels of AET and PET. For example, as seen in Table 3.5, the TDI under whole-class instruction was much higher than under independent work conditions. One possibility that may need to be investigated further for Sunny is that he is responsive to instructional processes when the teacher is highly engaged in direct instruction. Of course, drawing conclusions about what events in the classroom affect student performance must go beyond the effects of teacher instruction alone. It is very important to remember that other data collected during the interview and observed (somewhat anecdotally) during the systematic data collection may play critical roles in the student's academic performance. Perhaps most critical would be contingencies for work, such as feedback about accuracy, rewards, having to make up work, homework assignments, and so forth. The presence of these needs to be noted during the observation and considered during the analysis of the observational data.

Readers who are interested in learning the BOSS are encouraged to obtain the workbook that accompanies this text. One of the difficulties that can arise in using the BOSS or any direct, systematic observation technique, is the practical issues that emerge in conducting observations. The required use of a timing device that is not overly obtrusive, the necessity of a recording procedure such as data sheets, the use of a clipboard to hold the recording device, the need to conduct calculations of the data immediately following the observation, and the need to make sure that the data-collection procedure includes obtaining peer-comparison information, can make the process of conducting these observations difficult. One solution to the problem has been to place the data-collection process on a PDA such as a Palm™ or other handheld device. A version of the BOSS has been developed to conduct the entire process on a PDA. Those interested in the PDA version of the BOSS, can obtain this software from Harcourt Assessment, Inc. (*http://harcourtassessment.com*). The PDA version offers the evaluator a simple device that provides timing and cueing capabilities, data recording, calculations, and flexibility to modify the recording system to meet the examiner's requirements. Data from the PDA are easily synchronized with a personal computer, and reports can be generated showing the outcomes of the data-collection process. (Further descriptions of the BOSS software for the PDA can be found in the workbook that accompanies this text.)

STUDENT INTERVIEW

The perspective of the student is also important in gaining a full understanding of the academic environment. The degree to which students understand the instructions given by teachers for assignments, the degree to which students know how to access help if they are having problems answering questions, and knowledge of classroom rules are all critical to accurately interpreting the outcomes of direct observations. Additionally, students can provide an indication of possible sources of confusion in academic instruction that can offer potential targets for designing remediation strategies.

To learn more about student perspectives of the academic environment, an interview of the student is conducted in conjunction with the completion of a systematic direct observation. Questions are asked related to the degree to which the student understands the expectations of the teacher for the specific assignment that was completed during the observation, the student's self-confidence that he/she can complete the assigned work accurately, whether the student feels he/she is given sufficient time to complete the assignment, and the degree to which he/she feels included in classroom discussions.

Although many student interview formats are available, one provided by Shapiro (1996a, 1996b) has been found to be especially useful (see Figure 3.4). The student interview is conducted typically after the student has completed an independent work assignment, and is specific to a single area of academic performance. Questions on the form are asked in reference to the specific work assignment. In addition, more general questions are included, such as those on the bottom portion of Figure 3.4.

Student perspectives can offer very important considerations when designing intervention programs. For example, Figure 3.5 provides the outcome of an interview conducted with Sunny following a writing assignment. As one can see, Sunny indicates that he understands the teacher's expectations, feels he can do the assignments, likes the subject, and only complains about the amount of time given. He indicates that he likes writing (although not cursive), likes to do his own stories, and enjoys working with others when he is struggling. A comparison to Figure 3.3 shows that Sunny's teacher had a very different perspective on his writing performance. His teacher notes that he struggles greatly in the subject, does not really appear to like writing, and has difficulty with all components of the process. In designing an intervention in writing, it would be important that

STUDENT INTERVIEW FORM

Student name _____

Subject   _____

Date   _____

STUDENT-REPORTED BEHAVIOR

_____ None completed for this area

Understands expectations of teacher	☐ Yes	☐ No	☐ Not sure
Understands assignments	☐ Yes	☐ No	☐ Not sure
Feels he/she can do the assignments	☐ Yes	☐ No	☐ Not sure
Likes the subject	☐ Yes	☐ No	☐ Not sure
Feels he/she is given enough time to complete assignments	☐ Yes	☐ No	☐ Not sure
Feels like he/she is called upon to participate in discussions	☐ Yes	☐ No	☐ Not sure

General comments:

Questions used to guide interview:

Do you think you are pretty good in _____?

If you had to pick one thing about _____ you liked, what would it be?

If you had to pick one thing about _____ you don't like, what would it be?

What do you do when you are unable to solve a problem or answer a question with your assignment in _____?

Do you enjoy working with other students when you are having trouble with your assignment in _____?

Does the teacher call on you too often? Not often enough? In _____?

FIGURE 3.4. Student Interview Form.

STUDENT INTERVIEW FORM

Student name <u>Sunny</u>

Subject <u>Writing</u>

Date <u>4/10/03</u>

STUDENT-REPORTED BEHAVIOR

_____ None completed for this area

Understands expectations of teacher	☒ Yes	☐ No	☐ Not sure
Understands assignments	☒ Yes	☐ No	☐ Not sure
Feels he/she can do the assignments	☒ Yes	☐ No	☐ Not sure
Likes the subject	☒ Yes	☐ No	☐ Not sure
Feels he/she is given enough time to complete assignments	☐ Yes	☒ No	☐ Not sure
Feels like he/she is called upon to participate in discussions	☒ Yes	☐ No	☐ Not sure

General comments:

Not enough time to do writing because does not understand what she needs to do. Writing a letter take long time to figure out what to write. Can't do neat cursive since she just learned to do it.

Questions used to guide interview:

Do you think you are pretty good in <u>writing?</u> ?

Maybe, sometimes cursive is not too good.

If you had to pick one thing about _____ you liked, what would it be?

Do my own stories.

If you had to pick one thing about _____ you don't like, what would it be?

Writing stories in class.

What do you do when you are unable to solve a problem or answer a question with your assignment in _____?

Ask a friend.

Do you enjoy working with other students when you are having trouble with your assignment in _____?

Yes.

Does the teacher call on you too often? Not often enough? In _____?

A little too much.

FIGURE 3.5. Student Interview Form for Sunny.

Sunny gain a better understanding of his skills deficiencies prior to beginning any specific remediation plan, since Sunny would not understand the reason why writing was being targeted as an area of intervention.

PERMANENT PRODUCT REVIEW

The final step in an analysis of the instructional environment involves a review of permanent products. In almost every classroom, students produce materials as part of the learning process. These may be worksheets from workbooks, copied worksheets developed by the teacher, compositions, tests, quizzes, reports, and other such academic activities. All of these materials represent potentially important information that can assist the evaluator in learning more about a student's academic performance under the naturally occurring contingencies of the classroom. Analysis of these materials can offer valuable information about the areas of a student's strengths and weaknesses. In addition, because these materials are produced under naturally occurring classroom conditions, they may offer important insights into whether a student is performing differently on different types of tasks.

For example, Figure 3.6 shows the results of a first-grade student's attempt to complete a required written-language assignment. Looking at the top panel, it becomes evident that this student is using phonetic analysis in trying to write unknown words. The student also shows some letter reversals (backwards *p* in *play*), as well as poor letter formation (look at the lowercase *d*). Knowledge of irregular endings (such as *y* in *funny* and *play*) is not evident. However, the student does understand the concept of punctuation (notice the use of a comma after *TV*). Using these and many other such written-language activities, patterns of the student's strengths and weaknesses become evident.

A writing example from Sunny's assessment is shown in Figure 3.7. The writing occurred as part of an in-class assignment. Sunny's writing sample shows his difficulties in many aspects of mechanics, including poor spelling and lack of punctuation. His story also lacks creativity, detail, and depth.

A permanent product review can also be very useful when combined with systematic, direct observation. For example, a systematic observation during which a student is asked to complete a page of math problems using the BOSS may show that the student is passively engaged for over 90% of the intervals. However, an examination of the worksheet produced during that observation reveals that the student only completed 3 out of 20 problems. Thus, although the student is highly engaged, the rate of work completion is so slow that the student is likely to be failing mathematics tests. Clearly, the combination of permanent product reviews, along with other

On Saturdays, I like to . . .

Woc TV,
ANd GAWTSIA ANa
qLAe

I feel silly when . . .

WI MAc AfoNe
FAS

FIGURE 3.6. Example of written-language assignment used for permanent product review. Upper panel: "Watch TV, and go outside and play"; lower panel: "When I make a funny face."

On Saterday my sister Akira and I
had a fight it all started whin I was
fatloing her at the race track

and she got emade at me Akira

was gowing to say hiy to her

frind Dall and so was I but
Akira did not let me go.

FIGURE 3.7. Written language sample for Sunny.

data collected, can be a helpful method for evaluators to better understand the nature of the classroom demands and their outcomes on performance.

SUMMARY AND CONCLUSIONS

In this chapter, the initial portion of conducting an academic assessment has been presented. Specifically, procedures for a teacher interview, student interview, conducting direct observations, along with an examination of permanent products, combine to offer an assessment of the instructional environment. These data set the stage for designing effective interventions. The next portion of the assessment, evaluating a students' academic skills for purposes of instructional placement, is presented in Chapter 4.

TEACHER INTERVIEW FORM FOR ACADEMIC PROBLEMS

Student: _____   Teacher: _____

Birth date: _____   Date: _____

Grade: _____   School: _____

                                   Interviewer: _____

GENERAL

Why was this student referred? _____

_____

What type of academic problem(s) does this student have?

_____

READING

Primary type of reading series used   Secondary type of reading materials used

☐ Basal reader   ☐ Basal reader

☐ Literature-based   ☐ Literature-based

☐ Trade books   ☐ Trade books

                                            ☐ None

Reading series title (if applicable) _____

    Grade level of series currently placed _____

    Title of book in series currently placed _____

How many groups do you teach? _____

Which group is this student assigned to? _____

At this point in the school year, where is the average student in your class reading?

    Level and book _____

    Place in book (beg., mid., end, specific page) _____

    Time allotted/day for reading _____

How is time divided? (Independent seatwork? Small group? Cooperative groups? Large groups?)

_____

_____

How is placement in reading program determined? _____

_____

How are changes made in the program? _____

_____

Does this student participate in remedial reading programs? How much?

_____

Typical daily instructional procedures _____

_____

Contingencies for accuracy? _____

_____

Contingencies for completion? _____

_____

Types of interventions already attempted:

    Simple (e.g., reminders, cues, self-monitoring, motivation, feedback, instructions):

_____

_____

    Moderate (e.g., increasing time of existing instruction, extra tutoring sessions):

_____

_____

    Intensive (e.g., changed curriculum, changed instructional modality, changed instructional grouping, added intensive one-to-one):

_____

_____

Frequency and duration of interventions used:

_____

_____

Extent to which interventions were successful:

_____

_____

Daily scores (if available) for past 2 weeks _____

_____

Group standardized test results (if available) _____

_____

ORAL READING

How does he/she read orally compared to others in his/her reading group?

____ Much worse   ____ Somewhat worse   ____ About the same

____ Somewhat better   ____ Much better

In the class?

____ Much worse   ____ Somewhat worse   ____ About the same

____ Somewhat better   ____ Much better

WORD ATTACK

Does he/she attempt unknown words? _____

WORD KNOWLEDGE/SIGHT VOCABULARY

How does the student's word knowledge (vocabulary) compare to others in his/her reading group?

____ Much worse   ____ Somewhat worse   ____ About the same

____ Somewhat better   ____ Much better

In the class?

____ Much worse   ____ Somewhat worse   ____ About the same

____ Somewhat better   ____ Much better

How does the student's sight-word vocabulary compare to others in his/her reading group?

____ Much worse   ____ Somewhat worse   ____ About the same

____ Somewhat better   ____ Much better

In the class?

____ Much worse   ____ Somewhat worse   ____ About the same

____ Somewhat better   ____ Much better

COMPREHENSION

How well does the student seem to understand what he/she reads compared to others in his/her reading group?

_____ Much worse _____ Somewhat worse _____ About the same

_____ Somewhat better _____ Much better

In the class?

_____ Much worse _____ Somewhat worse _____ About the same

_____ Somewhat better _____ Much better

Areas of comprehension where student has success (+)/difficulty (–):

_____ Main ideas

_____ Prediction

_____ Recollection of facts

_____ Identifying plot

_____ Identifying main characters

_____ Synthesizing the story

_____ Other (describe):

_____

_____

BEHAVIOR DURING READING

Rate the following areas from 1 to 5 (1 = very unsatisfactory, 3 = satisfactory, 5 = superior).

Reading Group

a. Oral reading ability (as evidenced in reading group) _____
b. Volunteers answers _____
c. When called upon, gives correct answer _____
d. Attends to other students when they read aloud _____
e. Knows the appropriate place in book _____

Independent Seatwork

a. Stays on task _____
b. Completes assigned work in required time _____
c. Work is accurate _____
d. Works quietly _____
e. Remains in seat when required _____

Homework (if any)

a. Handed in on time   ____
b. Is complete   ____
c. Is accurate   ____

MATHEMATICS

Curriculum series _____

What are the specific problems in math? _____

_____

Time allotted/day for math _____

How is time divided? (Independent seatwork? Small group? Large group?

Cooperative groups?) _____

_____

Are your students grouped in math? _____

If so, how many groups do you have, and in which group is this student placed? _____

_____

For an **average** performing student in your class, at what point in the planned course
format would you consider this student at mastery?

    (See computational mastery form.) _____

_____

For an **average** performing student in your class, at what point in the planned course
format would you consider this student instructional?

    (See computational mastery form.) _____

_____

For an **average** performing student in your class, at what point in the planned course
format would you consider this student frustrational?

    (See computational mastery form.) _____

_____

For the **targeted** student in your class, at what point in the planned course format would
you consider this student at mastery?

    (See computational mastery form.) _____

_____

For the **targeted** student in your class, at what point in the planned course format would you consider this student instructional?

(See computational mastery form.) _____

_____

For the **targeted** student in your class, at what point in the planned course format would you consider this student frustrational?

(See computational mastery form.) _____

_____

How is mastery assessed? _____

Describe any difficulties this student has in applying math skills in these areas:

Numeration _____

Estimation _____

Time _____

Money _____

Measurement _____

Geometry _____

Graphic display _____

Interpretation of graph _____

Word problems _____

Other _____

How are changes made in the student's math program? _____

_____

Does this student participate in remedial math programs? _____

Typical daily instructional procedures _____

_____

_____

Contingencies for accuracy? _____

_____

Contingencies for completion? _____

_____

Types of interventions already attempted:

Simple (e.g., reminders, cues, self-monitoring, motivation, feedback, instructions):

_____

_____

Moderate (e.g., increasing time of existing instruction, extra tutoring sessions):

_____

_____

Intensive (e.g., changed curriculum, changed instructional modality,
changed instructional grouping, added intensive one-to-one):

_____

_____

Frequency and duration of interventions used:

_____

_____

Extent to which interventions were successful:

_____

_____

Daily scores (if available) for past 2 weeks _____

_____

Group standardized test results (if available) _____

_____

BEHAVIOR DURING MATH

Rate the following areas from 1 to 5 (1 = very unsatisfactory, 3 = satisfactory, 5 = superior)

Math Group (large)

a. Volunteers answers   ____
b. When called upon, gives correct answer   ____
c. Attends to other students when they give answers   ____
d. Knows the appropriate place in math book   ____

Math Group (small)

a. Volunteers answers   ____
b. When called upon, gives correct answer   ____
c. Attends to other students when they give answers ____
d. Knows the appropriate place in math book ____

Math Group (cooperative)

a. Volunteers answers   ____
b. Contributes to group objectives ____
c. Attends to other students when they give answers ____
d. Facilitates others in group to participate ____
e. Shows appropriate social skills in group ____

Independent Seatwork

a. Stays on task ____
b. Completes assigned work in required time ____
c. Work is accurate ____
d. Works from initial directions ____
e. Works quietly ____
f. Remains in seat when required ____

Homework (if any)

a. Handed in on time ____
b. Is complete ____
c. Is accurate ____

SPELLING

Type of material used for spelling instruction:

   ☐ Published spelling series

      Title of series _____

   ☐ Basal reading series

      Title of series _____

   ☐ Teacher-made materials _____

   ☐ Other _____

Level of instruction (if applicable) _____

At this point in the school year, where is the average student in your class spelling?

   Level, place in book _____

Time allotted/day for spelling _____

How is time divided? (Independent seatwork? Small group? Cooperative groups?)

_____

_____

How is placement in the spelling program determined? _____

_____

How are changes made in the program? _____

_____

Typical daily instructional procedures _____

_____

Types of interventions already attempted:

    Simple (e.g., reminders, cues, self-monitoring, motivation, feedback, instructions):

    _____

    _____

    Moderate (e.g., increasing time of existing instruction, extra tutoring sessions):

    _____

    _____

    Intensive (e.g., changed curriculum, changed instructional modality, changed instructional grouping, added intensive one-to-one):

    _____

    _____

Frequency and duration of interventions used:

_____

_____

Extent to which interventions were successful:

_____

_____

Contingencies for accuracy? _____

_____

Contingencies for completion? _____

_____

WRITING

Please describe the type of writing assignments you give? _____
_____

Compared to others in your class, does he/she have difficulty with (please provide brief descriptions):
☐ Expressing thoughts _____
☐ Story length _____
☐ Story depth _____
☐ Creativity _____

Mechanics:
☐ Capitalization
☐ Punctuation
☐ Grammar
☐ Handwriting
☐ Spelling
Comments: _____
_____

BEHAVIOR

Are there social–behavioral adjustment problems interfering with this student's academic progress? (be specific)
_____
_____

Check any item that describes this student's behavior:
_____ Distracted, short attention span, unable to concentrate
_____ Hyperactive, constant, aimless movement
_____ Impulsive aggressive behaviors, lacks self-control
_____ Fluctuating levels of performance
_____ Frequent negative self-statements
_____ Unconsciously repeating verbal or motor acts
_____ Lethargic, sluggish, too quiet
_____ Difficulty sharing or working with others

A COMPUTATION SKILLS MASTERY CURRICULUM

GRADE 1

1. Add two one-digit numbers: sums to 10
2. Subtract two one-digit numbers: combinations to 10

GRADE 2

3. Add two one-digit numbers: sums 11–19
4. Add a one-digit number to a two-digit number—no regrouping
5. Add a two-digit number to a two-digit number—no regrouping
6. Add a three-digit number to a three-digit number—no regrouping
7. Subtract a one-digit number from a one- or two-digit number—combinations to 18
8. Subtract a one-digit number from a two-digit number—no regrouping
9. Subtract a two-digit number from a two-digit number—no regrouping
10. Subtract a three-digit number from a three-digit number—no regrouping
11. Multiplication facts—0's, 1's, 2's

GRADE 3

12. Add three or more one-digit numbers
13. Add three or more two-digit numbers—no regrouping
14. Add three or more three- and four-digit numbers—no regrouping
15. Add a one-digit number to a two-digit number with regrouping
16. Add a two-digit number to a two-digit number with regrouping
17. Add a two-digit number to a three-digit number with regrouping from the 10's column only
18. Add a two-digit number to a three-digit number with regrouping from the 100's column only
19. Add a two-digit number to a three-digit number with regrouping from 10's and 100's columns
20. Add a three-digit number to a three-digit number with regrouping from the 10's column only
21. Add a three-digit number to a three-digit number with regrouping from the 100's column only
22. Add a three-digit number to a three-digit number with regrouping from the 10's and 100's columns
23. Add a four-digit number to a four-digit number with regrouping in one to three columns
24. Subtract two four-digit numbers—no regrouping
25. Subtract a one-digit number from a two-digit number with regrouping
26. Subtract a two-digit number from a two-digit number with regrouping
27. Subtract a two-digit number from a three-digit number with regrouping from the 10's column only

28. Subtract a two-digit number from a three-digit number with regrouping from the 100's column only
29. Subtract a two-digit number from a three-digit number with regrouping from the 10's and 100's columns
30. Subtract a three-digit number from a three-digit number with regrouping from the 10's column only
31. Subtract a three-digit number from a three-digit number with regrouping from the 100's column only
32. Subtract a three-digit number from a three-digit number with regrouping from the 10's and 100's columns
33. Multiplication facts—3–9

GRADE 4

34. Add a five- or six-digit number to a five- or six-digit number with regrouping in any columns
35. Add three or more two-digit numbers with regrouping
36. Add three or more three-digit numbers with regrouping
37. Subtract a five- or six-digit number from a five- or six-digit number with regrouping in any columns
38. Multiply a two-digit number by a one-digit number with no regrouping
39. Multiply a three-digit number by a one-digit number with no regrouping
40. Multiply a two-digit number by a one-digit number with no regrouping
41. Multiply a three-digit number by a one-digit number with regrouping
42. Division facts—0–9
43. Divide a two-digit number by a one-digit number with no remainder
44. Divide a two-digit number by a one-digit number with remainder
45. Divide a three-digit number by a one-digit number with remainder
46. Divide a four-digit number by a one-digit number with remainder

GRADE 5

47. Multiply a two-digit number by a two-digit number with regrouping
48. Multiply a three-digit number by a two-digit number with regrouping
49. Multiply a three-digit number by a three-digit number with regrouping

BLANK FORM FOR THE BEHAVIORAL OBSERVATION
OF STUDENTS IN SCHOOLS (BOSS)

Child Observed: _____   Academic Subject: _____

Date: _____   Setting: __ ISW:TPsnt   __ SmGp:TPsnt

Observer: _____   __ ISW:TSmGp   __ LgGp:TPsnt

Time of Observation: _____   Interval Length: _____   Other: _____

Moment	1	2	3	4	5*	6	7	8	9	10*	11	12	13	14	15*	S	P	T
AET																		
PET																		
Partial																		
OFT-M																		
OFT-V																		
OFT-P																		
TDI																		

Moment	16	17	18	19	20*	21	22	23	24	25*	26	27	28	29	30*	S	P	T
AET																		
PET																		
Partial																		
OFT-M																		
OFT-V																		
OFT-P																		
TDI																		

Moment	31	32	33	34	35*	36	37	38	39	40*	41	42	43	44	45*	S	P	T
AET																		
PET																		
Partial																		
OFT-M																		
OFT-V																		
OFT-P																		
TDI																		

Moment	46	47	48	49	50*	51	52	53	54	55*	56	57	58	59	60*	S	P	T
AET																		
PET																		
Partial																		
OFT-M																		
OFT-V																		
OFT-P																		
TDI																		

	Target Student			*Peer Comparison			Teacher	
	S AET	____	% AET	____	S AET	____	% AET	____	S TDI	____
Total	S PET	____	% PET	____	S PET	____	% PET	____	% TDI	____
Intervals	S OFT-M	____	% OFT-M	____	S OFT-M	____	% OFT-M	____	Total Intervals	
Observed	S OFT-V	____	% OFT-V	____	S OFT-V	____	% OFT-V	____	Observed ____	
____	OFT-P	____	% OFT-P	____	S OFT-P	____	% OFT-P	____		

CHAPTER 4

♦ ♦ ♦

Step 2: Assessing Instructional Placement

♦

After the teacher interview, rating scales, direct observation, student interview, and examination of permanent products have been completed, the evaluator is now ready to conduct the evaluation of student academic skills. This is done by administering a series of probes taken directly from curriculum materials. Materials for this part of the evaluation can be selected on the basis of the information gathered during the teacher interview and the review of permanent products. For example, examination of the last student mastery test in math (chapter test, unit test, end-of-book test) may provide indications of which types of computational probes need to be given. Likewise, teacher-reported information, such as the student's current placement in the reading series, helps to establish which level of reading probes to give. Data obtained about the expected and actual levels of performance will further guide the construction of test probes.

Assessment in some academic areas will be very similar across children; however, different types of probes may be used in different cases. For example, in reading, some cases may only involve administration of passages; other cases may require word lists and/or probes assessing phonemic awareness skills, such as phoneme segmentation, in addition to passages.

It is important to recognize that although the specific data collected on academic performance may vary according to the needs of an individual case, the procedures employed for the data-collection process should be the same. Described in the next section of this chapter are step-by-step instructions for assessing individual academic skills using curriculum-based assessment (CBA).

READING

Conducting an evaluation of reading has two major objectives:

1. To determine if the student is appropriately placed in the curriculum materials (i.e., finding a student's instructional level). Many times, students fail to master material but are passed on through the reading series without any remedial efforts.
2. To establish baseline reading levels that can serve as comparison points for monitoring progress through the reading curriculum.

The assessment of reading skills involves the administration of short, grade-based oral reading passages. Difficulty levels of passages are carefully controlled, so that reading assessments can determine how a student's performance compares against the expected performance of typical students at each grade level. Similar to an individual reading inventory (IRI), one critical difference of a reading CBA is that IRIs are not usually designed to be sensitive to continual measurement across time.

Using the Curriculum of Instruction versus Generic Passages

Most schools use literature-based reading series. A literature-based reading series is an anthology of literature. Materials are selected for their interest and motivation considering a student's grade level. Passages are not designed to be carefully controlled for vocabulary or skill development. As a result, a book used in the third grade of a series may vary widely in its readability. Instructional methods using these materials often involve combining the teaching of reading within the context of teaching language, which includes writing, skills development, and understanding. The emphasis in reading instruction is on students' obtaining meaning from reading.

Although passages can be taken from the reading series in which the student is being instructed, the difficulty level of the passages must be determined if they are to be used for a CBA. Given that literature-based reading series use anthologies, the difficulty levels of passages can vary greatly both across and within a reading series. As a result, it is recommended that generic passages already carefully controlled for difficulty level be used rather than developing passages from the reading series being used for instruction. Such passages are available commercially from several sources such as AIMSweb® (*http://www.aimsweb.com*), Scholastic

Fluency (*http://teacher.scholastic.com*), Children's Educational Services, Inc. (*http://www.readingprogress.com*), and Read Naturally (*http://readnaturally.com*). Materials for assessing prereading skills of emerging readers that include oral reading fluency passages up through sixth grade are also available (DIBELS: *http://dibels.uoregon.edu; http://sopriswest.com*).

If one does not want to use generically developed passages and wants to create a set of passages from curricular material, it is important that the passages be controlled for readability level, regardless of which reading series is used for instruction. It is often difficult to find passages from the curriculum of instruction that are always within the grade level that one is assessing. As such, passages are viewed as acceptable if they are no more than ±1 grade level from the level that the evaluator is assessing. In other words, if the evaluator is assessing grade 2, the passage should range in readability from grades 1–3.

Determining the readability of passages can be done with the use of current computer technology. Most word-processing programs (e.g., Microsoft Word) offer a built-in readability formula that can be accessed easily. In addition, programs are available commercially that offer calculations of readability across many different formulas (*http://www. readability-software.com*; OKAPI reading probe generator on *http://www.interventioncentral.org*). This particular product offers formulas that include the Dale–Chall, Spache, Fry, Flesch Grade Level, Flesch Reading Ease, SMOG, FORCAST, and Powers–Somner–Kearl. Each formula uses a somewhat different basis on which readability is determined. For example, the Spache formula is vocabulary-based and useful for elementary-level materials from primary through fourth grade. Similarly, the Dale–Chall and Flesch Grade Level formulas are vocabulary-based measures that are useful for assessing readabilities for upper-elementary and secondary-level materials. Similarly, other formulas, such as the FOG and the Flesch Reading Ease, examine the number of syllables within words and are used to rate materials used in business and industry, and other adult materials. The Fry index cuts across a wide range of materials from elementary- through college-level. Typically, the Spache, Dale–Chall, and Fry formulas are the most common in determining readability for material that would typically be used in developing a CBA.

Although readability formulas can be useful in providing general indicators of the difficulty levels of materials, they usually are based on only one aspect of the reading process, such as vocabulary or syllables in words. Another measure that simultaneously examines both vocabulary and sentence length in determining readability is the Lexile® formula (*http://www.lexile.com*). The application of this formula can provide a more precise metric for determining reading material difficulty. Lexile measures are available for a wide range of commercially available literature typically used in schools. In addition, passages available from AIMSweb and Scholastic Fluency have been graded based on the Lexile formula.

In general, the purpose of this step in the assessment process is to determine a student's instructional reading level within curricular materials. Because most reading instruction uses literature-based reading series, where material is not well controlled for difficulty, the assessment process requires the use of material that is outside the curriculum of instruction, such as well controlled generically developed reading passages. Given that the objective is to find out where in a graded set of materials a student's reading skills fall, this approach is perfectly acceptable. Evaluators should not be concerned about the apparent lack of a link to the curriculum of instruction, given that the reading material used for assessment is likely to be comparable to the instructional material. However, if an assessor wanted to create his/her own passages from material in which the student is being instructed, the next section describes the procedure.

Constructing Oral Reading Probes

1. For each book in a reading series, the evaluator should select three 150- 200-word passages (for first through third grades, 50- to 100-word passages): one from the beginning, one from the middle, and one from the end of the book. This will provide a total of three passages for each book in the reading series and reflect a reasonable range of the material covered in that grade level of the series. Readability of each of these passages is checked against a common formula (Spache for materials up to fourth grade, Dale–Chall for those above). Passages that do not fall within one (0.5 is better) grade level of the identified material are discarded. To facilitate the scoring process, the evaluator retypes the passage on a separate sheet with corresponding running word counts placed in the right-hand margin.

For preprimers and primers, shorter passages may be used. In addition, the differentiations between preprimers may not be salient enough to warrant separate probes for each individual book. In these cases, it is recommended that only the last of the preprimer books be used for purposes of assessment.

Another issue that sometimes emerges is that a reading series may have more than one level assigned to a single book. Although it is only necessary to assess by book, and not level within books, some examiners may wish to create a series of probes for each level within the book. This is a perfectly acceptable practice, but it may lengthen the assessment period considerably.

Passages selected should not have a lot of dialogue, should be text (not poetry or plays), and should not have many unusual or foreign words. It is not necessary to select passages only from the beginning of stories within the text.

2. The evaluator should make two copies of each passage selected. One passage will be for the child to read and the other copy will be used to score the child's oral reading. The evaluator may consider covering his or her copy with a transparency or laminating the probe, so that the copy can be reused.

3. For each probe, the evaluator should develop a set of five to eight comprehension questions. These questions should include both literal and inferential comprehension questions. Literal comprehension questions would be those that ask "who," "what," "where," or "why." For example, after reading "The Three Little Pigs," questions such as "What was the house of the second pig made of?" or "What did the Big Bad Wolf threaten to do to the pigs' house?" would be literal comprehension questions. Inferential questions would require a response that goes beyond the information contained in the passage. In "The Three Little Pigs" story, a question such as "Why would a house made of bricks be stronger than one made of straw?" would be an example of an inferential comprehension question. Although comprehension questions are developed for each probe, only one passage from each level of the series will be used in the assessment. Idol et al. (1996), Howell and Nolet (1999), and Blachowicz and Ogle (2001) offer excellent suggestions for developing comprehension questions.

The issue of whether to administer comprehension questions in a CBA is rather controversial. Results of a number of validation studies have consistently suggested that oral reading rate is a strong predictor of comprehension skills (e.g., Deno, Mirkin, & Chiang, 1982; Hamilton & Shinn, 2003; Hintze, Callahan, Matthews, Williams, & Tobin, 2002; Shapiro, Edwards, Lutz, & Keller, 2004). Correlations between measures of comprehension and oral reading rate are consistently higher than .60 in most studies. Many practitioners, however, are very uncomfortable with not assessing comprehension skills. Anyone working with students referred for academic problems has come across occasional students known as "word callers." These pupils have superb decoding skills and may read very fluently, yet have significant deficiencies in reading comprehension. Failure to assess comprehension skills for such a student could lead one to erroneous conclusions about the student's reading level. Many practitioners accurately point out that the process of reading itself is a matter of comprehension and not fluent oral reading. Essentially, these individuals are questioning the content validity of this measurement procedure.

Given the amount of time the assessment of comprehension adds to the evaluation process, this is not a small matter to resolve. There is a significant portion of the literature that would permit one to ignore the assessment of comprehension altogether. However, all of this literature is correlational in nature and is difficult to apply to individual cases. Clearly, one will miss the mark for some students if comprehension is not assessed.

The numbers of students who fall into the "word caller" category are probably quite small and do not justify the time it takes to add a full assessment of comprehension in every case. Typically, students who have poor oral reading skills have comprehension levels that are equal to or lower than their reading fluency levels. Thus, for those students who are referred for reading problems and found to have oral reading rates substantially below expectations, an assessment of comprehension is unnecessary and not recommended.

Despite the evidence that oral reading rate will typically reflect the level of reading comprehension, making an assessment of comprehension unnecessary, it is recommended that a *screen* for comprehension problems be part of the CBA. This is done by randomly selecting one of the three passages at each level of the series and administering a comprehension check only for that passage. In this way, the evaluator can feel more comfortable with the relationship between oral reading rate and comprehension. The comprehension screen will also provide the evaluator with additional information on the depth of a student's reading difficulties.

The comprehension screen is not designed to take the place of a needed full evaluation of a student's reading comprehension skills. The key indicator for when comprehension should be assessed is most likely found in comparing teacher interview data and the reason for referral against the observed oral reading rate. Should a student be referred for a reading problem and be found to have oral reading rates consistent with grade-level expectations, a full assessment of comprehension skills is necessary to confirm the suspected reading problem. Assuming that the reason for referral is valid, an assessment of comprehension skills should reveal a significant reading deficiency. If this is not found, then one needs to question the validity of the reason for referral. Using this as a guideline, one should find the need to assess comprehension to be infrequent.

Administration and Scoring of Oral Reading Probes

1. The evaluator should begin with the book in which the child is currently placed. (This should have been indicated during the teacher interview.)

2. For each book of the reading series, the evaluator administers first the probe from the beginning, then the one from the middle, and finally the one from the end.

Before beginning the assessment, the evaluator should tell the child that he or she is going to be asked to read and should do his or her best. If the evaluator is going to ask comprehension questions for that particular passage, the child should be told before beginning that he or she will be asked a few questions after the passage is read. The evaluator should then give a copy of the first probe to the child, make sure the stopwatch is ready, instruct the child to read aloud, and start the watch.

As the child reads, the evaluator should mark the following errors on the sheet:

a. *Omitted words.* An error of omission should be marked if the student leaves out an entire word. For example, if the line is "The cat drinks milk," and the student reads, "The drinks milk," the evaluator should mark an error. If the student omits the entire line, the evaluator should redirect the student to the line as soon as possible and mark *one* error. If the evaluator cannot redirect the student, the omission should be counted as one error and not as an error for each word missed.

b. *Substitution.* An error of substitution should be marked if the student says the wrong word. If the student deletes suffixes such as *-ed* or *-s* in speech patterns, the deletion should be noted and counted as an error.

c. *Mispronunciation.* If a student mispronounces a word, the evaluator should give the child the correct word, and instruct him/her to go to the next word if he or she hesitates.

d. *Insertions.* If a student adds a word that is not in the passage, this is noted but *not* scored as an error. For example, if the passage reads, "He ate at his grandmother's house," and the student reads, "He ate at his other grandmother's house," the insertion of the word other is noted but not scored as an error.

e. *Repetition.* Repetition of words should not be marked as errors.

f. *Self-corrections.* Self-correction should not be marked as an error.

g. *Pause.* After a pause of 3 seconds, the evaluator should supply the word and count the pause as an error.

Note. If comprehension questions are administered, the evaluator should proceed to paragraph 3a.

3. At the end of a minute, the evaluator should stop the child. If the child is in the middle of a sentence, he or she should be allowed to finish, but in either case, the evaluator should mark where the child is at the end of a minute on the probe.

4. The evaluator should count the number of words that the child gets correct in a minute, as well as the number of words incorrect. If the child reads for a minute, then the number of words (correct or incorrect) is the rate per minute. If the child finishes the passage or reads for more than one minute, the rate should be computed as follows:

$$\frac{\text{Number of words (correct or incorrect)}}{\text{Number of seconds read}} \times 60 = \text{Words per minute}$$

The evaluator should now proceed to paragraph 5.

3a. The evaluator should allow the child to finish reading the *entire probe*, marking where the child is at the end of each minute. The evaluator should allow the child to look at the probe while the comprehension questions are asked. It is important to make a note of whether the child rereads or scans the probe when answering the questions. This information may be useful in determining if the child has effective strategies for retrieving information recently read. The percentage of questions answered correctly is the comprehension score for that probe.

4a. The evaluator should count the total number of words read correctly and incorrectly in the passage. These numbers are divided by the total time the child takes to read the entire passage, using the following formula:

$$\frac{\text{Number of words (correct or errors)}}{\text{Number of seconds read}} \times 60 = \text{Words per minute}$$

5. Following the scoring procedures outlined, the evaluator should score each probe. The *median* correct, *median* incorrect, and the comprehension score are the child's scores on that book. The median score is the *middle* of the three scores on the probes.

The reason the median score is used, rather than the mean, is to control for any potential effects of difficulty of passages within a book that were not accounted for by the readability formula. Although there should not be significant changes across the three probes from a single book, one may have selected a passage that is either too easy or too hard in comparison to the overall level of the particular book. Using the median score helps to control for any variance that may be due to such an extreme score.

6. Using the criteria for placement, the evaluator should move either up or down the series and give the next set of three probes. A student may be instructional in words correct but frustrational in comprehension and/or words incorrect. The evaluator needs to look at all three measures and decide if the student's scores are within the instructional level. For example, if a student's median words correct and incorrect are well within the instructional level, but comprehension is below instructional level, the evaluator may decide that the student's oral reading fluency is instructional but that a more in-depth evaluation of comprehension skills is needed. Likewise, if the student's median words correct are in the instructional range and the error rate substantially exceeds instructional level, the evaluator

may view the student's performance as frustrational, especially if the comprehension level is less than expected. When the evaluator finds that the child is within the criteria for instructional level, the evaluator moves up the series; if not, the evaluator moves down.

There are several ways in which one can determine criteria for instructional level. The most accurate method would be to collect local norms within a particular district or school. The process for collecting these norms is complex, and interested readers should consult an excellent description of the procedure by Shinn (1988, 1989b). Examples of norms obtained from various settings are provided in Chapter 7 (see Tables 7.2, and 7.3). Setting instructional levels from local norms is usually done by using performance at the 25th percentile at either winter or spring assessments. Differences across districts can be substantial, especially if the districts draw from a different socioeconomic base. For example, Table 4.1 illustrates normative data in oral reading fluency collected in three school districts using the percentage of students in the district on free and reduced lunch as a measure of the overall socioeconomic level. The first is a suburban district

TABLE 4.1. Words Correct per Minute Scores
at the 25th Percentile across Three School Districts
from High, Moderate, and Low Socioeconomic Bases

	Fall	Winter	Spring
Grade 1			
High	4	29	59
Moderate	4	15	26
Low	1	2	6
Grade 2			
High	31	69	79
Moderate	31	55	67
Low	11	21	31
Grade 3			
High	68	86	102
Moderate	62	77	89
Low	36	38	44
Grade 4			
High	80	98	114
Moderate	83	96	104
Low	53	59	75
Grade 5			
High	103	113	121
Moderate	90	101	115
Low	77	83	88

with a high socioeconomic base, the second, a mixed urban–suburban district with a moderate-level socioeconomic base, and the third, a small urban district with a low socioeconomic base.

Using these data, one would set the instructional level for reading in a district with a moderate socioeconomic base by using the winter (midyear) data collection as the base marker for students starting in second grade. Given that first-grade students are still acquiring basic reading skills, the spring (May) assessment, which is taken at the end of the first grade period, would be a better indicator for those students. The data would suggest that scores of 55 words correct per minute would represent instructional level for second grade, 77 for third grade, and around 100 for fourth and fifth grades. By contrast, if the district were in a low socioeconomic level, oral reading fluency levels at the 25th percentile would be far less. In all districts, words incorrect would need to be at 4 or less (the accepted standard), with comprehension at approximately 80%. Mastery levels would be set in the same way using the 75th percentile. The norms in these tables are given for illustrative purposes only and should not be equally applied to all other settings.

An important distinction between the collection of local norms and those used by Fuchs and Deno (1982) is that the norming of CBA in a district may not be able to suggest the best place in which a child should be instructed. Table 4.2 provides recommended reading levels for mastery, instructional, and frustrational levels based on a "best guess" approach for instruction. Where a student is expected to begin instruction should be at a point at which material has not yet been completely mastered (mastery level), but also is not too difficult (frustration). Thus, although a student may be found to be in the 25th percentile in reading according to local norms, the decision as to where instruction should begin is made by seeing where the student's oral reading rates fall in comparison to students in other grades. For example, if a fourth-grade student's reading places him at the 10th percentile compared to other fourth graders, but at the 38th percentile compared to third graders, and at the 75th percentile compared to second graders, it seems that placement at the third-grade level would be meaningful. If local norms are not available, however, decisions based on the Fuchs and Deno criteria for instructional level are acceptable.

One of the problems that can arise in deciding whether a student's reading level is instructional occurs when a student is moved from the second- to third-grade-level materials. As seen in Table 4.2, a student reading in third-grade material at 70 words correct per minute (WCPM) is considered to be at the instructional level. In second-grade material, 40 WCPM is instructional. Thus, for example, a third-grade student who is found to read at 60 WCPM in third-grade materials is at a frustrational level. The

TABLE 4.2. Revised Placement Criteria for Direct Reading Assessment

Grade level of materials	Level	Words correct per minute	Errors per minute
1–2	Frustration	< 40	> 4
	Instructional	40–60	4 or less
	Mastery	> 60	4 or less
3–6	Frustration	< 70	> 6
	Instructional	70–100	6 or less
	Mastery	> 100	6 or less

Note. From Fuchs and Deno (1982). Reprinted by permission of the authors.

same student, when tested in second-grade material, may be found to read at 70 WCPM, which is mastery. The problem is that the student appears not to have an instructional level. In this case, one would interpret these findings in light of the change in difficulty of material that occurs between second and third grade, along with the ensuing increase in expected performance. This student would be viewed as having an instructional level somewhere between grade 2 and grade 3 material.

7. The evaluator should continue to give probes until the median scores are instructional, *and* the one above them is frustrational.

The optimal pattern would be something like this:

- Level 7: Frustrational
- Level 6: Instructional
- Level 5: Instructional
- Level 4: Mastery

Often, this exact pattern will not be obtained. Some children never reach a mastery level and will have a long series of instructional levels. Some may have only one instructional level, and others may have a series of frustrational levels, never reaching instructional level even when assessed at first grade. When students do not reach instructional levels in first-grade materials, assessment of prereading skills will be necessary (see discussion below on the DIBELS). If one finds two consecutive instructional levels, it is unnecessary to continue further. *The child's placement is at the highest instructional level.* The evaluator also may have to use his or her judgment about instructional, frustration, and mastery levels. The criteria provided are not specific cutoffs, but should be viewed as gradual changes. For example, a child scoring at 48 WCPM (where 50 is mastery) on one level and 51 on the next is probably close to mastery on both levels.

Interpreting Reading Probe Data

The results of the reading assessment should provide an indication of the level in the reading series where instruction would be most profitable. Defined as the "instructional level," this is the place in the curriculum series where a student is likely to be challenged but make progress if he or she is taught at that level. In contrast, placement in curriculum materials that are at a higher level would be frustrational and too difficult for students to learn effectively. Placement in curriculum materials at a lower level would be at mastery and not present sufficient challenge to the student. This is an important issue, because children many times are being asked to read at levels and in materials that have high probabilities of failure. It is recognized that one cannot always expect a teacher to move a student down to a reading level far below the lowest student in the class. This presents significant practical problems that cannot be addressed easily. Often, consultants need to be creative about this problem and offer suggestions that may be more acceptable within the present classroom structure. For example, if it is found that a fourth-grade student should be in a second-grade book, according to the instructional criteria, then one may suggest to the teacher the possibility of moving only to the third-grade book, but providing some type of additional individual instructional time with the student. The use of peer tutoring can often significantly assist the teacher when this type of problem arises. For example, a peer who is reading at a higher level may provide sight-word drill for the targeted student. This additional effort can be provided while the student remains in his or her current reading group. Recommendations such as this are discussed in more detail in Chapter 5. Regardless of the recommendations made based on the identification of the student's instructional level in reading, these data provide diagnostic information to the evaluator about why a student may be having difficulty in grade-level assigned reading material.

A second important finding based on the reading assessment is the identification of potential goals for reading achievement during the ensuing instructional period. On the basis of current oral reading rates, the teacher can set weekly, biweekly, monthly, and yearly goals for both oral reading rates and numbers of pages covered. When reading probes taken from the year-end goal are readministered, progress on the student's performance across time can be monitored. Again, more detail on this use of CBA data in general, and reading in particular, is included in Chapter 6.

Performance in Reading Below First-Grade Level

When a student's performance on a measure of oral reading fluency falls below instructional level at the first grade, it is necessary to assess the student's prereading skills. In the same way that the oral reading fluency metric is a key index that reflects a student's overall performance in reading, a set of skills has also been found to be a strong predictor of early literacy development. Skills that need to be assessed include the areas of phonemic awareness, phonics, and understanding of the alphabetic principle.

Many measures have been developed that are designed to assess these types of skills. For example, Good and his colleagues (Good & Kaminski, 1996, 2002; Kaminski & Good, 1996) developed measures to be in line with recommendations made by the National Reading Panel (2000) and the National Research Council (1998) for assessing early literacy. Specifically, the measures entitled *Dynamic Indicators of Basic Early Literacy Skills* (DIBELS) assess skills in the areas of phonemic awareness, phonics, fluency, vocabulary, and comprehension. The measures are designed to be used primarily for students in grades K–3, and only certain skills areas are assessed at each grade level. The measures blend into a measure of oral reading fluency that continues through the sixth-grade level.

Figure 4.1 shows each of the skills domains assessed in grades K–3, the measure used to assess that domain, and the grade at which they are administered. All measures assess the student's performance within a specified period of time, resulting in a score depicting the number of items cor-

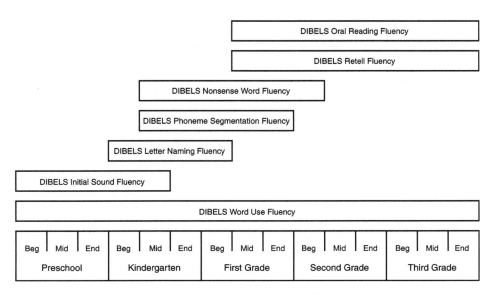

FIGURE 4.1. Sequence of skills areas assessed in the DIBELS. Adapted from Good and Kaminski (2002). Copyright 2002 by Dynamic Measurement Group, Inc. Adapted by permission.

rect per minute. For example, whereas Word Use Fluency (WUF) is assessed across grades K–3, Initial Sound Fluency (ISF), designed to assess early sound–letter recognition, is assessed only during kindergarten, since students by midkindergarten should master this skill. Likewise, Phoneme Segmentation Fluency (PSF) begins with assessment at midkindergarten and continues through the fall and winter of first grade. Empirically derived benchmarks for student performance at each assessment session identify students who have deficient, emerging, and established levels of those skills. The DIBELS measures are available currently in three formats. A version (6th edition; Good & Kaminski, 2002) is available for free download through the DIBELS official home page (*http://dibels.uoregon.edu/*). Commercial versions of the measures (6th and subsequent editions) are also available for purchase through Sopris West (*http://www.sopriswest. com*).

Another set of early literacy measures designed to be used at kindergarten- and first-grade levels is offered for purchase by AIMSweb through a subscription service (*http://www.aimsweb.com*). Specifically, measures of PSF, Nonsense Word Fluency, Letter Naming Fluency, and Letter–Sound Fluency are included.

Although the full description of the assessment measures is beyond the scope of this text, an example of one of the skills assessed from those available from AIMSweb, Nonsense Word Fluency, is provided in Figure 4.2. In the example, students are shown a set of nonsense words consisting of one syllable and asked to pronounce each of these. Students are given one minute to complete the task, and the number of syllables correct in one minute represents the score on the task.

Outcomes from the assessment of these early literacy measures indicate to evaluators the nature of the deficiencies in student reading skills that may need to be the focus of remediation. Good and Kaminski (2002) have developed benchmarks for each measure to provide users with indicators of level of risk for academic failure in reading. Figure 4.3 shows the established DIBELS benchmarks for kindergarten. Knowledge of student performance on these measures, along with expected benchmarks for success, allows evaluators to set goals for expected future performance as well.

MATHEMATICS

Assessing mathematics begins by obtaining the sequence of instruction for computational skills for your school district. If this is not available, the evaluator may use the list of objectives given in Chapter 3 (see Appendix 3B). There is not much deviation from district to district in the order in which these skills are taught.

hak	hez	mus	mol	jas
sem	mep	mez	sif	lat
non	kos	mib	tud	hap
tig	zam	luj	kaf	wef
sel	tuj	tic	lul	woz
fuv	sim	hib	rab	jut
en	fav	vuf	pic	saf
yud	jej	nof	raj	num
lod	tol	oc	tup	yif
iz	hil	hip	vuv	wob
sij	tut	kaj	dov	zeb
kef	yej	bim	jit	fub
joc	rij	dif	nes	zos
dep	kul	pel	lob	joj
tem	zod	bep	az	lop

FIGURE 4.2. AIMSweb® Nonsense Word Fluency Progress Monitoring Assessment. Copyright 2003 by Edformation, Inc. Reprinted by permission.

Kindergarten

	Beginning of Year		Middle of Year		End of Year	
Variable	Performance	Status	Performance	Status	Performance	Status
DIBELS Initial Sound Fluency	ISF < 4	At Risk	ISF < 10	Deficit		
	4 ≤ ISF < 8	Some Risk	10 ≤ ISF < 25	Emerging		
	ISF ≥ 8	Low Risk	ISF ≥ 25	Established		
DIBELS Letter Naming Fluency	LNF < 2	At Risk	LNF < 15	At Risk	LNF < 29	At Risk
	2 ≤ LNF < 8	Some Risk	15 ≤ LNF < 27	Some Risk	29 ≤ LNF < 40	Some Risk
	LNF ≥ 8	Low Risk	LNF ≥ 27	Low Risk	LNF ≥ 40	Low Risk
DIBELS Phoneme Segementation Fluency			PSF < 7	At Risk	PSF < 10	Deficit
			7 ≤ PSF < 18	Some Risk	10 ≤ PSF < 35	Emerging
			PSF ≥ 18	Low Risk	PSF ≥ 35	Established
DIBELS Nonesense Word Fluency			NWF < 5	At Risk	NWF < 15	At Risk
			5 ≤ NWF < 13	Some Risk	15 ≤ NWF < 25	Some Risk
			NWF ≥ 13	Low Risk	NWF ≥ 25	Low Risk

FIGURE 4.3. DIBELS benchmark goals for kindergarten. Adapted from Good and Kaminski (2002). Copyright 2002–2003 by Dynamic Measurement Group, Inc. Adapted by permission.

At the same time that skills in computation are being developed, skills development in mathematics requires that students can accurately apply computation to mathematical skills such as time, geometry, money, measurement, and other applications of concepts in mathematics. Additionally, students need to be able to effectively solve word problems and use graphic displays. The assessment of skills in concepts and applications of mathematics are a needed addition to the assessment of computation.

Over the last several years, there has been a trend in the instruction of mathematics toward the teaching of problem-solving skills, while de-emphasizing the teaching of computational competencies. Although obtaining data on a student's skills in problem-solving and other noncomputational aspects of mathematics (e.g., estimation) is certainly considered important, CBA still emphasizes computational objectives as the foundation upon which success in other aspects of mathematics is built. Even the solution of mathematics problems in time or money will require underlying competency in computation.

Math probes can be made for the assessment of either a single skill (such as two-digit addition with regrouping in the 10's column only or interpreting data from graphs), or multiple skills (such as all addition and subtraction facts with results less than 10, or skills in graphic interpretation, estimation, numeration, and measurement). Single-skill probe sheets are very useful for providing very specific recommendations regarding deficient and mastered math skills, and are typically used in the assessment of instructional placement phase of the academic skills evaluation. These sheets can also be valuable in monitoring the acquisition of newly taught skills during the instructional modification phase of the assessment. Multiple-skills sheets offer the advantage of assessing a broader range of skills at the same time. These sheets are typically used when conducting progress monitoring of student performance (the final phase of the CBA). These are also excellent for determining where additional assessment may be necessary.

Single-Skill Probes

1. The evaluator should define the specific types of math problems that are of interest. This can be determined either by examination of a recent end-of-book (or end-of-level) test (if available), by administering a multiple-skills probe that cuts across the entire set of objectives expected for the grade, or through the teacher interview. During the teacher interview, it is recommended that the teacher mark on the list of computational skills where the student has attained mastery, where the student is being instructed, and where the student is having significant difficulties. By look-

ing at the range of items between the teacher's rated mastery and frustration levels of the student's computation skills, the evaluator can select the possible types of computational skills to be assessed. It is not necessary to assess every single computational objective between the mastery and frustration levels. Instead, three or four objectives should be selected that will allow the evaluator to assess the range of items between these two points. In selecting these objectives, the evaluator should try to choose those that require different operations (e.g., addition and subtraction), if both types of objectives are listed between mastery and frustration points.

2. The evaluator should write (or type) several sheets of problems of the same type, leaving enough room for computation, if necessary (e.g., in the case of long division). For simpler problems, 30–35 problems to a sheet would be good (e.g., single-digit fact families). Several sheets of the same computational type may be needed, with the same format but different numbers. The evaluator should be sure to provide a good sample of all numbers within the parameters that are set and be careful about using zeros.

There are several excellent computer programs available that will automatically generate specific math probes. Mathematics Worksheet Factory, available from Schoolhouse Technologies (*http://www.schoolhousetech. com*), offers a very flexible program that includes both single- and multiple-skill problems across both computation and concepts–applications. Another program that is free is Aplus math (*http://www.aplusmath.com*). This program also offers worksheets for both single- and multiple-skills problems. A program available free-of-charge that will generate both single- and multiple-skill problems can be found on the Intervention Central website (*http://www.interventioncentral.org*). The math worksheet generator here is divided by specific computation objectives, similar to those found in Appendix 3B. The worksheets are in the basic math operations of addition, subtraction, multiplication, and division, and can be customized to develop worksheets that are both specific to addition, subtraction, multiplication, and division, and combine problems across these operations.

Multiple-Skills Probes

Three types of multiple-skill probes can be developed. When using multiple-skill probes at the instructional placement phase of the evaluation to identify specific strengths and deficiencies in computational skills, the evaluator should define the upper skill of interest and determine how many skills will be assessed at once. A number of problems of each type should be devised, as noted earlier. For each sheet, the evaluator should select two or three of each computational skill and place them onto a probe sheet. An example of a multiple-skills probe, adding and subtracting two- and three-digit numbers without regrouping, is given in Figure 4.4.

Assessments of student concepts–applications of mathematics principles for purposes of instructional placement require that evaluators have some knowledge of both skills with which students struggle and those with which they are successful. During the teacher interview, questions are asked about these skills areas. From these questions, single-skill probes of these areas could certainly be generated. However, given the wide range of concepts–applications that are often covered across a mathematics curriculum, it is usually better to administer a multiple-skills probe of grade-based skills that cut across the concepts–applications likely to be embedded in the instruction. An excellent commercial resource for such worksheets is available from Pro-Ed (L. S. Fuchs, Hamlett, & Fuchs, 1999). An example of these worksheets is provided in Figure 4.5. Based on performance on these worksheets, more single-skill probe worksheets in that area can be developed.

When the objective of assessment is to monitor progress, as in the final phase of the CBA, the third type of multiple-skills probe is developed. These probes reflect all the curriculum objectives that are identified for that grade. In other words, if the evaluator is monitoring progress across curriculum objectives for a third-grade student, the multiple-skills probe needs to contain problems that sample all the skills to be taught across the third-grade curriculum. *Monitoring Basic Skills Progress* (2nd edition; Fuchs, Hamlett, & Fuchs, 1999a) is an excellent and well-researched set of blackline masters that offer 30 probes per grade level for both computation and concepts–applications. In addition, the software programs mentioned previously, such as those available on Intervention Central, Aplusmath, or through commercial products such as the Mathematics Worksheet Factory, have the capacity to allow evaluators to develop multiple-skill worksheets.

27	45	520	462
+ 70	− 34	+ 277	− 252
20	78	703	748
+ 22	− 11	+ 274	− 626
44	566	51	520
− 32	− 263	+ 27	+ 453

FIGURE 4.4. Multiple skills math probe for addition and subtraction of 2- and 3-digit numbers without regrouping.

Column E   Applications 3   Column F

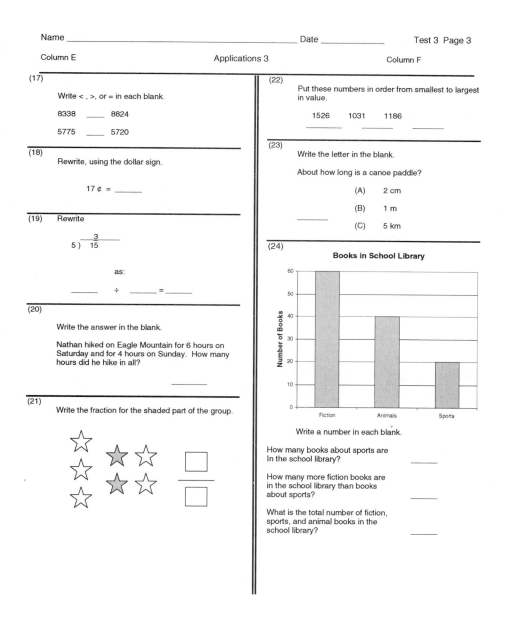

(17)

Write < , >, or = in each blank.

8338 _____ 8824

5775 _____ 5720

(18)

Rewrite, using the dollar sign.

17 ¢ = _____

(19) Rewrite

$$5 \overline{)\ \begin{array}{c} 3 \\ 15 \end{array}}$$

as:

_____ ÷ _____ = _____

(20)

Write the answer in the blank.

Nathan hiked on Eagle Mountain for 6 hours on Saturday and for 4 hours on Sunday. How many hours did he hike in all?

_____

(21)

Write the fraction for the shaded part of the group.

(22)

Put these numbers in order from smallest to largest in value.

1526   1031   1186

_____   _____   _____

(23)

Write the letter in the blank.

About how long is a canoe paddle?

(A)   2 cm

(B)   1 m

_____   (C)   5 km

(24)

Books in School Library

Write a number in each blank.

How many books about sports are in the school library?   _____

How many more fiction books are in the school library than books about sports?   _____

What is the total number of fiction, sports, and animal books in the school library?   _____

FIGURE 4.5. Example of problems from a concepts/application probe. From L. S. Fuchs, Hamlett, and Fuchs (1999c). Copyright 1999 by Pro-Ed. Reprinted by permission.

Administration and Scoring of Math Probes

1. Generally, no more than two different probe sheets for each skill or cluster of skills are administered. The evaluator should give the probe to the child and tell him or her to work each problem, going from left to right without skipping. If the child does not know how to do a problem, he or she should go on to the next one. For probes in addition or subtraction, the student is stopped after 2 minutes. For probes involving multiplication and/or division, the student is stopped after 5 minutes.

2. If the child's score on the probe sheet is significantly below instructional level, the evaluator should move downward in the curriculum to a less challenging probe. If the evaluator feels the student's performance on the probe was not indicative of the student's best efforts, a second probe of the same skills can certainly be administered. Likewise, if the evaluator finds the student highly frustrated by the skill being assessed, he or she can stop the student short of the time permitted for the probe, and does not need to administer a second probe at the same level. It is important, however, to note the exact time the student worked on the math probe. If the child scores close to or within the instructional or mastery level, the evaluator should administer one additional probe of those same skills.

3. Each of the probes should be scored as follows: The evaluator should count the separate digits in an answer. For all skills except long division, only digits *below the answer line* are counted. For example, in a two-digit addition problem with regrouping, digits written above the 10's column are not counted.

The evaluator should count the number of digits correct and incorrect for each probe. If the child completes the worksheet before time is up, the evaluator should divide the number of digits by the total number of seconds and multiply by 60. This equals the digits correct (or incorrect) per minute. The *mean* score for all probes of the same skills serves as the score for that skill or cluster.

A problem encountered in scoring the math probes may occur when students are doing double-digit multiplication. An error in multiplication will result in incorrect scores when the student adds the columns. Even though all operations are correct, a single mistake in multiplication can result in all digits being incorrect. When a student makes an error in multiplication, digits should be scored as correct or incorrect if the addition operations are performed correctly. For example, the problem

$$
\begin{array}{r}
45 \\
\times\ 28 \\
\hline
360 \\
90 \\
\hline
1260
\end{array}
$$

has 10 digits correct (9 digits plus the place holder under the 0). Suppose the problem has been completed as follows:

$$
\begin{array}{r}
45 \\
\times\ 28 \\
\hline
350 \\
80 \\
\hline
1150
\end{array}
$$

The problem is scored as having 8 digits correct (7 digits plus the place holder under the 0), because the student multiplied incorrectly but added correctly.

In addition to scoring the math problems for digits correct and incorrect, it may also be helpful to score the probes for the percentage of problems completed correctly. This is a more commonly used metric in classrooms and may be helpful in communication to the teacher.

When scoring concepts and applications, many problems have multiple part answers (see Figure 4.5). Scoring of these worksheets involves counting each of the blanks to be answered by students as a point, and dividing the number of correct answers by the total possible answers, giving a percentage of possible points

Criteria for Instructional Level

Setting criteria for frustrational, instructional, and mastery levels in math is less clear than in reading. Table 4.3 offers a set of guidelines for determining instructional level for computation. These data come from early work of Deno and Mirkin (1977) and are reasonable data for establishing levels for students when using single-skill probes and when scoring of computation, described previously, for digits below the answer line. However, methods of teaching computation, especially multiplication, have changed significantly since these data were developed. For example, many students are taught to multiply using the lattice method, a procedure which breaks multiplication into a combination of simple two-digit multiplication facts and additive components. As a result, students do not always conduct double digit multiplication using the typical algorithm that was prescribed previously. Counting digits below the answer line for students using the lattice method would result in fewer digits counted compared to students who use the more typical, multiply, carry, and add algorithm.

As a function of the change in instruction, another way of calculating instructional level is to use digits in the *answer only*, rather than all digits below the answer line. In this method of scoring, only the final set of digits representing the answer would be scored correct or incorrect, and all other digits ignored.

TABLE 4.3. Placement Criteria for Direct Assessment
of Math Computation

Grade	Level	Criterion Median digits correct per minute	Median digits incorrect per minute
1–3	Frustration	0–9	8+
	Instructional	10–19	3–7
	Mastery	20+	≤ 2
4+	Frustration	0–19	8+
	Instructional	20–39	3–7
	Mastery	40+	≤ 2

Note. The data are from Deno and Mirkin (1977). The table is from Shapiro and Lentz. Copyright 1986 by Lawrence Erlbaum Associates. Reprinted by permission.

When using digits in the answer only, the guidelines for determining instructional level need to be different from those shown in Table 4.3. Normative data for computation using the answer-only approach to scoring are reported in Table 4.4. The data come from two school districts, one a suburban, high socioeconomic level population, and the other a mixed urban–suburban moderate socioeconomic level population. Table 4.4 provides data that use the 25th percentile at each grade during the spring assessment on multiple-skills probes one grade level below the student's actual grade (i.e., third graders were given second-grade material; fourth graders were

TABLE 4.4. Instructional Level for Math Computation across Two School Districts from High and Moderate Socioeconomic Bases and Concepts–Applications in the Moderate Socioeconomic Base District

Grade	High	Moderate
	Computation[a]	
2–3	10 dcpm	10 dcpm
4	17 dcpm	13 dcpm
5	21 dcpm	13 dcpm
	Concepts/applications[b]	
2–3		25%
4–5		28%

[a]Digits correct per minute (dcpm).
[b]Percentage of possible points.

given third-grade material). Given the spiraling nature of mathematics curricula, where skills introduced at one grade are not typically fully acquired until subsequent grades, assessing math skills one grade level below the student's assigned grades is logical.

No specific recommendations for establishing instructional levels for concepts/applications can be made at this time. Some normative data has been reported in one mixed urban/suburban district, and these are offered as guidelines in Table 4.4.

There are clear discrepancies between these sets of data for instructional level. Based on research and clinical experience, it is recommended that the set of data for either the high or moderate district be used when normative data for districts are not available. As was the case with reading, the data recommended here may be valuable as best guesses.

Interpreting Data from Math Probes

Mathematics typically is taught at a single level across students within a classroom. Although students may be divided into math groups, the differences between groups may be reflected more in depth of content than in actual curricular material covered. As such, deciding instructional placement of a student into a particular level of the curriculum is not of interest.

Much more important here are decisions regarding the particular computational and concepts–application skills present or absent in the student's repertoire. A fourth-grader who is asked to do division and multiplication, but who does not have mastery of basic addition and subtraction facts, clearly needs to have additional and substantial instruction on those basic facts before he or she can be expected to learn the material being instructed in the classroom. A second grader who does not understand principles of estimation may have difficulty with more complex word problems. By contrast, a student who attains high levels of accuracy on expected levels of performance, but at rates that are below expectations, needs improvement in his/her fluency with the material; however, the basic concepts have been learned. For example, a student may know the concept of regrouping (borrowing), but cannot perform the computations fast enough to be at a mastery level. A student who understands the strategies to interpret graphs, but is very slow in applying these strategies, will not reach desired instructional levels. The key outcomes of assessing for instructional level are to facilitate descriptions of acquired knowledge and to make specific recommendations for future interventions. On the basis of these data, it should be possible to tell a teacher the specific skills on which instruction should be focused.

As with reading data, the results of the assessment of instructional placement in math can serve as a mechanism for setting short- and long-term goals. The repeated administration of these measures over time permits progress toward these goals to be evaluated. Again, more details on this use of the data are discussed in Chapters 7.

WRITTEN EXPRESSION

The purpose of assessing written expression is to determine the level and type of skills that students have attained. In contrast to reading and math, it is unlikely that there are any particular curricular objectives to which the written expression assessment can be linked. Instead, the procedure employed is a more general technique that is used across grades.

Construction, Administration, and Scoring of Probes

1. A series of "story starters" should be constructed that can be used to give the initial idea for students to write about. In developing story starters, consideration is given to the type of discourse that is being assessed. Expressive or narrative starters relate to creative writing of fictional stories (e.g., "I'll never forget the night I heard that strange sound outside my window"). Explanatory or expository discourse are starters that are subject oriented and ask the writer to write about an area of fact (e.g., "When the air pressure is rising, the forecast is usually for better weather"). Persuasive discourse is writing that is audience related and asks for the writer to provide a specific, convincing argument, such as in an advertisement (e.g., "The data are convincing that increased exercise lowers blood pressure"). Although any of these types of starters can be used, the most typical use of assessing written language is done by using narrative story starters. These starters should contain items that most children will find of sufficient interest to generate a written story. Table 4.5 offers an extensive list of possible story starters. During the assessment, the evaluator may choose to give two or three story starters, again using the median scores.

2. The evaluator should give the child a copy of the story starter and read the starter to him or her. The evaluator then tells the student that he or she will be asked to write a story using the starter as the first sentence. The student should be given a minute to think about a story before he or she will be asked to begin writing.

3. After 1 minute, the evaluator should tell the child to begin writing, start the stopwatch, and time for 3 minutes. If the child stops writing before the 3 minutes are up, he or she should be encouraged to keep writing until time is up.

4. The evaluator should count the number of words that are correctly written. "Correct" means that a word can be recognized (even if misspelled). Capitalization and punctuation are ignored. The title is also

TABLE 4.5. List of Possible Narrative Story Starters

I just saw a monster. The monster was so big it . . .

I made the biggest sandwich in the world.

Bill and Sue were lost in the jungle.

One day Mary brought her pet skunk to school.

One day it rained candy.

Tom woke up in the middle of the night. He heard a loud crash.

Jill got a surprise package in the mail.

One time I got very mad.

The best birthday I ever had . . .

I'll never forget the night I had to stay in a cave.

The most exciting thing about my jungle safari was . . .

When my video game started predicting the future, I knew I had to . . .

I never dreamed that the secret door in my basement would lead to . . .

The day my headphone radio started sending me signals from outer space, I . . .

The worst part about having a talking dog is . . .

When I moved to the desert, I was amazed to find out that cactuses . . .

When I looked out my window this morning, none of the scenery looked familiar.

I've always wanted a time machine that would take me to that wonderful time when
. . .

I would love to change places with my younger/older brother/sister, because . . .

The best thing about having the robot I got for my birthday is . . .

I always thought my tropical fish were very boring until I found out the secret of
their language . . .

I thought it was the end of the world when I lost my magic baseball bat, until I
found an enchanted . . .

The best trick I ever played on Halloween was . . .

I was most proud of my work as a private detective when I helped solve the case of
the . . .

If I could create the ideal person, I would make sure that he or she had . . .

You'll never believe how I was able to escape from the pirates who kept me prisoner
on their ship . . .

TABLE 4.6. Normative Data for Words Written per 3 Minutes from a Suburban, High-Socioeconomic-Base School District

Grade	Ranks	Fall	Winter	Spring
1	75	7	17	20
	50	4	13	16
	25	3	8	12
2	75	27	33	38
	50	21	25	28
	25	14	18	22
3	75	41	48	50
	50	33	41	42
	25	27	34	33
4	75	53	57	60
	50	45	48	57
	25	36	40	39
5	75	60	65	69
	50	51	55	57
	25	43	45	45

TABLE 4.7. Means and Standard Deviations for Grade-Level Local Norms for Total Words Written for Two Midwestern Districts

Grade	District	Fall	Winter	Spring
2	A	11.7	16.7	24.7
		(7.3)	(10.0)	(11.5)
	B	—	—	—
3	A	22.9	27.8	33.8
		(10.3)	(11.9)	(12.4)
	B	—	—	—
4	A	32.7	36.4	41.4
		(12.9)	(12.4)	(12.9)
	B	26.1	36.9	41.6
		(12.1)	(12.2)	(12.5)
5	A	40.3	44.6	46.4
		(14.5)	(13.7)	(13.6)
	B	36.8	38.8	41.5
		(11.7)	(14.7)	(12.5)
6	A	47.4	47.5	53.3
		(13.8)	(14.3)	(15.4)
	B	—	—	—

Note. From Shinn (1989b, p. 112). Copyright 1989 by The Guilford Press. Reprinted by permission.

counted if the student writes a title. The rates of correct and incorrect words per 3 minutes are calculated. If the child stops writing before the 3 minutes are up, the number of words correct should be divided by the amount of actual time (in seconds) spent in writing, and this should be multiplied by 180 for the number of words correct per 3 minutes.

5. Table 4.6 provides normative data for written performance per 3 minutes from the same high socioeconomic level school district reported previously in discussions about reading and math computation. Table 4.7 provides the norms reported by Shinn (1989b) from large urban (District A) and rural (District B) Midwestern school districts, representing data on approximately 1,000 students from grades 1 to 5 across 15 different elementary schools.

The criteria for these probes may be best determined by taking a local sample. For example, 5–10 other children in the same grade, who are considered not to have any difficulty, could be administered the same story starters as the target students, and the data from those 5–10 children aggregated to form a classwide norm. Alternatively, a teacher may administer the story starters to an entire class to determine a local norm. Written expression probes can also be scored and examined for spelling, punctuation, capitalization, and grammatical usage.

Interpreting Written Expression Probes

Different types of data are obtained from the assessment of written expression. Other than determining where the student's written expression falls relative to that of his or her peers, the probe also offers opportunities to explore related problems, such as spelling, grammatical usage, and mechanics of writing. Furthermore, the assessment allows one to examine the creativity a student can generate. Although there are no norms for such a subjective area, stories that reflect imagination and insight can suggest certain capabilities of students. In addition, one can examine the stories for structure (beginning, plot, end) and make specific suggestions to teachers for written expression goals. Similar to other parts of the CBA, written expression can offer indications of ongoing progress in meeting goals across the school year.

Although total words written can be used as a reflection of overall performance in writing, the metric does not account for meaningful connections in the writing process. Espin and colleagues (Espin et al., 1999; Espin et al., 2000), have used the method of scoring "Correct Word Sequences" within story starters. The measure counts the number of meaningful links between words. Credit is given for word sequences that consider correct spelling, punctuation, grammar, and syntax. Figure 4.6 shows an example of a sentence scored using correct word sequences.

^I woud drink ^ water ^ from ^ the ^ ocean	5
^ and ^ I woud eat ^ the ^ fruit ^ off ^ of	6
^ the ^ trees ^.^ Then ^ I woud bilit a	5
^house ^ out ^ of ^ trees, ^ and ^ I woud	6
gather ^ firewood ^ to ^ stay ^ warm^.^ I	6
woud try ^ and ^ fix ^ my ^ boat ^ in ^ my	6
^ spare ^ time^.	3
Correct Word Sequences	37

FIGURE 4.6. Scoring of a story starter using correct word sequences. Carrot symbols indicate correct links between words and/or punctuation.

The advantage of correct word sequences over words written is that the scoring accounts for the important elements that embody effective writing while maintaining the efficiency of a fluency metric. The metric also permits an analysis of the strengths and weaknesses in the writing process. Several distinct disadvantages must also be considered. First, no normative data has been reported in the literature, so the expected outcomes for students across grades is not known. Likewise, how the metric will perform over time and its sensitivity to outcomes of writing interventions is also unknown. Espin et al. (1999) did offer some data support for the use of the measure in discriminating good from poor writers among 10th-grade students. However, the applicability of the metric to younger students is still unknown. Finally, the metric takes much longer to score, compared to words written. Estimates from the personal experience of the author have found the metric to take three or four minutes per writing probe, as compared to less than 15 seconds for counting words written.

SPELLING

The assessment of spelling is often taken directly from the instructional curriculum. It is important to note, however, that there often is not substantial overlap between the reading and spelling series (Serenity & Kundert, 1987). Examination of the teacher interview data should show whether spelling is being taught from a separate series, from the reading series, or by using teacher-generated word lists. Although probes can be constructed from the same curricular material in which the student is being instructed, the nature of spelling instruction in schools does not allow for careful control of material across grades. Most schools today do not teach spelling apart from reading and other language arts activities. As such, words being taught and assessed in weekly spelling lessons may not be linked to any specific grade-based spelling curriculum. Given that the objective of this part of the assessment process is to determine a student's instructional placement and find specific skills areas where the student may be deficient, it is recommended that the spelling CBA use a more standard set of spelling words that are more carefully controlled for word difficulty across the grades, such as the Harris-Jacobson word list (Harris & Jacobson, 1972). In addition, AIMSweb (*http://www.aimsweb.com*) also offers such materials.

Constructing, Administering, and Scoring Spelling Probes

1. The evaluator should select three sets of 20 words taken from the text or material used to assess spelling for the purpose of instructional placement.

2. Words should be dictated to the student at the rate of one word every 10 seconds for first or second graders (12 words), and one word every 7 seconds for third graders and up (20 words).

3. The evaluator should dictate from successive grade-level probes until the following criteria are met:

- Grades 1–2: 20–39 letter sequences correct per 2 minutes
- Grades 3–6: 40–59 letter sequences correct per 2 minutes, 20 seconds

4. The evaluator should count the correct letter sequences. Spelling is scored in terms of correct letter sequences. The procedure for scoring is as follows:

a. A "phantom" character is placed before and after each word. For example, the word

__ B U T T E R __
has seven possible letter sequences.

b. If the word BUTTER is spelled as

__ B U T E R __ has five letter sequences correct.
__ B U T T A R __ has five letter sequences correct.
__ B A T T A R __ has three letter sequences correct.

Interpreting Spelling Probe Data

In spelling, most instruction is done with an entire group. Thus, recommendations regarding instructional level in spelling may not be that meaningful. Results of the CBA in spelling will be helpful in recommending when students need to have additional drill and practice on words previously instructed but not mastered. In addition, the data may show the types of errors typically made by the student (e.g., consistently missing middle vowels, but getting beginning and ending consonants correct; correctly identifying all components of words except ending sounds; spelling all words phonetically). These types of error analyses will allow for specific instructional recommendations.

SUMMARIZING THE DATA-COLLECTION PROCESS

CBA, as described here, incorporates the first two phases of the assessment process: collection of data about the instructional environment, and the student's instructional placement within the curriculum. Information is obtained through the teacher interview, rating scales, direct observation, examination of permanent products, student interview, and administration of skill probes. Decisions that can be made from these data include those pertaining to instructional level and correct placement in the curriculum, potential variables affecting academic performance within the teaching and learning process, recommendations for interventions, relative standing compared to peers on academic skills, setting long- and short-term goals, assessment of progress on goals, and evaluation of the effectiveness of designed interventions. In addition, the data can and have been used in making eligibility decisions (Germann & Tindal, 1985) as well as in program evaluation (Deno, 1985; Shinn, 1998).

To facilitate the process of integrating the data from the various data sources, a form is available that provides places to report all the data from each part of the evaluation. A copy of this form is given in Appendix 4A, with an expanded version available in the workbook accompanying this text. Places are available for recording results of skills probes, teacher interview data, student interview data, direct observation data, and any relevant comments about the examination of permanent products. The form has been used across hundreds of cases and has been reported as very useful in integrating the information from the assessment. Evaluators are encouraged to copy and employ this form as they conduct CBA.

The final two steps in the academic assessment process involve the development and implementation of instructional modifications based on the data collected through the assessment of the academic environment and evaluation of instructional placement, and the monitoring of the student's progress using these modifications over time. Chapters 5 and 6 discuss possible interventions that may be applicable to alter academic performance. The final step in the assessment process, progress monitoring, is then described.

DATA SUMMARY FORM FOR ACADEMIC ASSESSMENT

Child's name: _____

Teacher: _____

Grade: _____

School: _____

School district: _____

Date: _____

READING—SKILLS

Primary type of reading series used
- ☐ Basal reader
- ☐ Literature-based
- ☐ Trade books

Secondary type of reading materials used
- ☐ Basal reader
- ☐ Literature-based
- ☐ Trade books
- ☐ None

Title of curriculum series: _____

Level/book—target student: _____

Level/book—average student: _____

Results of passages administered:

Grade level/ book	Location in book	WC/ min	Words incorrect/ min	% correct	Median scores for level WC	ER	%C	Learning level (M, I, F)
	Beginning							
	Middle							
	End							
	Beginning							
	Middle							
	End							
	Beginning							
	Middle							
	End							
	Beginning							
	Middle							
	End							

READING—ENVIRONMENT

Instructional Procedures:

Primary type of reading instruction:
☐ Basal readers   ☐ Whole-language
☐ Other (describe)

Number of reading groups: _____

Student's reading group (if applicable): _____

Allotted time/day for reading: _____

Contingencies: _____

Teaching procedures: _____

_____

_____

Observations: _____ None completed for this area

System used:
   ☐ BOSS
   ☐ Other _____

Setting of observations:
☐ ISW:TPsnt   ☐ SmGp:Tled   ☐ Coop
☐ ISW:TSmGp   ☐ LgGp:Tled   ☐ Other _____

BOSS results:

Target	Peer	Target	Peer
AET% _____	AET% _____	OFT-M% _____	OFT-M% _____
PET% _____	PET% _____	OFT-V% _____	OFT-V% _____
		OFT-P% _____	OFT-P% _____
	TDI% _____		

Intervention Strategies Attempted:

_____ Simple _____

_____

_____ Moderate _____

_____

_____ Intensive _____

_____

TEACHER-REPORTED STUDENT BEHAVIOR

Rate the following areas from 1 to 5 (1 = very unsatisfactory, 3 = satisfactory, 5 = superior)

Reading Group

a. Oral reading ability (as evidenced in reading group) _____
b. Volunteers answers _____
c. When called upon, gives correct answer _____
d. Attends to other students when they read aloud _____
e. Knows the appropriate place in book _____

Independent Seatwork

a. Stays on task _____
b. Completes assigned work in required time _____
c. Work is accurate _____
d. Works quietly _____
e. Remains in seat when required _____

Homework (if any)

a. Handed in on time _____
b. Is complete _____
c. Is accurate _____

STUDENT-REPORTED BEHAVIOR   _____ None completed for this area

Understands expectations of teacher	☐ Yes	☐ No	☐ Not sure
Understands assignments	☐ Yes	☐ No	☐ Not sure
Feels he/she can do the assignments	☐ Yes	☐ No	☐ Not sure
Likes the subject	☐ Yes	☐ No	☐ Not sure
Feels he/she is given enough time to complete assignments	☐ Yes	☐ No	☐ Not sure
Feels like he/she is called upon to participate in discussions	☐ Yes	☐ No	☐ Not sure

MATH—SKILLS

Curriculum series used: _____

Specific problems in math: _____

Mastery skill of target student: _____

Mastery skill of average student: _____

Instructional skill of target student: _____

Instructional skill of average student: _____

Problems in math applications: _____

Results of math probes:

Probe type	No.	Digits correct/min	Digits incorrect/min	% problems correct	Learning level (M, I, F)

MATH—ENVIRONMENT
Instructional Procedures:

Number of math groups: _____

Student's group (high, middle, low): _____

Allotted time/day: _____

Teaching procedures: _____

_____

Contingencies: _____

Observations: _____ None completed for this area

System used:
  ☐ BOSS
  ☐ Other _____

Setting of observations:
☐ ISW:TPsnt   ☐ SmGp:Tled   ☐ Coop
☐ ISW:TSmGp   ☐ LgGp:Tled   ☐ Other _____

BOSS results:

Target	Peer	Target	Peer
A% _____	AET% _____	OFT-M% _____	OFT-M% _____
PET% _____	PET% _____	OFT-V% _____	OFT-V% _____
		OFT-P% _____	OFT-P% _____
	TDI% _____		

Intervention Strategies Attempted:

_____ Simple _____

_____

_____ Moderate _____

_____

_____ Intensive _____

_____

TEACHER-REPORTED STUDENT BEHAVIOR

Rate the following areas from 1 to 5 (1 = very unsatisfactory, 3 = satisfactory, 5 = superior)

Math group (large)

a. Volunteers answers   _____
b. When called upon, gives correct answer   _____
c. Attends to other students when they give answers   _____
d. Knows the appropriate place in math book   _____

Math Group (small)

a. Volunteers answers   _____
b. When called upon, gives correct answer   _____
c. Attends to other students when they give answers   _____
d. Knows the appropriate place in math book   _____

Math Group (cooperative)

a. Volunteers answers   _____
b. Contributes to group objectives   _____
c. Attends to other students when they give answers   _____
d. Facilitates others in group to participate   _____
e. Shows appropriate social skills in group   _____

Independent Seatwork

a. Stays on task   _____
b. Completes assigned work in required time   _____
c. Work is accurate   _____
d. Works from initial directions   _____
e. Works quietly   _____
f. Remains in seat when required   _____

Homework (if any)

a. Handed in on time   _____
b. Is complete   _____
c. Is accurate   _____

STUDENT-REPORTED BEHAVIOR   _____ None completed for this area

Understands expectations of teacher	☐ Yes	☐ No	☐ Not sure
Understands assignments	☐ Yes	☐ No	☐ Not sure
Feels he/she can do the assignments	☐ Yes	☐ No	☐ Not sure
Likes the subject	☐ Yes	☐ No	☐ Not sure
Feels he/she is given enough time to complete assignments	☐ Yes	☐ No	☐ Not sure
Feels like he/she is called upon to participate in discussions	☐ Yes	☐ No	☐ Not sure

SPELLING—SKILLS

Type of material used for spelling instruction:

☐ Published spelling series

    Title of series _____

☐ Basal reading series

    Title of series _____

☐ Teacher-made materials

☐ Other _____

Curriculum series (if applicable): _____

Results of spelling probes:

Grade level of probe	Probe no.	LSC	% words correct	Median LSC for grade level	Level (M, I, F)
	1				
	2				
	3				
	1				
	2				
	3				
	1				
	2				
	3				
	1				
	2				
	3				

SPELLING—ENVIRONMENT

Instructional Procedures:

Allotted time/day: _____

Teaching procedures: _____

Contingencies: _____

Observations: _____ None completed for this area

System used:
   ☐ BOSS
   ☐ Other _____

Setting of observations:

☐ ISW:TPsnt   ☐ SmGp:Tled   ☐ Coop

☐ ISW:TSmGp   ☐ LgGp:Tled   ☐ Other _____

BOSS results:

Target	Peer	Target	Peer
AET% _____	AET% _____	OFT-M% _____	OFT-M% _____
PET% _____	PET% _____	OFT-V% _____	OFT-V% _____
		OFT-P% _____	OFT-P% _____
	TDI% _____		

Intervention Strategies Attempted:

_____ Simple _____

_____

_____ Moderate _____

_____

_____ Intensive _____

_____

STUDENT-REPORTED BEHAVIOR   _____ None completed for this area

Understands expectations of teacher	☐ Yes	☐ No	☐ Not sure
Understands assignments	☐ Yes	☐ No	☐ Not sure
Feels he/she can do the assignments	☐ Yes	☐ No	☐ Not sure
Likes the subject	☐ Yes	☐ No	☐ Not sure
Feels he/she is given enough time to complete assignments	☐ Yes	☐ No	☐ Not sure
Feels like he/she is called upon to participate in discussions	☐ Yes	☐ No	☐ Not sure

WRITING—SKILLS

Types of writing assignments: _____

Areas of difficulty:

Content:
- ☐ Expressing thoughts
- ☐ Story length
- ☐ Story depth
- ☐ Creativity

Mechanics:
- ☐ Capitalization
- ☐ Punctuation
- ☐ Grammar
- ☐ Handwriting
- ☐ Spelling

Results of written expression probes:

Story starter	Words written	Instructional level?	Comments

WRITING—ENVIRONMENT

Instructional Procedures:

Allotted time/day: _____

Teaching procedures: _____

_____

Observations: _____ None completed for this area

System used:
- ☐ BOSS
- ☐ Other _____

Setting of observations:
- ☐ ISW:TPsnt
- ☐ ISW:TSmGp
- ☐ SmGp:Tled
- ☐ LgGp:Tled
- ☐ Coop
- ☐ Other _____

BOSS results:

Target	Peer	Target	Peer
AET% _____	AET% _____	OFT-M% _____	OFT-M% _____
PET% _____	PET% _____	OFT-V% _____	OFT-V% _____
	TDI% _____	OFT-P% _____	OFT-P% _____

STUDENT-REPORTED BEHAVIOR

_____ None completed for this area

Understands expectations of teacher	☐ Yes	☐ No	☐ Not sure
Understands assignments	☐ Yes	☐ No	☐ Not sure
Feels he/she can do the assignments	☐ Yes	☐ No	☐ Not sure
Likes the subject	☐ Yes	☐ No	☐ Not sure
Feels he/she is given enough time to complete assignments	☐ Yes	☐ No	☐ Not sure
Feels like he/she is called upon to participate in discussions	☐ Yes	☐ No	☐ Not sure

◆ ◆ ◆

CHAPTER 5

Step 3: Instructional Modification I
General Strategies

◆

BACKGROUND

The selection of interventions to remediate academic problems has long been dominated by attempts to match specific characteristics of student learning styles to specific methods of instruction. Based on the idea that effective matching of learning style and instructional method would result in the most effective and efficient learning, significant efforts have been devoted to both identifying these critical, underlying processes and developing intervention programs aimed at remediating these processes. Effective teaching was felt to be based on identification of aptitude–treatment interactions (ATIs) that were evident for the referred child.

Two general approaches to designing treatment interventions resulted from this model. One strategy was to identify the deficient processes and design interventions that would assist students in compensating for the problem. For example, students with numerical memory problems might be given concrete cues to assist them in the computation process. Those with poor written expression might be permitted to submit responses on a test by dictating or audiotaping their answers. The second approach to deriving interventions based on the ATI model was to determine the students' modality strengths in learning and to teach specifically to those strengths. For example, students found to be deficient in auditory analysis (phonics) would be taught using a sight-oriented approach to reading. Those students found to be stronger at simultaneous than at sequential processing would be instructed in more holistic means of learning basic skills.

Although the ATI approach to remediating academic problems has intuitive and logical appeal, as well as a long, deep-rooted history in the educational process, there really is little empirical support for the continued use of this strategy. Historically, significant efforts were devoted to developing assessment and remediation programs based on this approach (e.g., Barsch, 1965; Frostig & Horne, 1964; Johnson & Myklebust, 1967; Kephart, 1971; Wepman, 1967). Typically, these programs involved the administration of tests to determine deficient psychological processes underlying acquisition of basic academic skills. Tests attempted to identify within-child processes such as sequential memory, figure–ground perception, auditory perception, and visual–motor integration; training programs aimed at remediating the specific deficiencies were then provided. Substantial reviews of the literature concerning the empirical support for the assessment instruments, as well as their related instructional training programs, have clearly suggested that such approaches to remediating academic problems are likely to fail (Arter & Jenkins, 1979; Cronbach & Snow, 1977; Kavale & Forness, 1987; Tarver & Dawson, 1978; Ysseldyke & Mirkin, 1982).

Several individuals have suggested reasons why the search for ATIs is doomed to fail. Cronbach and Snow (1977) have suggested, after reviewing over 90 studies examining ATIs, that no ATI is so well replicated that it can guide the development of instructional strategies. Gordon et al. (1985) noted that many investigators find it hard to dismiss the ATI model because of its intuitive appeal, despite its current lack of empirical validation. Messick (1970), in an early paper, felt that existing assessment technology cannot effectively identify the complexities of interactions that occur during the learning process.

Perhaps another reason why the ATI model will not succeed in the development of instructional interventions can be seen in the nature of ATI findings. These studies are almost exclusively based on analysis of large groups of students. Conclusions drawn from these findings may not always be applicable to individual students, even if the assessment methodologies suggest that a student has specific deficiencies. In other words, even though studies may suggest that students with strong sequential processing skills, as assessed on the Kaufman Assessment Battery for Children (K-ABC), would best be instructed in math by a stepwise approach to computation, these results may not be directly applicable to a specific, individual student. Although there have been some significant calls for use of large-group, randomized designs to establish the effectiveness of intervention strategies in education (Shavelson & Towne, 2002), some serious questions have been raised about the use of group design methodologies in general for decision making about effective interventions (e.g., Kratochwill, 1985a; Shapiro, 1987b).

Despite the substantial problems with ATI models for designing academic interventions, the use of these strategies continues to permeate the literature. Continued efforts in assessment measures, such as the K-ABC and the Cognitive Assessment System (CAS), to identify underlying psychological processes and link them to intervention programs, unfortunately, reinforce the idea that there is empirical support for such efforts.

An alternative to the ATI model attempts to examine the *functional* rather than *structural* relationships between individual learners and their academic performance. Instructional strategies are based on empirical data suggesting which procedures are most effective in improving academic skills. Specifically, the targeted problem is identified and divided into component skills needed to acquire the behavior, and these components are taught using a wide variety of techniques designed to facilitate generalization (Zigmond & Miller, 1986). The strategies include practice, rehearsal, increased opportunities to respond, use of feedback and reinforcement principles, and other techniques consistent with effective teaching. Setting short- and long-term goals, monitoring student performance, and adjusting components of instruction are all part of the process. As one can see, these procedures are not related to any particular structural characteristic inherent to individuals.

The important aspect of this model of effective teaching is that instructional procedures remain maximally sensitive to their functional relationship to behavior change. Those procedures that produce improvement in a specific student's performance are retained. Those interventions not found to result in the desired change are discarded, *but only for that individual.* Another student, who may appear equally deficient, may be responsive to the same procedure that failed for a former student. In other words, the procedures remain sensitive to individual differences in student *performance*, but unrelated to any structural differences.

Efforts to describe effective remediations for academic problems based on functional relationships to behavior are not new. For example, Staats, Minke, Finley, Wolf, and Brooks (1964) demonstrated in numerous studies that reading skills of children could be modified through contingent reinforcement programs. Hall, Lund, and Jackson (1968) showed that teacher attention could affect study behavior. Lovitt and Curtiss (1969) found that manipulation of points awarded for academic performance could improve performance on a wide variety of mathematics, reading, and language arts tasks. Broussard and Northrup (1995), Northrup et al. (1994), March and Horner (2002), Roberts et al. (2001), Dunlap, Kern, and Worcester (2001), Daly and Murdoch (2000), Hendrickson, Gable, Novak, and Peck (1996), Daly et al. (1997), and Cooper et al. (1990) all showed examples of how a functional analysis of behavior can be applied to academic problems of both general education and special education classrooms.

Clearly, the functional approach to selection of interventions for academic problems is linked closely to behavioral assessment procedures. Methods for monitoring the performance of students on the areas targeted for change and for facilitating decisions about altering instructional strategies play critical roles in the model. In addition, the particular interventions that may be effective at improving a child's academic performance are partially evident from the assessment process. Whether interventions need to concentrate on antecedent or consequent events surrounding academic performance (e.g., changing the teacher's pacing of instruction and feedback mechanisms), or on the curricular material itself (e.g., changing the student's placement in reading material), will be based on the data gathered through the teacher interviews, direct observations, teacher rating scales, reviews of permanent products, student interviews, and the administration of direct skill probes.

Despite the direct link between the assessment process and the monitoring of interventions, the selection of the particular intervention strategy may not be based entirely on the assessment data. In addition to the data collected, teacher skills, knowledge, and clinical experience may all play an important part in choosing an appropriate intervention. In other words, on the basis of all the information obtained, a decision is made to *try* a specific intervention strategy for any of a number of reasons, including the following: (1) It has been effective with other students with similar problems before; (2) the research suggests that this may be effective; (3) the teacher is comfortable with this strategy over other possible strategies; (4) the teacher is skilled with using this type of approach; or (5) the data suggest that this procedure would manipulate a critical variable for improvement. What is crucial is that although logical analysis is used to select the intervention strategy, evaluation of the intervention's effectiveness occurs through ongoing data collection.

Intervention strategies based on functional approaches to academic skills remediation can be conceptualized as a continuum from simple to complex. As can be seen in Figure 5.1, at the simple level, no major changes are made to the instructional processes themselves. The focus of interventions at this level is on student motivation, feedback, instructions, timing or location of the intervention process, and other strategies aimed at improving aspects of the academic environment in which learning takes place. These interventions are usually very easy to implement and take minimal time and resources, but they can have a substantial impact on student performance. Some examples of these types of strategies would be having students graph their own data; providing reminder cues, such as highlighting signs of math computation problems; or changing the location of instruc-

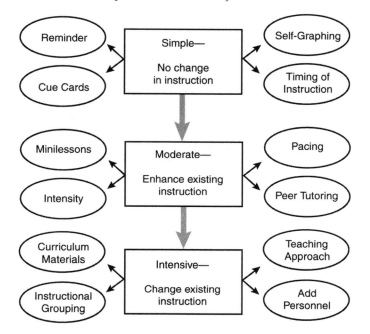

FIGURE 5.1. Levels of intervention development.

tion from late afternoon (when the student may be more fatigued) to the morning. The specific simple interventions recommended are based primarily on data collected through Step 1 of the assessment process, where aspects of the academic environment that may not be maximized are identified.

When simple interventions fail to be successful, those considered moderately complex are implemented. These interventions focus on the *enhancement* of existing instruction. Such interventions will increase the intensity, frequency, and/or duration of instructional interventions already in place rather than change the instruction itself. For example, if a student is showing difficulties in blending and segmenting of words in reading, a strategy that may be considered at the level of moderate complexity would be to have the teacher for a specified period of time conduct a series of intensive minilessons focused exclusively on these specific skills. Another potential strategy at the level of moderate complexity would be to have teachers increase the pacing and focus of instruction in specific skills areas, reducing any down time that may occur during the instructional lessons. In all cases, the intention of moderately complex interventions fits these interventions within existing instructional time by maximizing student responsiveness to instruction. These interventions require modest additional resources, such as allowing teachers the additional time to conduct mini-lessons or reducing distractions from the instructional process.

If interventions at simple or moderate levels of complexity fail, then those considered at the intensive level of complexity would be implemented. These strategies involve changes in which the typical instruction itself is altered. Changes in the instructional materials and grouping of the students for instruction, or changes in the entire curriculum are put into place. Using one-on-one instruction with materials beyond the typical instructional process would be considered to be intensive interventions. These types of interventions require substantial and potentially new resources, as well as time. Teachers often need extensive supports and consultation to implement such interventions, as well as, potentially, additional professional development.

Many, many interventions for academic problems based on functional relationships at each of the three levels of intervention exist. The literature contains literally thousands of research articles that document the value of all types of procedures for all types of academic problems. Specific journals are devoted only to the publication of effective instructional interventions (e.g., *Learning Disabilities Forum*; *Learning Disabilities Research and Practice*; *Teaching Exceptional Children*; *Remedial and Special Education*). I attempt in this chapter to describe several general strategies that have been broadly applied across different types of academic skills. Those chosen for review represent strategies with substantial empirical databases (Rathvon, 1999; Thomas & Grimes, 2002); they include self-management, peer tutoring, performance feedback, direct instruction–precision teaching, and cooperative learning. (Selected procedures from the literature described specifically for remediating basic skills in reading, mathematics, spelling, and written language are described in Chapter 6). Clearly, in this volume, descriptions of the procedures cannot be comprehensive or exhaustive. It is strongly suggested that interested readers examine the numerous source materials listed for each method before trying to implement these strategies.

GENERAL STRATEGIES FOR ACADEMIC PROBLEMS

Self-Management

Significant efforts have been made to design and evaluate behavior-change strategies that place control of the specified contingencies in the hands of the individual whose behavior is being changed. These procedures have substantial appeal, since they potentially may result in generalization across time and setting (e.g., Holman & Baer, 1979). In addition, the procedures may be more efficient, since they require only minimal involvement of significant others. This may be particularly important in school settings, where teachers often legitimately complain that class size inhibits the potential for interventions with individual students. A related advantage of self-management is the potential for these procedures to teach students to be responsible for their own behavior. For many students with developmental disabilities, this may be a particularly important issue (e.g., Fowler, 1984; Hughes et al., 2002; Koegel, Harrower, & Koegel, 1999; Shapiro, 1981; Shapiro & Cole, 1994).

Several authors have offered varying definitions of self-management (Browder & Shapiro, 1985; Fantuzzo & Polite, 1990; Fantuzzo, Rohrbeck, & Azar, 1986; Mace & West, 1986). Although these definitions emphasize different aspects of the process, the model of self-management suggested by Kanfer (1971) seems to have broad-based appeal. His model contains three primary components: self-monitoring, self-evaluation, and self-reinforcement. Self-monitoring includes both self-observation and self-recording of behavior. At times, this process alone may be reactive and result in behavior change (e.g., Nelson, 1977). Once behavior is monitored, the individual must evaluate his/her response against a known criterion. The process of self-evaluation leads directly to self-reinforcement, because the individual must now decide whether he/she has met the criteria for self-reinforcement and, if so, must apply the appropriate consequences. Although there have been significant questions regarding the mechanisms operating in self-management (e.g., Bandura, 1976; Brigham, 1980; Hughes & Lloyd, 1993; Mace & Kratochwill, 1985; Mace & West, 1986), Kanfer's model has fairly wide acceptance among researchers (Karoly, 1982).

Self-management procedures can be roughly divided into two categories (Roberts & Dick, 1982; Shapiro & Cole, 1994). One set of procedures is based on principles of contingency management and is designed primarily to manipulate the consequences of behavior. These procedures usually involve self-monitoring of behavior and rewards for attaining specified criteria. The other type of procedure is based more on control of conditions antecedent to behavioral events—specifically, the manipulation of cognitive variables. These procedures typically employ some form of verbal mediation strategy.

Contingency Management Procedures

Self-management procedures based on principles of contingency management are usually straightforward. Individuals are taught to self-monitor (self-observe and self-record) the presence or absence of a specified response. The actual recording mechanism can involve mechanical devices, such as response counters, or tally marks using paper and pencil. The individual can be cued to self-monitor via audio signals (e.g., prerecorded beeps) or via the signaling of others (e.g., teacher's announcement that it is time to record). Individuals may also be taught to self-monitor the completion of a task (such as a worksheet in school) rather than using an external cueing device. The variety of mechanisms available for setting up a self-monitoring program have been extensively described (e.g., Gardner & Cole, 1988; Nelson, 1977; Shapiro, 1984; Shapiro & Cole, 1994, 1999).

Setting up a self-monitoring program requires that the response to be monitored be clearly defined for the student. For example, if students are to monitor their on-task behavior at a given cue, they may have to be trained to discriminate between those behaviors defined as "working" and those defined as "not working." Many studies employing self-monitoring procedures include a training period that precedes the actual implementation of the technique. Usually, it does not take long for students to learn the needed discrimination. Studies of children with developmental disabilities, as well as autism (e.g., Copeland, Hughes, Agran, Wehmeyer, & Fowler, 2002; Hughes, Korinek, & Gorman, 1991; Koegel et al., 1999; Newman, Reinecke, & Meinberg, 2000; Shapiro, Browder, & D'Huyvetters, 1984); preschool children (e.g., Connell, Carta, & Baer, 1993; de Haas-Warner, 1991; Fowler, 1986; Harding, Howard, & McLaughlin, 1993); students with LD (e.g., Bryan, Burstein, & Bryan, 2001; Hallahan et al., 1982; Reid, 1996; Smith, Young, Nelson, & West, 1992; Trammel, Schloss, & Alper, 1994); students with ADHD and other behavioral–emotional disorders (e.g., Dunlap, Clarke, Jackson, & Wright, 1995; Levendowski & Cartledge, 2000; Shapiro, DuPaul, & Bradley-Klug, 1998; Shimaburkuro et al., 1999); and students at-risk for academic failure (e.g., Wood, Murdock, & Cronin, 2002) have all demonstrated successful self-monitoring, with relatively little time needed for training.

Once the target behavior is identified, a procedure to cue students when to self-monitor is needed. In some cases, external cues, such as audiotaped beeps, can be employed (e.g., Maag et al., 1993). In at least one case, a 1 minute interlude of music was played to cue students to self-monitor for on-task behavior (Shapiro, McGonigle, & Ollendick, 1981). In some settings, however, use of externally cued signals may be both disruptive to others in the classroom and interfere with instructional processes. In such cases, it is possible to teach students to self-monitor very specific events, such as the completion of a worksheet, or an individual problem on a worksheet. These types of cueing mechanisms may require some initial instruction but rarely are disruptive to others or to the teacher.

Selection and design of the self-monitoring device are also important considerations. The procedure chosen should be as simple as possible and require the least amount of effort on the student's part. For younger students, use of a "countoon" (Jenson, Rhode, & Reavis, 1994; Kunzelmann, 1970) may be helpful. This is simply a form with stick figure or icon drawings representing the desired behavior already printed on the form. For example, if a student were to self-monitor in-seat behavior, a series of stick figures of a child sitting in a seat might be drawn on a form. The child simply crosses out the figure as a form of self-monitoring.

Self-monitoring alone may be reactive and result in behavior change. Although there is an extensive literature on the reactive effects of self-monitoring (e.g., Nelson & Hayes, 1981; Shapiro & Cole, 1994), it is clear that the task of simply observing one's own behavior may be sufficient to alter the behavior in the desired direction. It is therefore logical to use self-monitoring alone as an intervention procedure. Many times, students will show desired changes without any additional backup rewards. In such cases, the positive behavioral changes and associated reinforcers (better grades, fewer teacher reprimands, pleased parents) are probably functioning to sustain the observed behavior change. Although reactive self-monitoring is desirable, it does not always occur. Numerous studies have been reported in the literature, in which additional rewards were required to facilitate the behavior-change process. One should therefore not be discouraged by the failure of self-monitoring alone to be reactive.

Another important aspect of any self-management program is making sure that student reports of self-monitored behavior are accurate. Some studies have found that teacher checking of the accuracy of students' self-monitored behavior is necessary to maintain desired levels of behavior change (e.g., Lam et al., 1994; Rhode, Morgan, & Young, 1983; Santogrossi, O'Leary, Romanczyk, & Kaufmann, 1973; Smith et al., 1992). Teachers should plan on "surprise" checks of self-monitoring accuracy throughout the implementation of an intervention program. Obviously, these checks will need to be frequent in the beginning portion of the self-management treatment. Robertson, Simon, Pachman, and Drabman (1980), Rhode et al. (1983), Shapiro and Cole (1994), Smith et al. (1992), Smith, Young, West, Morgan, and Rhode (1988), and Young, West, Smith, and Morgan (1991) offer descriptions for how to gradually reduce the needed teacher-checking procedure.

Applications of contingency-based self-management procedures for academic skills have most often used forms of self-monitoring as the intervention strategy. Many of these investigations have targeted academic skills indirectly by having students self-monitor on-task behavior or its equivalent. For example, in a series of studies conducted as part of the University of Virginia Institute for Research in Learning Disabilities (Hallahan et al., 1982), elementary-age students with LD were taught to self-monitor their on-task behavior ("Was I paying attention?") at the sound of a beep emitted on a variable-interval, 42-second (range 11–92 seconds) schedule. Data on the number of math problems completed correctly on a series of three assigned sheets of problems were also recorded. Results of their study showed significant improvements in on-task behavior, but only modest changes in the number of problems completed correctly. Other studies by these same authors produced similar results (e.g., Hallahan, Marshall, & Lloyd, 1981; Lloyd, Hallahan, Kosiewicz, & Kneedler, 1982). In looking more carefully at this issue, Lam et al. (1994) compared the relative effects of self-monitoring on the on-task behavior, academic accuracy, and disruptive behavior of three students with severe behavior disorders. Of special interest in our study was the collateral effect of the self-monitoring of one of these behaviors upon the other. Results showed that in the specific behavior for which self-monitoring was applied (i.e., on-task behavior, academic accuracy, or disruptive behavior), substantial improvement was evident. However, the most improvement in the collateral behaviors was present when self-monitoring was applied to academic accuracy over the other two behaviors. Similar outcomes were found in several other studies (Carr & Punzo, 1993; Harris et al., 1994; Maag et al., 1993; Reid & Harris, 1993). In all cases, self-monitoring was reactive, without any additional contingencies on performance.

McLaughlin, Burgess, and Sackville-West (1982) had six students with behavioral disorders record whether they were studying or not studying during an individual reading instruction period at random intervals determined by the students. The procedure was employed within a classroom already using a classwide token economy procedure. In a subsequent phase, students had to match teacher recordings to earn the appropriate points. Results showed that self-monitoring of study behavior significantly improved the percentage of problems completed correctly, with particular gains when teacher matching was required.

Prater, Hogan, and Miller (1992), working with an adolescent student with learning and behavior disorders, used self-monitoring supported by audio and visual prompts to increase on-task behavior and academic performance. After the procedure was implemented in a resource room, a modified version of the self-monitoring procedure, using only visual prompts, was then implemented in two mainstream classrooms (mathematics and English). Results for improvements in on-task behavior were commensurate with the implementation of the self-monitoring procedures in all three settings. Similarly, Shimaburko et al. (1999) demonstrated that having students with LD and ADHD self-monitor and graph their performance on tasks of reading comprehension, mathematics, and written expression significantly improved both on-task and academic performance in all areas.

The use of self-management procedures derived from contingency management principles clearly has applicability in designing intervention strategies for academic problems. Although the procedure has been used more often to target on-task behavior and its equivalents, it can be used successfully with academic targets per se. Indeed, literature reviews have shown that the most significant gains in academic performance are related to strategies (not just self-management) that directly target academic performance rather than treating academic skills as collateral variables to on-task behavior (Hoge & Andrews, 1987; Skinner & Smith, 1992).

Cognitive-Based Interventions

Procedures developed for the modification of cognitions have typically employed varied forms of self-instruction. Originally described by Meichenbaum and Goodman (1971), self-instruction involves having individuals talk aloud as they perform a task. The self-instructions are designed to refocus the individual's thoughts and teach effective problem solving. Although the technique was first described by Meichenbaum and Goodman for reducing impulsive behavior in children, the procedure has since been applied to many problems, including increasing on-task behavior (e.g., Bornstein & Quevillon, 1976; Manning, 1990), social skills (e.g., Cartledge & Milburn, 1983; Combs & Lahey, 1981; Lochman & Curry, 1986; Maag, 1990), and academic skills (e.g., Fox & Kendall, 1983; Mahn & Greenwood, 1990; Roberts, Nelson, & Olson, 1987; Swanson & Scarpati, 1984).

Johnston et al. (1980) provided an excellent example of a typical self-instruction training program. Three children with mild mental retardation were taught to add and subtract with regrouping by training them to make specific self-statements related to performing the task accurately. Training was conducted in a 20- to 30-minute session, during which the children were given problems to complete. The instructor then modeled the use of self-instruction by asking and answering a series of questions. The self-instruction training was conducted following guidelines established by Meichenbaum and Goodman (1971) and involved the following: (1) The trainer first solved the problem using the self-instructions, while the subject watched; (2) the child performed the task, while the trainer instructed aloud; (3) the child spoke aloud, while solving the problem with the help of the trainer; (4) the child performed the self-instructions aloud, without trainer prompting; and finally, (5) the child performed the task using private speech. Figure 5.2 shows an example of the self-instructions actually employed in the study. Results of this study demonstrated that self-instruction training can be an effective strategy for teaching such skills. Similar results were found in a follow-up study (Whitman & Johnston, 1983).

Shapiro and Bradley (1995) provided another example of using a self-instruction training procedure to improve the skills of a 10-year-old, fourth-grade boy, Ray, who was having significant problems in math. Specifically, Ray was having difficulties learning to conduct subtraction with regrouping. Using a self-instruction training methodology, a four-step "cue

Q. What kind of a problem is this?   36
                                                                    + 47

A. It's an add problem. I can tell by the sign.

Q. Now what do I do?

A. I start with the top number in the 1's column and I add. Six and 7 (the child
points to the 6 on the number line and counts down 7 spaces) is 13. Thirteen
has two digits. That means I have to carry. This is hard so I go slowly. I put
the 3 in the 1's column (the child writes the 3 in the 1's column in the
answer) and the 1 in the 10's column (the child writes the 1 above the top
number in the 10's column in the problem).

Q. Now what do I do?

A. I start with the top number in the 10's column. One and 3 (the child points
to the 1 on the number line and counts down 3 spaces) is 4. Four and 4 (the
child counts down 4 more spaces) is 8 (the child writes the 8 in the 10's column in the answer).

Q. I want to get it right so I check it. How do I check it?

A. I cover up my answer (the child covers the answer with a small piece of
paper) and add again starting with the bottom number in the 1's column.
Seven and 6 (the child points to the 6 on the number line and counts down
7 spaces) is 13 (the child slides the piece of paper to the left and uncovers
the 3; the child sees the 1 which he or she has written over the top number
in the 10's column in the problem). Got it right. Four and 3 (the child points
to the 4 on the number line and counts down 3 spaces) is 7. Seven and 1
(the child counts down 1 more space) is 8 (the child removes the small piece
of paper so the entire answer is visible). I got it right so I'm doing well. (If, by
checking his or her work, the child determines that he or she has made an
error, he or she says, "I got it wrong. I can fix it if I go slowly." The child
then repeats the self-instruction sequence starting from the beginning.)

FIGURE 5.2. Example of self-instruction training sequence for addition with
regrouping. From Johnston, Whitman, and Johnson (1980, p. 149). Copyright
1980 by Pergamon Press, Ltd. Reprinted by permission.

card" was used to teach Ray how to solve two-digit minus one-digit subtraction problems with regrouping (see Figure 5.3). Individual sessions
were held between Ray and his teacher three times per week across a 4-
week period. As seen in Figure 5.4, Ray showed an immediate response to
the procedure, with increased performance over the 4-week period.

A very similar approach to cognitive-behavioral modification was
described by Cullinan, Lloyd, and Epstein (1981) and entitled "academic
strategy training." The first step of strategy training involves the design of
the approach. To design an attack strategy, tasks are divided through task
analysis into several component steps. Figure 5.5 provides an example of

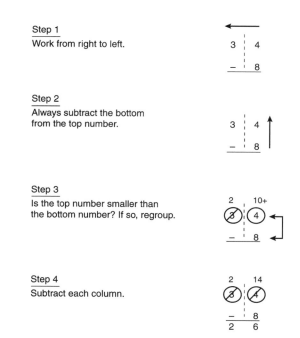

Step 1
Work from right to left.

Step 2
Always subtract the bottom
from the top number.

Step 3
Is the top number smaller than
the bottom number? If so, regroup.

Step 4
Subtract each column.

FIGURE 5.3. Example of self-instruction training sequence for subtraction with regrouping. From Shapiro and Bradley (1995, p. 360). Copyright 1995 by The Guilford Press. Reprinted by permission.

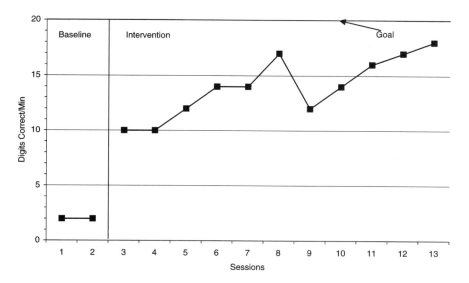

FIGURE 5.4. Results of self-instructional intervention. From Shapiro and Bradley (1995, p. 361). Copyright 1995 by The Guilford Press. Reprinted by permission.

TASK CLASS FOR MULTIPLICATION FACTS

Description: Multiplication of any number (0-10) by any number (0-10)

Examples: $0 \times 6 =$ _____ ; $3 \times 9 =$ _____ ; $7 \times 4 =$ _____ ; $8 \times 8 =$ _____ ;
$10 \times 1 =$ _____

Objective: Given a page of unordered multiplication problems written in horizontal form with factors from 0 to 10, the student will write the correct products for the problems at a rate of 25 problems correct per minute with no more than 2 errors per minute.

ATTACK STRATEGY FOR MULTIPLICATION FACTS

Attack Strategy: Count by one number the number of times indicated by the other number.

Steps in Attack Strategy:	Example:
1. Read the problem.	$2 \times 5 =$
2. Point to a number that you know how to count by.	Student points to 2.
3. Make the number of marks indicated by the other number.	$2 \times 5 =$
4. Begin counting by the number you know how to count by and count up once for each mark, touching each mark.	///// "2, 4 . . . "
5. Stop counting when you've touched the last mark.	" . . . 6, 8, 10"
6. Write the last number you said in the answer space.	$2 \times 5 = 10$

TASK ANALYSIS SHOWING PRESKILLS FOR MULTIPLICATION ATTACK STRATEGY

1. Say the numbers 0 to 100.
2. Write the number 0 to 100.
3. Name $\times$ and $=$ signs.
4. Make the number of marks indicated by numerals 0 to 10.
5. Count by numbers 1 to 10.
6. End counting-by sequences in various positions.
7. Coordinate counting-by and touching-marks actions.

FIGURE 5.5. Task class, attack strategy, and task analysis of preskills for multiplication facts. From Cullinan, Lloyd, and Epstein (1981, pp. 43–44). Copyright 1981 by Pro-Ed, Inc. Reprinted by permission.

an attack strategy used for teaching multiplication facts. Once designed, the strategy is taught directly to students, using multiple examples of appropriate and inappropriate application. Students practice the strategy until they demonstrate mastery, at which time they should be able to perform the task correctly with any items from the response class of the task.

Studies investigating strategy training have shown the procedure to be effective in teaching handwriting and composition skills (e.g., Blandford & Lloyd, 1987; Graham & Harris, 1987, 2003; Kosiewicz, Hallahan, Lloyd, & Graves, 1982), word reading accuracy (Lloyd, Hallahan, et al., 1982), reading comprehension (e.g., Blachowicz & Ogle, 2001; Lysynchuk, Pressley, & Vye, 1990; Miller, Giovenco, & Rentiers, 1987; Schunk & Rice, 1992), and arithmetic (e.g., Case, Harris, & Graham, 1992; Cullinan et al., 1981; Montague, 1989; Montague & Bos, 1986). Conceptually, these procedures are identical to self-instruction training and appear to be applicable across academic areas.

Deshler and Schumaker (1986) described another set of procedures called the "strategies intervention model," designed to facilitate the performance of secondary-level students with mild handicaps. The purpose of these procedures is not to teach specific skills areas, as with self-instruction training and strategy training, but to teach students how to learn. For example, an instructional goal in the strategies intervention model would be to teach students skills for summarizing and memorizing material for a social studies test, rather than teaching them actual social studies content. The goal of the approach is to teach strategies that are broadly applicable across content areas.

The strategies intervention model begins by identifying the curriculum demands that the student lacks (e.g., note taking, writing well-organized paragraphs). Once these deficiencies are identified, a specific teaching strategy is taught. Different strategy programs have been developed for various types of problems and have been packaged into the learning strategies curriculum (Schumaker, Deshler, Alley, & Warner, 1983). The first strand of the curriculum includes the word-identification strategy (Lenz, Schumaker, Deshler, & Beals, 1984) and is aimed at teaching decoding of multisyllabic words. Other strategies are used to teach related skills, such as the visual imagery strategy (Clark, Deshler, Schumaker, & Alley, 1984), the self-questioning strategy (Clark et al., 1984), and the paraphrasing strategy (Schumaker, Denton, & Deshler, 1984). Finally, the multipass strategy (Schumaker, Deshler, Alley, & Denton, 1982) is used for attacking textbooks by using methods similar to the SQ3R (Survey, Question, Read, Recite, Review) method of study. The second strand of the curriculum concentrates on note taking and memorization skills, and the final strand of the curriculum emphasizes written expression and demonstrations of competence.

Significant field testing and evaluation of the strategies intervention model have been conducted through the University of Kansas Institute for Research in Learning Disabilities and reported in a large number of published journal articles and technical reports (e.g., Deshler & Schumaker, 1986, 1993; Deshler, Schumaker, Alley, Warner, & Clark, 1982; Deshler, Schumaker, Lenz, & Ellis, 1984; Ellis & Lenz, 1987; Ellis, Lenz, & Sabournie, 1987a, 1987b; Tralli, Colombo, Deshler, & Schumaker, 1966). Results have consistently shown that before training, students showed limited use of these strategies and poor performance on the related academic skills. After training, students showed marked improvements in academic performance. At present, the learning strategies curriculum is being implemented by a wide range of school districts across the country. Deshler and Schumaker (1986) and Schumaker and Deshler (2003) report that although the strategies intervention model has enjoyed substantial success in reports of student outcome, there appear to be significant relationships between the level of staff training implementing the model and academic gains of adolescents. Clearly, caution is warranted for interested readers to secure appropriate and effective training in this model before implementing the procedures in their own districts.

Conclusions

Self-management appears to be a promising intervention for remediating academic problems. Procedures such as self-monitoring are rather simple to employ and may result in significant gains. In particular, the possibility of achieving generalization across tasks, time, and behaviors is exciting.

Equally appealing is the use of cognitive-based procedures such as self-instruction training. Although these procedures obviously require more effort on the part of trainers, they clearly have the potential for teaching academic skills to students. Even more encouraging are the examples of efforts such as those of the researchers from the University of Kansas, who have taken the basic concepts of self-instruction training and cognitive-behavioral modification, and applied them to the development of a curriculum for teaching adolescent students with LD how to solve problems for academic tasks.

Peer Tutoring

Another strategy with wide applications across academic content areas has been the use of peer tutoring. Although numerous examples have been reported in the literature, systematic efforts both to demonstrate use of peer tutoring and to investigate specific variables that affect academic performance have emerged from the work of Greenwood and his associates at the

Juniper Gardens Children's Project in Kansas City, Kansas (e.g., Delquadri, Greenwood, Whorton, Carta, & Hall, 1986; Greenwood, 1991; Greenwood, Delquadri, & Carta, 1997; Greenwood et al., 1989; Greenwood, Carta, et al., 1992; Greenwood, Terry, et al., 1992; Greenwood, Terry, Utley, Montagna, & Walker, 1993). The broad applicability of the classwide peer tutoring (CWPT) procedure has been shown through a range of studies demonstrating successful outcomes for students who are second language learners (Greenwood et al., 2001), for teaching health and safety information to students with developmental disabilities (Utley et al., 2001), as well as a modified version for students with autism (Kamps, Dugan, Potuchek, & Collins, 1999).

The underlying conceptual framework for the origination of the development of the CWPT procedures was significant literature suggesting that rates of student engagement in academic tasks are uniformly low across regular and special education settings (Berliner, 1979; Greenwood, 1991; Greenwood et al., 1985; Haynes & Jenkins, 1986; Leinhardt et al., 1981). Hall et al. (1982) and Greenwood et al. (1981) operationalized academic engagement as opportunities to respond. Specifically, they reasoned that a necessary condition for academic progress is the frequent presentation of antecedents for student responding in academic performance. These concepts were demonstrated and replicated empirically in several studies (Greenwood, 1996; Greenwood, Delquadri, & Hall, 1984; Greenwood, Dinwiddie, et al., 1984; Greenwood, Horton, & Utley, 2002; Greenwood, Terry, et al., 1994; Greenwood et al., 1987).

CWPT was employed as a logical mechanism for increasing students' opportunities to respond. In particular, the strategies developed were designed to be employed within larger, general education classes that contained students identified as LD or slow-learners. Typical classroom instruction provided by a teacher, even to a small group of students, involves asking a single question and calling upon a single student to respond. When a peer-tutoring procedure is employed, half the students in the class (assuming dyad tutoring) can respond in the same amount of time as a single student using teacher-oriented instruction. Elliott, Hughes, and Delquadri (cited in Delquadri et al., 1986) reported that some children improved their academic behavior from 20% to 70% as a result of peer-tutoring procedures.

Greenwood (1991) reported the long-term impact of time spent engaged in academic instruction across 416 first-grade students who were followed for 2 years. Complete data were collected on a total of 241 of these students at the end of the third grade. Students were divided into three groups: (1) an at-risk group of students with low socioeconomic status (SES) for whom teachers implemented a CWPT program from the second half of first grade through second grade; (2) an equivalent group of at-risk students for whom no peer tutoring was implemented; and (3) a nonrisk group of students from average- to high-SES backgrounds. Data collected on time spent in academic engaged time and scores on the Metropolitan Achievement Tests (MAT) favored the group receiving the CWPT program and the nonrisk group.

It is important to remember that the peer-tutoring procedures described by Greenwood and his associates involve same-age tutors and are classwide procedures. Other investigators have used cross-age (Beirne-Smith, 1991; Cochran, Feng, Cartledge, & Hamilton, 1993; Topping & Whiteley, 1993; Vaac & Cannon, 1991) and cross-ability (Allsopp, 1997; Arblaster, Butler, Taylor, Arnold, & Pitchford, 1991; Gilberts, Agran, Hughes, & Wehmeyer, 2001; Kamps et al., 1999) peer tutoring, all showing similar positive effects. Indeed, Rohrbeck, Ginsburg-Block, Fantuzzo, and Miller (2003) in a meta-analysis of peer-assisted learning procedures with elementary school students, reported effect sizes in achievement of 0.59, finding that these procedures were most effective with young, urban, low-income students from minority backgrounds. Although the procedures to be described here are those described by Greenwood and colleagues for same-age CWPT, these strategies are very similar for other types of peer-tutoring procedures.

Procedures for Classwide Peer Tutoring

The procedure for peer tutoring involves the use of (1) weekly competing teams; (2) tutor–tutee pairs within teams; (3) points earned for correct responding; (4) a modeling error-correction procedure; (5) teacher-mediated point earning for correct tutor behavior; (6) switching of tutor–tutee at midsession; (7) daily tabulation of point totals and public posting on a game chart; (8) selection of a winning team each day and each week; and (9) regular teacher assessments of students' academic performance, independent of tutoring sessions. For most subject areas, the tutoring sessions are divided into 30-minute blocks—10 minutes of tutoring for each student, and 5–10 minutes for adding scores and posting team outcomes. Additional information on the specifics of implementing a program in CWPT is available in a manual published by Sopris West (Greenwood, Delquadri, & Carta, 1997) and on the Classwide Peer Tutoring—Learning Management Systems (CWPT-LMS) website (*http://www.lsi.ku.edu/ jgprojects/cwptlms/html2002/index.htm*). Described below is a typical CWPT process, although modifications of the exact procedures are certainly made for individual classroom situations. Readers interested in pursuing the full implementation of CWPT should examine the CWPT-LMS (Greenwood et al., 2001; Greenwood, Hou, Delquadri, Terry, & Arreaga-Mayer, 2000), which represents the compilation of a system of peer tutoring that incorporates what is known to work best in classrooms, how CWPT can be applied schoolwide, how CWPT can be sustained over time, and how to use computer technology to enhance the outcomes of CWPT.

Each Monday, students are paired through a random selection process. Individual ability levels of students are not considered in the assignment of tutors. Children remain in the same tutor–tutee pairs for the entire week. Each pair of students is also assigned to one of two teams for the week.

When tutoring sessions begin, a timer is set for 10 minutes, and the tutee begins the assigned work. The specific academic skill assigned can be reading sentences aloud, reading words from a word list, spelling dictated words, completing assigned math problems, or any other academic task desired by the teacher. For example, in reading sentences, the tutee begins reading sentences aloud to the tutor. Tutors give 2 points for reading each sentence without errors. One point is earned for successfully correcting an error identified by the tutor. Tutors are instructed to correct errors by pronouncing the correct word or words and having the tutee reread the sentence until it is correct. In spelling, points are based on tutees' orally spelling each word and then writing the word three times, if not correct. Throughout the tutoring session, the teacher circulates around the room, providing assistance to tutors and tutees and awarding bonus points to pairs for cooperative tutoring. Tutees are also given bonus points for responding immediately when asked questions by the tutors.

After 10 minutes, tutors and tutees reverse roles, and the same procedures are followed. At the end of all tutoring sessions for that day, individual points are summed and reported aloud to the teacher. Individual points are recorded on a large chart in the front of the classroom, and team totals are determined. No rewards other than applause for winning efforts are provided to the teams.

On Fridays, the week's tutoring is assessed by the teacher. Each child is assessed using curriculum-based measures in the academic skills tutored that week. Students who continue to have difficulties with certain skills may then be directly instructed outside of tutoring sessions by the teacher.

Before students can begin the tutoring process, they must be trained. Training is conducted using explanation, modeling, role playing, and practice. During the first day of training, the teacher presents a brief overview of the tutoring program, demonstrates with a teacher aide or consultant how errors are to be corrected, how points are administered by tutors, and how they are recorded on student point sheets, and has students practice tabulating points and reporting these results to the teacher. In the second day of training, students actually practice tutoring, with feedback from the teacher and consultant regarding identifying errors, using the correction procedure, using praise, and tabulating points. If needed, a third day of practice is held for students to learn the tutoring process. Typically, students learn the procedures quickly and can begin tutoring after the first or second day. It may be necessary to continue to train younger students for a few more days, however.

The teacher's role during tutoring sessions involves initially determining dyads, timing the sessions, monitoring tutoring and awarding bonus points for correct tutoring, answering questions as needed, and tabulating and posting points. After each session, the teacher reviews point sheets to assess student accuracy and honesty in reporting and assesses academic progress using curriculum-based measures once each week, usually on Fridays.

Conclusions

Procedures for establishing peer tutoring are easy and can be applied to a wide range of academic areas. As demonstrated in the work of Greenwood and colleagues, it is not necessary to be concerned about matching students of differing ability levels. Indeed, some studies have demonstrated that peer tutoring may result in academic improvements in tutors as well as tutees (e.g., Cochran et al., 1993; Dineen, Clark, & Risley, 1977; Franca, Kerr, Reitz, & Lambert, 1990; Houghton & Bain, 1993). After all, one of the best ways to learn something is to try to teach it to someone else!

Beyond the work of Greenwood and colleagues, other investigations have demonstrated generalized effects of peer tutoring in mathematics (DuPaul & Henningson, 1993; Fantuzzo, King, & Heller, 1992; McKenzie & Budd, 1981), the acquisition of peer tutoring through observation of peer models (Stowitschek, Hecimovic, Stowitschek, & Shores, 1982), combining an in-school peer-tutoring procedure with a home-based reinforcement system (Trovato & Bucher, 1980), and using preschool- or kindergarten-age students as peer tutors (Eiserman, 1988; L. S. Fuchs, Fuchs, & Karns, 2001; L. S. Fuchs, Fuchs, Thompson, et al., 2001; Tabacek, McLaughlin, & Howard, 1994; Young, Hecimovic, & Salzberg, 1983). Scruggs, Mastropieri, Veit, and Osguthorpe (1986), Gumpel and Frank (1999), and Franca et al. (1990) examined the relationship of peer tutoring to social behaviors for students with behavior disorders. Johnson and Idol-Maestas (1986) showed that access to peer tutoring can serve as an effective contingent reinforcer. Fuchs and her colleagues (Fuchs, Fuchs, Phillips, et al., 1995; Phillips et al., 1993, 1994) have combined CWPT strategies with curriculum-based measurement as a method for individualizing student instruction. Their procedure, entitled Peer Assisted Learning Strategies (PALS), has been found to be successful at improving young students' skills in reading (Mathes, Grek, Howard, Babyak, & Allen, 1999), high school students' serious reading problems (L. S. Fuchs, Fuchs, & Kazdan, 1999), and mathematics skills of elementary-age students, with and without identified learning disabilities (L. S. Fuchs, Fuchs, Hamlett, Phillips, & Karns, 1995) as well as computation and concepts–applications among high school students with skills significantly below grade level (Calhoun & Fuchs, 2003). Clearly, there are substantial empirical and clinical reports for the effectiveness of peer tutoring to improve academic performance of students. More importantly, these studies have demonstrated that peer-tutoring procedures can be applied across all academic areas, with students of varied academic levels, and from elementary through high school.

Performance Feedback

A simple procedure that has been found to be effective in modifying a variety of academic behaviors is the provision of response-contingent feedback about performance. Van Houten and Lai Fatt (1981) examined the impact of public posting of weekly grades on biology tests with 12th-grade high school students. Results of the first experiment revealed that the effects of public posting plus immediate feedback and praise increased accuracy from 55.7% to 73.2% across the 47 students in the study. In a replication of the study, Van Houten and Lai Fatt showed that public posting alone with biweekly feedback increased student performance. These results were consistent with earlier studies examining the use of explicit timing and public posting in increasing mathematics and composition skills in regular elementary school students (Van Houten & Thompson, 1976; Van Houten et al., 1975). Kastelen, Nickel, and McLaughlin (1984) also showed that public posting of grades, immediate feedback, and praise improved the percentage of task completion in reading among 16 eighth-grade students. In addition, some generalization to spelling and writing tasks were evident.

In another study of public posting in the classroom, Bourque, Dupuis, and Van Houten (1986) compared the posting of student names versus coded numbers for weekly spelling test results in four third-grade classrooms. Results showed performance to be the same regardless of whether student names or codes were used. Other simple forms of public posting, such as placing pictures of students on a bulletin board as a reward for achieving significant improvement on weekly spelling tests, have been successful (Gross & Shapiro, 1981).

Systems for providing contingent feedback to students can be developed in many ways. Typically, a chart is created on which student progress is posted. These charts can vary from simple recording of test scores to some form of visual aid. For example, the use of bar graphs can be particularly helpful for students who have difficulty deciphering daily test scores. It is extremely important, however, that any public posting of scores be done in a positive, constructive manner. Van Houten and Van Houten (1977) described a system in which individual student accomplishments were compared to accomplishments of students as part of a team. Results of their study showed that although increases in performance were present under both conditions, significantly more improvement was present during the team phase.

Not surprisingly, the use of feedback systems and public posting of individual performance can result in significant improvement in academic skills. The procedure can be applied to many academic skills and across age and grade levels of students.

Direct Instruction

The term "direct instruction" has been applied in two related but different ways within the literature. Rosenshine (1979) has used the term "direct instruction" (not capitalized) to refer to instructional strategies that enhance a student's academic engaged time. Specifically, he considers techniques that result in frequent student responses, fast-paced instruction, teacher control of material, and other such methods designed to increase engaged time as indicative of direct instruction. No emphasis is given to the specific curriculum materials.

"Direct Instruction" (capitalized) is the instructional approach conceptualized by Englemann and his colleagues (e.g., Englemann & Carnine, 1982), and implemented and evaluated through Project Follow-Through in the late 1960s and 1970s. Although Direct Instruction includes all of the characteristics described by Rosenshine (1979), it also includes very specific curricular materials that contain explicit, systematic, step-by-step instructions for teaching.

The underlying principle in the Direct Instruction materials is that for *all* students to learn, materials and teacher presentation must be clear and unambiguous (Englemann, Becker, Carnine, & Gersten, 1988; Gersten, Woodward, & Darch, 1986). Although this sounds simple, many instructional programs, particularly basal reading materials, have not been designed with sufficient precision to allow students with mild handicaps to succeed. Direct Instruction curricula have been developed so that students initially acquiring a skill are presented with questions for which there can only be one, correct response. In addition, materials are generated that offer simple but elegant strategies for application (Gersten et al., 1986). For example, after students are taught to discriminate short and long vowel sounds of three vowels (O, A, I), they are taught a rule: "If the last letter is E, you'll hear a letter *name* in the word. You'll hear the name of the letter that is underlined." Practice using the rule is then implemented, with students constantly being asked to recite the rule as the skill is mastered.

Development of the Direct Instruction model was based on two guiding principles: "Teach more in less time" and "Control the details of what happens" (Becker & Carnine, 1981). All instructional activities are designed to increase academic engaged time and to focus on teaching the general case. For example, rather than teaching single sounds sequentially through the curriculum, 40 different sounds may be taught, with rules provided for linking them together. In this way, general decoding skills can be taught quickly and efficiently. To control the instructional environment, all lessons are scripted for the teacher. What the teacher is to say and do is written out within the teaching manuals. Student progress is monitored using criterion-referenced progress tests, and the methods for obtaining these data are explicitly described in the manuals.

The teaching techniques of the Direct Instruction model vary according to the skill levels of the students (Becker & Carnine, 1981). Whereas initial acquisition of skills in reading relies heavily on small-group instruction and unison responding, later skills are taught through more independent and large-group instruction. In addition, less reliance on unison responding occurs in later grades. Feedback mechanisms also change across grades, with children in the early grades receiving immediate feedback and older children getting delayed feedback. The overriding emphasis in the model is on mastery instruction. Students being instructed in small groups are not advanced until *all* students in the group achieve mastery on the skill being taught. For example, Stein and Goldman (1980) compared performance of students with LD (ages 6–8) being instructed in either the Direct Instruction (DISTAR) reading curriculum or the Palo Alto series. Although the two series are very similar in content, a critical difference in teaching strategy is the insistence of the DISTAR curriculum that each student in the group master the skills at one level before proceeding to the next. By contrast, the Palo Alto curriculum allows teachers to proceed when most students have acquired the instructed skill. Results of their study showed that the mean gain for DISTAR was 15 months (over the 9 month period) compared to a gain of 7 months for the Palo Alto curriculum.

The Direct Instruction model contains at least seven basic principles for teaching strategies. Each of these is presented briefly. Readers interested in more detailed descriptions should see Englemann and Carnine (1982).

Scripted Presentations

Each lesson is scripted for the teacher. The exact words to be used in presenting materials, along with appropriate sequencing of teacher questions and responses to student performance, are offered. Becker and Carnine (1981) stated that this feature of the model is frequently criticized; critics object that scripted lessons may stifle teacher creativity and initiative. The authors point out, however, that the use of scripts allows teachers to use a pretested strategy with proven effectiveness. Scripts also reduce the time needed for teachers to prepare lessons. Furthermore, scripted lessons make the monitoring of student performance easier, since lessons are standardized.

Small-Group Instruction

Much of the teaching in the model, particularly at the earlier grades, is done in small groups. This structure permits frequent student responses, more direct adult contact, teacher-controlled instruction, and opportunities for modeling by other students. These groups often consist of 5–10 students and occur throughout the instructional day. In upper grades, reliance on small groups is reduced, and increased large-group and independent instruction are employed.

Unison Responding

During the small-group instruction, students are frequently asked to respond in unison. This creates an atmosphere of fast paced, high intensity, and active participation.

Signals

Another important component of the Direct Instruction model is the use of signals within the instructional process. Signals are used throughout a lesson to help pace students as to when responses should be given. For example, in sounding out a word, students may be told to say a sound aloud as long as a teacher touches a signal for that sound. This procedure ensures that students blend correctly as the teacher moves from sound to sound across the word. Effective use of signals can also provide opportunities to allow students who need a few extra seconds to formulate a response that is not dominated by the more able students in a group.

Pacing

Through the use of signals, unison responding, and small-group instruction, the pacing of instruction is clearly controlled. Becker and Carnine (1981) point out that students are likely to be more attentive to fast-paced presentation. However, the use of a fast-paced instructional strategy does not mean that teachers rush students into giving responses when more time is needed to formulate answers. Carnine (1976), in some early research on Direct Instruction, demonstrated that students answer correctly about 80% of the time when in a fast-paced condition (12 questions per minute) but answer correctly only 30% of the time in a slow-rate condition (5 questions per minute).

Corrections

Correcting errors is an important part of the process of Direct Instruction. Research on correcting errors, although limited, suggests that students need to attend to the feedback and rehearse the corrected strategies for the results of error correction to be effective (Fink & Carnine, 1975). In addition, modeling of correct responses can be effective, but the correction needs to be applied in subsequent situations (Stromer, 1975).

Praise

Not surprisingly, the use of praise within the small-group, fast-paced instructional sessions is a critical component of the Direct Instruction model. The relationship of teacher attention to increasing student attentiveness is well documented (e.g., Cossairt, Hall, & Hopkins, 1973; Hall, Lund, & Jackson, 1968). It is interesting to note, however, that the role of praise alone within the Direct Instruction model has not been investigated (Becker & Carnine, 1981).

Summary of Direct Instruction

The Direct Instruction model was one of the major models of compensatory education evaluated through Project Follow-Through in the 1970s. Although the evaluation conducted by the Abt Associates (1976, 1977) has been questioned in regard to the fairness of the measures employed, the adequacy of the sample, and the appropriateness of the analysis, the evaluation did provide direct comparisons of eight different models of compensatory education. Each model was based on a different instructional philosophy; their emphases included child self-esteem, child language development, parent education, child cognitive development, behavior analysis, and direct instruction. Comparisons were made using measures of basic skills (word knowledge, spelling, language, math computation), cognitive and conceptual skills (reading, math concepts, math problem solving, Raven's Progressive Matrices), and affective measures (the Coopersmith Self-Esteem Inventory and Intellectual Achievement Responsibility Scale). These measures were combined into a measure entitled the Index of Significant Outcomes (ISO).

Results of the Abt report are clear. Examination of overall ISO scores found that the Direct Instruction model ranked first across cognitive, affective, and basic skills measures. Moreover, in none of the subareas examined did it rank less than third (Becker & Carnine, 1981). The Abt report also compared the models on four subtests of the MAT: Total Reading, Total Math, Spelling, and Language. In all areas, the Direct Instruction model far outscored all other models, with scores across the four basic skills areas ranging from the 40th percentile in Reading to the 50th percentile in Spelling and Language. Total Math scores fell into the 48th percentile.

Data obtained by Becker and Englemann (1978) at the Direct Instruction sites provide even stronger evidence of the success of the model. Scores obtained on the Wide Range Achievement Test (WRAT), given at the prekindergarten and third-grade periods, found students at or above the 50th percentile on the Reading, Arithmetic, and Spelling subtests. In further follow-up data, Becker and Gersten (1982) reported WRAT and MAT scores for all students who had been in the 3-year Direct Instruction sites and were now in the fifth and sixth grades. Results showed that students who attended the Project Follow-Through programs outperformed a matched group of students who did not. These effects were particularly strong in reading, math problem solving, and spelling. Effects on the MAT Science, Math Concepts, Math Computation, and Word Knowledge subtests were somewhat less. In no case, however, did any comparison favor the control group. One finding of the follow-up study, however, was that, compared to a national norm sample, these children began to lose ground after Project Follow-Through ended. This suggests that without continued instruction using similar strategies, children are unlikely to compete effectively against their peers.

Gersten, Keating, and Becker (1988) presented the results of two long-term studies of the Direct Instruction model. Academic achievement scores of 1,097 students in the fifth and sixth grade who had received direct instruction in grades 1–3 were compared against 970 students who had received traditional education. The second study followed students through high school who had received or not received Direct Instruction. Outcomes from these studies showed that the fifth- and sixth-grade students performed better on standardized achievement tests in reading, spelling, and mathematics. Students from the second study followed up at high school performed better in reading and math, had been retained in grades fewer times, and had a higher rate of college acceptance than the comparison groups.

The results of the Abt studies and the strong showing of Direct Instruction should not be surprising. Indeed, significant research since Project Follow-Through has continued to demonstrate the superiority of Direct Instruction to other strategies for teaching basic skills to learners with mild handicaps (Gersten et al., 1986; White, 1988). Furthermore, the research on academic engaged time (Greenwood, 1991; Rosenshine, 1981;

Rosenshine & Berliner, 1978), opportunities to respond (Greenwood et al., 1985), and other time variables related to educational gains (Gettinger, 1984; Rich & Ross, 1989) has clearly demonstrated that educational processes resulting in increased student engaged time will result in increased student performance.

Perhaps the greatest criticisms of the Direct Instruction model comes from those who feel that the method results in stifled creativity and failure to consider individual differences in learning. Although these criticisms may be justified when considering the instructional process for high-achieving students, they seem inappropriate if aimed at students with handicaps or low achievement. These individuals most often are the focus of remedial programs and would therefore benefit most from Direct Instruction approaches.

Future research issues related to Direct Instruction do not need to center upon demonstrations of its effectiveness. These data exist and are convincing. More importantly, efforts need to be devoted to examining how these strategies can be more widely adopted into the educational system for students with handicaps. It is unfortunate that the technology and resources that exist for accelerating the performance of low-achieving youngsters apparently continue to go untapped.

Cooperative Learning and Group Contingencies

Traditional goals in classrooms implicitly assume competition rather than cooperation. Students are compared to each other; this results in discouraging student–student interaction, which might improve performance (Johnson & Johnson, 1985), and it clearly places low achievers at a disadvantage (Slavin, 1977). Several researchers have described and field-tested successful strategies for improving academic skills that are based on principles of cooperation rather than competition (Johnson & Johnson, 1985, 1986; Slavin, 1983a, 1983b).

Several reviews have been published substantiating the effectiveness of cooperative learning strategies (e.g., Axelrod & Greer, 1994; Cosden & Haring, 1992; Johnson, Maruyama, Johnson, Nelson, & Skon, 1981; Maheady, Harper, Mallette, & Winstanley, 1991; Nastasi & Clements, 1991; Slavin, 1980, 1983a). These procedures have been applied across all academic subjects, have occurred in both the United States and other countries, and have incorporated both individual and group reward systems. Of the 27 studies reported by Slavin (1980), 24 (89%) showed significant positive effects on achievement when rewards were based on individual performance of group members, in comparison with control groups. Indeed, typical educational lessons at all levels of instruction consider cooperative learning techniques to be a routine, expected part of the learning process.

Within cooperative learning strategies, group contingencies play a significant part (Slavin, 1991). Litow and Pumroy (1975) identified three types of group contingencies: (1) dependent, in which the group's attainment of a reward requires that the performances of a target student or students meet a specified criterion; (2) interdependent, in which the group's attainment of a reward requires that every member of the group meet a specified criterion or, alternatively, that the group's average performance exceed the criterion; and (3) independent, in which each member of the group's attainment of the reward requires that his or her own performance meet the specified criterion. Several studies have used these contingencies for managing academic skills (Chadwick & Day, 1971; Evans & Oswalt, 1968; Fantuzzo, Polite, & Grayson, 1990; Goldberg, 1998; Goldberg & Shapiro, 1995; McLaughlin, 1981; Shapiro & Goldberg, 1986, 1990; Turco & Elliott, 1990).

Procedures for Cooperative Learning

Although cooperative learning can be applied in several ways, Slavin, Madden, and Leavey (1984) provide an excellent example. Team-assisted individualization (TAI) consists of several procedures designed to combine cooperative learning strategies and individualized instruction. Students are first assigned to four- or five-member teams. Each team is constructed such that the range of abilities in that skill is represented across team members.

After team assignment, students are pretested on mathematics operations and are placed at the appropriate level of the curriculum, based on their performance. Students then work on their assignments within the team by first forming pairs or triads. After exchanging answer sheets with their partners, students read the instructions for their individualized assignments and begin working on the first skill sheet. After working four problems, students exchange sheets and check their answers. If these are correct, students move to the next skill sheet. If incorrect, the students continue in blocks of four problems on the same skill sheet.

When a student has four in a row correct on the final skill sheet, the first "checkout," a 10-item quiz, is taken. If the student scores at least 8 correct out of 10, the checkout is signed by the teammate, and the student is certified to take the final test. If the student does not score 80%, the teacher is called to assist the student with any problems not understood; a second checkout is taken, and if the criterion is met, the student is again certified to take the final test.

At the end of the week, team scores are computed by averaging all tests taken by team members. If the team reached the preset criterion, all team members receive certificates. Each day, teachers work with students who were at the same point in the curriculum for 5–15 minutes. This provides opportunities for teachers to give instruction on any items that students may find difficult.

Conclusions and Summary

Cooperative learning and group contingencies have a significant logical appeal. Concerns are often raised about mainstreamed students and their social acceptance by peers; greater social acceptance of such students may result from placing them in close, cooperative contact with other students. In addition, the strategies appear to be consistent with other approaches such as peer tutoring, which are based on increasing student engagement rates in classrooms.

Despite these very positive aspects of cooperative learning strategies, there appear to be a number of potential problems in using these procedures. We (Elliott & Shapiro, 1990) noted that in cooperative strategies in which interdependent or dependent group contingencies are employed, low-achieving members of a group may be criticized by high-achieving members. In addition, some strategies (not Slavin's) deemphasize the individualization of instruction. This would be a significant problem for students with handicaps.

Although some questions can be raised about cooperative learning strategies, the procedures clearly have documented effectiveness and acceptability (e.g., Elliott, Turco, & Gresham, 1987; Goldberg, 1998; Goldberg & Shapiro, 1995; Shapiro & Goldberg, 1986, 1990; Turco & Elliott, 1990). These procedures, again, can be employed as classwide techniques, not specifically aimed at students with academic deficiencies. As such, they become excellent preventive recommendations for students who remain in regular education classes.

SUMMARY

The many and varied strategies discussed in this chapter represent intervention techniques that can be broadly applied across types of academic problems, age ranges, handicapping conditions, and school settings. An extensive database supporting each of the strategies exists, along with significant evidence of field testing. Practitioners with limited experience in using these procedures are strongly encouraged to seek out detailed descriptions of the methods and to experiment with them in their own settings. Although some adaptations of procedures may be needed for specific settings, most techniques can be easily implemented, with few modifications. Furthermore, much of the literature cited in this chapter contains descriptions of methods that can be read, understood, and directly implemented.

CHAPTER 6

♦♦♦

Step 3:
Instructional Modification II
Specific Skills Areas

♦

Literally hundreds of intervention procedures have been reported in the literature as successful techniques to improve performance in the basic skills of reading, math, spelling, and written language. In addition, a large number of interventions have appeared in the literature designed to improve skills in content areas (e.g., biology, history) and more complex forms of skills, such as critical thinking or creative writing. Any attempt to provide a comprehensive review of these procedures in any single source would be impossible. This chapter presents a variety of strategies for each academic area that are known to address the key components of developing competence. Those that have repeatedly appeared in the literature in different forms are given the most attention. The choice of particular strategies is partially based on my own experience of success across a wide age range of students and types of academic problems. Readers are directed to several excellent resources that provide somewhat more in-depth analyses of many of the procedures discussed (e.g., Elliott, DiPerna, & Shapiro, 2001; Howell & Nolet, 1999; Kame'enui, Carnine, Dixon, Simmons, & Coyne, 2002; Mayer, 2002; Rathvon, 1999; Shinn, Walker, & Stoner, 2002).

READING

Probably the most frequently encountered academic difficulties are related to reading and language arts. Indeed, the report of the National Reading Panel (2000) found that over 17.5% of the nation's schoolchildren will encounter reading problems within their first 3 years of school. This amounts to over 10 million children nationwide. Approximately 75% identified as having reading problems by third grade are found to be struggling in reading at ninth grade (Francis, Shaywitz, Stuebing, Shaywitz, & Fletcher, 1996; Shaywitz, Escobar, Fletcher, & Makuch, 1992). These facts are not surprising given the complexity of skills needed to master reading. A student must understand rules of phonetic analysis, be capable of effective integration of sounds, be fluent enough to derive meaning from the material, and perform these skills at an automatic level. Breakdowns at any single level of skill may have "ripple effects" on the acquisition of subsequent skills. In addition, after learning all the rules for effective decoding, students using the English language must then learn all the exceptions. It is no wonder that reading remains the most difficult academic skill to master.

The development of competence in reading starts with the development of prereading skills, which are the foundations for subsequent skill development. Assuming these prereading skills develop adequately, reading performance then must include the development of fluency, vocabulary, and comprehension. Having become fluent readers, children must then learn to use these skills in reading material in content areas such as history, geography, science, and other subjects. These skills are interrelated, with the development of some skills (e.g., fluency and vocabulary) serving as necessary but not sufficient developers of other skills (e.g., comprehension).

At the prereading level, phonemic awareness and understanding the alphabetic principle are key building blocks for the development of reading. Indeed, Kame'enui et al. (1997) noted that the relationship between the development of phonemic awareness and acquisition of reading is one of the most well-documented findings in the literature. Phonemic awareness is the ability to hear and manipulate the sounds in spoken words. Understanding that syllables are made of these sequences of sounds is essential to establishing phonemic awareness (Yopp, 1992). The skill is critical, since letters represent sounds in a writing system, and without the ability to translate these letters to sounds, reading makes little sense. If a child cannot effectively hear that *bank* and *baby* begin with the same sounds, or effectively blend individual sounds together such as /cccccccaaaaaaaatttttt/ to make the word *cat,* the development of reading competence is unlikely to ever occur.

The alphabetic principle, working with print, is the ability to associate sounds with letters and use these sounds to form words. The principle consists of two components. First, alphabetic understanding develops the concepts that words consist of letters, and letters represent specific sounds. Second, phonological recoding is the ability to use relationships between letters and sounds to translate the sounds into meaningful words. Many subskills embedded in the alphabetic principle include but are not limited to developing an understanding of decoding, sight-word reading, sounding out words, word analysis, and recognizing word patterns (Texas Center for Reading and Language Arts, 1998).

Assuming that students have the necessary prereading skills, such as letter recognition, letter–sound association, and basic phonemic analysis skills, effective interventions for reading problems must concentrate on the acquisition of three related skills: reading fluency, vocabulary building, and comprehension. Although these skills are closely interrelated, acquiring fluency alone does not always improve comprehension. We have all come across students who have mastered reading fluently but cannot meaningfully synthesize what they have read (i.e., "word callers"). Although there is always some question whether such students can be effectively identified by teachers (Hamilton & Shinn, 2003), there certainly appear to be students who meet the definition of word callers. Students who have still not mastered the prerequisite skills of letter identification, sound–symbol association, and basic phonemic analysis need interventions aimed at teaching these essential reading skills.

Each of the five areas of developing reading skills has an extensive literature documenting interventions. Attempts to present all of these interventions are well beyond the scope of this volume. In the next section, I present intervention strategies that are representative of the many strategies available to address the skills area presented. It is important to remember that these skills must be explicitly taught. Skills development requires directly teaching each skill and recognizing that some of the skills serve as prerequisites to the development of subsequent skills. Readers are urged to seek out specific references and sources that can offer a fuller array of strategies in each of the areas. A particular website that offers a superb overview and references for teaching reading, particularly for the development of early literacy skills, can be found at the Institute for the Development of Educational Achievement (*http://reading.uoregon.edu*).

Phonemic Awareness and Alphabetic Principle

The ability to recognize and manipulate spoken sounds is a critical feature of developing phonemic awareness. For example, the word *sun* has three phonemes: /s/u/n/. In teaching phonemic awareness, children first need to learn sounds in isolation (i.e., *sun* begins with the sound "ssssssss"). They then must learn to blend these sounds together: /sss/–/uuu/–/nnn/ = *sun*. Finally, they must be able to segment the sounds, such as recognizing that the word *sun* consists of three sounds: /sss/–/uuu/–/nnn/.

Phonemic awareness is taught and developed in a progression from less to more complex skills. At the least complex level are skills such as teaching children to compare words and rhyme, moving to sentence segmentation, syllable segmentation, and blending, onset-rime blending and segmentation, and finally blending and segmenting individual phonemes, along with phoneme deletion and manipulation. Table 6.1 shows examples of the types of skills at each of these steps of developing phonemic awareness. Normally taught in kindergarten and first grades, these skills are taught in a specific instructional sequence using scaffolded instruction, where each step of the process builds on the preceding step, gradually removing the supporting elements, while maintaining student performance over time. For example, Figure 6.1 shows a curriculum map for teaching phonemic awareness in kindergarten students. Each skill is identified, along with the months of the school year when these skills are expected to be mastered.

There are many curricula available for effectively teaching phonemic awareness, and many use teacher-made materials. Smith, Simmons, and Kame'enui (1998) identified eight critical features of materials used for teaching phonemic awareness. First, as noted previously, one progresses from easier to more complex and difficult skills. Second, the focus is on the

TABLE 6.1. Descriptions of Skills for Developing and Teaching Phonemic Awareness

Skill	Description
Sound and word discrimination	What word doesn't belong with the others? *hit, mit, bit, sit, ran?*
Rhyming	What word rhymes with *sun*? **fun**
Syllable splitting	The onset of *hat* is /h/; the rime is /at/.
Blending	What word is made up of the sounds /h/ /a/ /t/? **hat**
Phonemic segmentation	What are the sounds in *hit*? **/h/ /i/ /t/**
Phoneme deletion	What is *hit* without the /h/? **it**
Phoneme manipulation	What word would you have if you changed the /h/ in hit to an /s/? **sit**

Note. Adapted from *Phonemic Awareness in Beginning Reading,* website at Institute for the Development of Educational Achievement, University of Oregon (*http://reading.uoregon.edu*). Copyright 2002–2003. Adapted by permission.

Mapping of Instruction to Achieve Instructional Priorities
Kindergarten

Instructional Priority: **Phonemic Awareness**	1	2	3	4	5	6	7	8	9
Focus 1: Sound and Word Discrimination									
1a: Tells whether words and sounds are the same or different	×	×							
1b: Identifies which word is different		×	×						
1c: Identifies different speech sound			×	×					
Focus 2: Rhyming[b]									
2a: Identifies whether words rhyme	×								
2b: Produces a word that rhymes		×	×						
Focus 3: Blending									
3a: Orally blends syllables or onset-rimes			×	×					
3b: Orally blends spearate phonemes					×	×	×		
Focus 4: Segmentation									
4a: Claps words in sentences	×								
4b: Claps syllables in words		×	×						
4c: Says syllables				×	×				
*4d: Identifies first sound in 1-syllable words		×	×	×	25				
*4e: Segments individual sounds in words					×	×	×	×	35[a]

*High-priority skill
[a]Sounds per minute
[b]Optimal time for rhyme instruction not established

FIGURE 6.1. Curriculum map for teaching phonemic awareness in kindergarten. From "Teaching Phonemic Awareness: Sequencing Phonemic Awareness Skills," website at Institute for the Development of Educational Achievement, University of Oregon (*http://reading.uoregon.edu*). Copyright 2002–2003. Reprinted by permission.

combination of blending and segmenting. Third, instruction starts with larger linguistic units, such as words and syllables, and progresses toward smaller units, such as phonemes. Fourth, instruction begins with short phonological units, such as the words *at, bit,* or *run*. Fifth, students are taught beginning (*sat*), ending (*sat*), and then medial (*sat*) sounds in words. Sixth, continuous sounds such as *m, s,* or *r,* are introduced before the stop sounds, such as *t, b,* or *d*. Seventh, once children demonstrate early phonemic awareness, instruction in letter–sound correspondence should be added to phonological awareness interventions. Finally, instruction in phonemic awareness needs to be done in short sessions of only 15–20 minutes repeated daily over 9–12 weeks.

Although materials can be teacher-made, commercially available curricula that accomplish the objectives of developing phonemic awareness and have research in support of their effectiveness include Phonological Awareness Training for Reading (Torgesen & Bryant, 1994), Phonemic Awareness in Young Children (Adams, Foorman, Lundberg, & Beeler, 1998), Ladders to Literacy (O'Connor, Notari-Syverson, & Vadasy, 1996), Road to the Code (Blachman, Ball, Black, & Tangei, 1999), and Project OPTIMIZE (Simmons & Kame'enui, 1999). The Institute for the Development of Educational Achievement offers superb recommendations for selection criteria in identifying effective curricular programs for developing early literacy skills (*http://reading.uoregon.edu*).

Beyond acquiring phonemic awareness, children need to understand the principle that words are composed of letters, and that these letters represent sounds. They also need to be able to recode letters and sounds, and to manipulate these sounds. Moats (1999) noted that the critical skill to be learned is decoding. Good readers must be able to effectively decode given that our language is far too complex to rely primarily on word identification or other memory strategies alone. In addition, there is a very strong relationship between effective decoding and the comprehension of written material. Foorman, Francis, Fletcher, and Lynn (1996) found the correlation between decoding and comprehension across grades to be consistently at 0.60 and higher.

Teaching the alphabetic principle begins in kindergarten. Students must learn to blend sounds together to form words, as well as take words apart to identify their individual sounds. The skill must be taught explicitly, while linking the learning of the skill to everyday reading experiences. Three explicit skills that need to be taught are letter–sound correspondence, sounding out words, and reading connected text. In teaching all skills, teachers need to design instruction that includes conspicuous strategies, mediated scaffolding, and strategic instruction. Figure 6.2 provides an illustration of the instructional design considerations when teaching letter-sound correspondence, the first of these skills.

When teaching students to sound out words, it is important to move through specific steps as students learn the skill. Beginning with producing sounds in words, students must learn to blend these sounds together to make whole words, and then produce the blended sounds to complete words. Teaching of the skill must carefully control for the types of letter sounds that are taught as well as the complexity of the words used. For example, one starts with the simplest vowel–consonant (VC) or consonant–vowel–consonant (CVC) letter combinations and progresses toward longer words (four- or five-phoneme words). One does not progress to teaching consonant blends until CVC and VC combinations are mastered. The words used in instruction are those with which students are familiar, pro-

Conspicuous strategies

- Teacher actions should make the task explicit. Use consistent and brief wording.

Mediated scaffolding

- Separate auditorily and visually similar letters.
- Introduce some continuous sounds early.
- Introduce letters that can be used to build many words.
- Introduce lowercase letters first unless uppercase letters are similar in configuration.

Strategic integration—simple before complex

1. Once students can identify the sound of the letter on two successive trials, include the new letter–sound correspondence with 6–8 other letter sounds.
2. When students can identify 4–6 letter–sound correspondences in 2 seconds each, include these letters in single-syllable, CVC, decodable words.

Review cumulatively and judiciously

Use a distributed review cycle to build retention:

NKNKKNNKKKKN

N = new sound; K = known sound

Example (r = new sound; m, s, t, i, f, a = known sounds): r m r s t r r i f a m r

FIGURE 6.2. Instructional design for teaching letter–sound correspondence. Adapted from "Teaching the Alphabetic Principle: Critical Alphabetic Principle Skills," website at Institute for the Development of Educational Achievement, University of Oregon (*http://reading.uoregon.edu*). Copyright 2002–2003. Reprinted by permission.

gressing toward those with which students have less familiarity. Instruction progresses students from simply sounding out words to saying whole words to sounding words out in their heads. Throughout the process, students are constantly practicing previously learned skills.

The teaching of reading connected text emerges as the third skill in the sequence of teaching the alphabetic principle. One should not assume that learning letter–sound correspondence or sounding out words will automatically transfer to reading connected text. Once students have shown that they can decode CVC or VC combinations, words made up of these combinations should be introduced in short, controlled passages. The teaching of reading connected text starts with teacher prompts to have students "figure out the word by saying the sounds to themselves." Once students have consistently accomplished this task, prompting to figure out sounds is eliminated. Finally, the pace of reading is gradually increased, giving students less time to decode words as they read.

When first introducing connected text, it is important that students are given passages in which they can read most of the words at a rate of at least one word every 3 seconds. Repeated opportunities with short sessions are required for students to constantly practice and gain fluency. Words are taught first from word lists, before they are introduced into the passages. Both sounding out and sight recognition skills are used as the student reads.

Teaching of the alphabetic principle, which occurs throughout grades K–3, requires careful sequencing of the varying skills. Using a curriculum map, teachers can carefully control the pace of instruction and through scaffolded instruction, build student skills toward attaining the foundational skills needed for becoming competent readers. Figure 6.3 shows an

Mapping of Instruction to Achieve Instructional Priorities
Second Grade

Instructional Priority: **Alphabetic Principle**	1	2	3	4	5	6	7	8	9
Focus 1: Letter–Sound Knowledge									
*1a: Produces dipthongs and digraphs	×	×							
Focus 2: Decoding and Word Recognition									
*2a: Identifies whether words rhyme	×	×	×	×					
2b: Reads compound words, contractions, possessives, inflectional endings			×	×	×	×			
2c: Reads multisyllablic words					×	×	×		
Focus 3: Sight-Word Reading									
*3a: Reads more sight words accurately	×	×	×	×	×	×	×	×	×
Focus 4: Reading Connected Text									
4a: Reads 90–100 wpm	40–60	×	×	×	×	×	×	×	90–100
4b: Reads with phrasing and expression			×	×	×				
4c: Listens to fluent oral reading and practices increasing oral reading fluency	10[a]	10	10	15	15	20	20	20	20
4d: Reads and rereads to increase familiarity	×	×	×	×	×	×	×	×	×
4e: Self-corrects word recognition errors	×	×							

*High-priority skill
[a]Minutes of practice per day

FIGURE 6.3. Curriculum map for teaching the alphabetic principle to second-grade students. Adapted from "Teaching the Alphabetic Principle: Sequencing Alphabetic Principle Skills," website at Institute for the Development of Educational Achievement, University of Oregon (*http://reading.uoregon.edu*). Copyright 2002–2003. Reprinted by permission.

illustration of a curriculum map for second grade in teaching the alphabetic principle.

Reading Fluency and Building Vocabulary

Children who do not read with sufficient fluency almost inevitably have severe comprehension problems, typically related to the inability to decode words quickly and automatically. Dysfluent readers will spend significant amounts of time struggling through text, only to discover at the end of the passage that they cannot remember a thing they have read.

Achieving success in fluency requires that students have repeated opportunities to practice while receiving corrective feedback. Practice sessions should be brief (15–20 minutes) but occur often within and across instructional days. Such practice should extend from school to home and represent an important component of teaching the reading process. By the end of second grade, students should be able to read connected text at levels of 90–100 words correct per minute. This includes learning to read both irregular and regular words fluently.

Among the procedures that appear to have substantial support for improving the oral reading fluency of students is *previewing,* defined by Rose (1984) as any method that provides the opportunity for a learner to read or listen to a passage prior to instruction and/or testing. Three types of previewing procedures have been identified: (1) oral previewing, or having the learner read the assigned selection aloud prior to the reading lesson; (2) silent previewing, or having the learner read the passage to him- or herself prior to the lesson; and (3) listening previewing, in which the teacher reads the assigned passage aloud and the learner follows silently (Hansen & Eaton, 1978).

The previewing procedures are really quite simple. Materials for instruction and data collection are typically selected from the student's present curriculum. Silent previewing involves asking the student to read the assigned passage silently and then aloud to the teacher. In listening previewing, students are asked to follow along as the teacher reads the passage. Students then read the passage aloud to the teacher. This type of previewing can also be done by tape-recording the passages ahead of time (Rose & Beattie, 1986). Oral previewing requires a student to read the passage aloud once before instruction, and then again after instruction.

Many researchers have found previewing to be a powerful strategy for improving reading skills. For example, Rousseau, Tam, and Ramnarain (1993) compared the use of presenting key words and previewing to improve the reading comprehension of five Hispanic, 11- and 12-year-old students. Using an alternating treatments design, the key word, listening previewing alone, and the combined interventions were compared. They found that the key word technique resulted in higher oral reading rates and reading comprehension scores than previewing alone, but that the combination of key word presentation and listening previewing had the best performance. O'Donnell, Weber, and McLaughlin (2003) reported that having a student discuss key words and listen to a passage prior to reading significantly increased the student's rate of reading fluency, as well as his/her comprehension of the passage. Skinner, Cooper, and Cole (1997) compared rapid and slow oral previewing procedures, and found that students read best when the adult previewing the material reduced his/her rate of reading. Skinner, Bamberg, et al. (1993), in comparing the effects of three different forms of previewing on the oral reading rates of 12 junior and senior high school students with LD found that significantly fewer errors were made under slow—compared to fast—rate previewing. Tingstrom et al. (1995) found that inclusion of listening previewing as a component in a repeated reading technique resulted in higher reading fluency rates for some students.

Another procedure for improving reading fluency has been described by Freeman and McLaughlin (1984). Students are asked to read aloud a word list simultaneously with a tape recording of the word list being read at a significantly higher reading rate. The idea behind the procedure is for students to model higher reading rates. This procedure is felt to be especially valuable in working with secondary-age students, who may fail to acquire fluency when reading in content areas, because they lack the necessary sight vocabulary.

In the Freeman and McLaughlin (1984) procedure, all students reading below 50 words correct per minute (WCPM) were asked to read aloud with a tape that presented the word lists at 80 WCPM. After reading the words with the tape recorder, students were then assessed on the same list. Results of the study were impressive, with all students showing substantial gains in oral reading rates on the word lists after the intervention was begun.

One of the most critical findings of the research on previewing and the taped-word procedure is the relationship of increased practice and opportunities to respond on fluency. For example, Hargis, Terhaar-Yonker, Williams, and Reed (1988) determined that students with mild handicaps need an average of 46 repetitions for a word to reach a level of automatic recognition. Two related techniques that have been developed are especially aimed at improving reading fluency through drill and practice: "folding-in" (also known as "incremental rehearsal"; Tucker, 1989) and the "drill sandwich." Full and detailed descriptions of the folding-in technique can be found in the workbook accompanying this text.

The folding-in technique is based on two well-established principles of learning: arranging an instructional match and providing for enough repetitions for material to move from unknown status to mastery. The instructional match, or instructional level, is the optimal condition under which a student will learn. When being taught at the instructional level, the student is sufficiently challenged, with a realistic opportunity for success. If the level of material becomes too difficult (frustrational), the student is likely to fail, and learning will be minimal. Likewise, if the material is too easy, the lack of challenge will result in little gain over current functioning. Gickling and Havertape (1981) and Gickling and Rosenfield (1995) identified the ratio of known to unknown information that must be established to teach students at their instructional level. Table 6.2 displays the instructional levels for reading comprehension and other practice-related activities.

As a drill procedure, the folding-in technique is based on having students learn new words by never allowing more than 15–30% of the material presented to be unknown. Here are the steps in using the technique:

1. Select a passage that the evaluator wishes to have the student read. The passage should be one that the student is currently working on in class. It is important that the passage contain no more than 50% unknown material.

2. Have the student read a portion of the passage (usually a paragraph or two) aloud and time the reading. Mark where the student was in the passage at the end of 1 minute. The number of words read correctly in this minute is designated as the presession reading fluency.

3. As the student reads, note at least three words that the student has difficulty with or does not seem to understand. On 3″ × 5″ index cards, write the two words. These words are designated as "unknowns."

4. On 3″ × 5″ index cards, select seven words from the passage that the student does seem to know. These should be words that are meaningful to the passage, not simply sight words such as *and, the,* or other non-meaningful expressions.

5. Begin the session by presenting the first unknown word. The evaluator should define the word for the student and use it in a sentence. Next, the evaluator should ask the student to repeat the definition and use it in a different sentence.

TABLE 6.2. Instructional Levels as Defined by Gickling's Model for CBA

Reading	Practice
93–97% known material	70–85% known material
3–7% unknown material	15–30% unknown material

6. Now the folding-in begins. After the unknown word is presented, one of the known words is presented. The student is asked to say the word aloud. Next, the unknown word is again presented, followed by the known word previously presented, and then a new known word. This sequence of presentation, unknown followed by knowns, is continued until all seven knowns and the one unknown word have been presented.

Next, the second unknown word is presented in the same way as the first, with its definition given and its use in a sentence, first by the evaluator and then by the student. This second unknown word is then folded-in among the other seven known words and one unknown word. In the course of the multiple presentations of the words, the student is asked to repeat the unknown word's definition and to use it in a sentence whenever he or she hesitates or incorrectly pronounces the word. Finally, the third unknown is folded-in among the other nine words (two unknown, seven known). Given that the other words were assessed as being known at the starting point, the student should not have any difficulty with these words.

7. Upon completion of the folding-in intervention, the student is asked to reread the passage. The evaluator again marks the word the student was reading at 1 minute. It is important that the student read only to the same point of the passage that he or she read to at the beginning of the session. The number of words read correctly in 1 minute is considered the student's postsession reading score.

8. Both the pre- and postsession scores are graphed (usually by the student).

9. The teacher begins the next session by having the student read the next portion of the passage. Following the reading, a review of the 10 words (eight known, two unknown) that were used in the previous session are reviewed. A mark is placed on one of the unknown words to designate that the student knew the word without hesitation during this session.

10. As each new unknown word is added to the drill procedure, one of the original known words is removed from the list. The original unknown words selected on the first session remain in the list, until eight additional unknown words are added. By the time the 11th new unknown word is added, the word that is removed has far exceeded the number of repetitions necessary for new material to reach mastery level.

The folding-in technique provides high levels of repetition with guaranteed success. Given that the student already knows at least 70% of the material throughout the intervention session, he or she is likely to maintain high levels of motivation and to concentrate on learning the new items that are being presented. Over time, this technique should result in the student learning more new material faster and retaining it longer than with more traditional techniques.

A technique that is very similar to folding-in is the drill-sandwich procedure. Described by Coulter and Coulter (1991), the intervention is based on the same principles of instructional match and frequent repetition. The drill sandwich begins in the same way as folding-in, by selecting three unknown and seven known words. However, instead of folding in the unknown words among the known, the total group of 10 words is presented sequentially, with the known words placed in the third, sixth, and eighth positions. The set of words are then presented multiple times (usually five times through the pack per session), with the words being shuffled at the end of each time through the set. Rearranging the words prohibits students from simply memorizing the upcoming word in the pack, rather than really reading the word off the index card. The passage is then reread at the end of the session.

I (Shapiro, 1992) have provided an illustration of the use of this procedure to improve the reading fluency of four students (ages 6–9). Results of the pre- and postsession fluency for one of the students is shown in Figure 6.4. As shown, the student's performance was consistently higher during

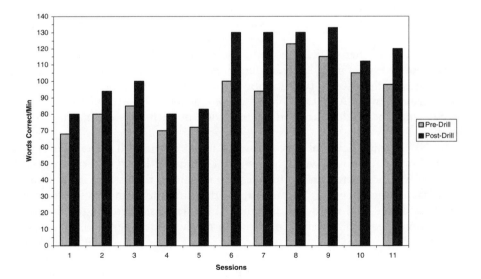

FIGURE 6.4. Oral reading rates of Anthony before and after drill session using the folding-in technique. From Shapiro (1992, p. 172). Copyright 1992 by the National Association of School Psychologists. Reprinted by permission.

postsession reading, with increases of reading fluency from 80 to 120 WCPM across the 11 sessions of treatment.

Several studies have examined the importance of the recommended instructional ratios of known to unknown items. For example, Neef, Iwata, and Page (1980) demonstrated that interspersing known items at a ratio of 50% during spelling instruction of new words resulted in superior performance in acquisition and long-term retention relative to other conditions. Roberts and her colleagues (Roberts & Shapiro, 1996; Roberts, Turco, & Shapiro, 1991) examined the degree to which one must remain within the specific 70% known, 30% unknown ratio suggested by Gickling and Havertape (1981). In these studies, the drill-sandwich procedure was used with children scoring in the average to low-average ranges on the reading subtest of the California Test of Basic Skills. In the first study (Roberts et al., 1991), students were randomly assigned to one of four conditions: (1) 90% known to 10% unknown; (2) 80% known to 20% unknown; (3) 60% known to 40% unknown; and (4) 50% known to 50% unknown. Based on the predictions of Gickling and Harertape (1981), it was expected that the best student performance would be evident for the 80% known to 20% unknown condition. At the end of 8 weeks of the intervention, results indicated that students acquired new information best in the most frustrating condition (50% known to 50% unknown); however, retention of learned words and the effect on untaught material was highest in the condition predicted by Gickling. In the second study, the ratio of known to unknown was stretched to 90% unknown to 10% known, 50% known to 50% unknown, and 80% known to 20% unknown. Results again indicated that although student acquisition of new information was best in the highly frustrating 90% unknown condition, students retained the information best when they were taught within the ratios recommended by Gickling.

Burns and his colleagues have provided a series of studies that have examined Gickling's recommended procedures for CBA. MacQuarrie et al. (2002) compared the drill-sandwich and folding-in techniques (called "incremental rehearsal" by Burns) in teaching words and vocabulary building. They found that the folding-in technique consistently led to more words retained. Burns (2001) examined the reliability of using acquisition and retention rates as a metric for determining the impact of the folding-in technique for students in third and fifth grade, and found acquisition correlations greater than .91 between material recalled 1 and 14 days after instruction. Correlations for retention were somewhat lower but still exceeded .87 for grades 3 and 5. Burns et al. (2000) also provided confirming evidence in support of Gickling's recommended instructional ratios. Although some research has not always substantiated Gickling's instructional ratios (e.g., Cooke, Guzaukas, Pressley, & Kerr, 1993), there does appear to be enough support for the use of the drill-sandwich and folding-in techniques to make strong suggestions that practitioners consider using them.

Probably the most effective way to improve reading skills is to have students increase their time for reading. Using an oral rather than a silent reading strategy, although somewhat controversial (e.g., Taylor & Conner, 1982), does assure the observer that the student is actively engaged in reading behavior. Procedures described in Chapter 5, such as Direct Instruction or peer tutoring, specifically emphasize repeated and frequent practice in their instructional methodologies. Indeed, the folding-in or drill-sandwich techniques can easily be adapted for use under peer-tutoring conditions.

Clearly, for students to learn to read fluently, they must develop a rich and functional vocabulary. Both expressive and receptive vocabulary skills are necessary. These skills require students to both produce and to associate meaning to words. Children generally learn new vocabulary by listening to storybooks (Elley, 1989). However, the teaching of vocabulary, as with other reading skills, needs to be explicit. Teaching techniques, such as pre-instruction of the meanings of critical words prior to reading, modeling of concepts when words cannot adequately describe the meaning (words such as *over*, *between*), or using synonyms to teach unknown words (*damp* means a little wet), are examples of the types of instructional strategies useful for teaching vocabulary. As with other skills, specific skill sequences are important to consider when vocabulary is the objective. Readers are encouraging to examine the excellent resources for teaching vocabulary (as well as all reading skills) outlined by the Institute for the Development of Educational Achievement (*http://reading.uoregon.edu*).

Comprehension and Content-Area Reading

Whether students master the skills of reading depends not only on their fluency but also, equally important, on their ability to comprehend the material they have read. It is important to recognize that comprehension is a skill to be taught, just as phonetic analysis and letter identification are skills to be instructed. Teaching comprehension is typically accomplished using either prereading or postreading strategies.

Postreading techniques tend to be straightforward. These often involve having students complete workbook pages and usually require students to respond to questions, such as identifying the main idea, sequence, and inferences from a previously read passage. Assignments are then graded, and feedback is offered.

Many examples can be found in the literature in which various aspects of postreading have been manipulated. For example, Swanson (1981) found that the use of self-recording, together with free time contingent on improvements in responses to questions asked after reading passages, resulted in increased performance on the comprehension task. This was in contrast to targeting error rates and silent reading rates, which resulted in no observable changes on comprehension measures.

Another useful postreading technique is retelling activities. These strategies typically ask students to repeat in their own words the meaning of what they had just read. Student retelling can be examined for the inclusion or exclusion of key components of a passage, such as main idea, plot, sequence, critical events, and so forth. Retelling can be completed after silent or oral reading if one is interested in determining whether reading aloud facilitates or interferes with student performance. Likewise, one can gradually increase the prompting process during retelling to determine whether students are using contextual cues to impact their understanding. For example, after reading a passage and being asked to retell what they read in their own words, students could be told to "scan the passage carefully as you retell the story" to determine if a simple instruction to examine material previously read is an effective strategy to improve comprehension. Figure 6.5 shows a form I have used to facilitate the retelling process. Full discussion of the retelling procedure is provided in the workbook.

A student's ability to recall information correctly in order to respond to a question is probably a function of memory as much as understanding of what the student read. Howell et al. (1993) accurately pointed out that we typically read materials because we have specific questions in mind that we would like to have answered. What we read depends much on what we want to get from the material we are reading. Thus, prereading strategies of instruction may be much more logical in teaching comprehension skills.

Howell et al. (1993) provided an excellent example of the difference between pre- and postreading activities. If a week after the student has read a passage, a teacher asks the student, "How old was Joy in that story?", the teacher is likely not to receive an accurate reply. Suppose, however, the teacher tells the student before he or she reads the passage, "Read this paragraph to find out how old Joy is." Obviously, the latter procedure seems to be more a measure of comprehension than of memory. In a typical prereading exercise, the teacher begins by reviewing the content of the passage and presenting new vocabulary. The student is then given the comprehension questions and asked to read the passage to find the answers. To assist the student in finding the answers, specific problem-solving or learning strategies may be taught.

Idol (1987) and Idol-Maestas and Croll (1987) have described a procedure called "story mapping" to teach comprehension skills. The procedure involves bringing the reader's attention to important and interrelated parts of the passage. Students are taught to organize the story into specific parts, including the setting, problem, goal, action, and outcome. Figure 6.6 illus-

QUANTIFICATION OF RETELLING FOR NARRATIVE TEXT

Student's Name: _____

Book/Page: _____   Date: _____

Directions: Place a 1 next to each item the student includes in his/her retelling. Credit the gist, as well as the obvious recall. Place an * if you ask the child questions to aid recall.

		Level				
		A	B	C	D	
Story sense						
Theme:	Main idea or moral of story	☐	☐	☐	☐	(1)
Problem:	Difficulty to overcome	☐	☐	☐	☐	(1)
Goal:	What the character wants to happen	☐	☐	☐	☐	(1)
Title:	Name of the story (if possible)	☐	☐	☐	☐	(1)
Setting						
	When and where the story occurs	☐	☐	☐	☐	(1)
Characters						
	Name the main characters	☐	☐	☐	☐	(1)
Events/episodes						
	Initiating event	☐	☐	☐	☐	(1)
	Major events (climax)	☐	☐	☐	☐	(1)
	Sequence: retells in structural order	☐	☐	☐	☐	(1)
Resolution						
	Name problem solution for the goal	☐	☐	☐	☐	(.5)
	End the story	☐	☐	☐	☐	(.5)

TOTAL ___ ___ ___ ___

FIGURE 6.5. Form for retelling narrative text.

MY STORY MAP

Name: _____ Date: _____

| The Setting |
| Characters: Time: Place: |

↓

| The Problem |

↓

| The Goal |

| Action |

| The Outcome |

FIGURE 6.6. Form for completing story-mapping exercises. From Idol (1987, p. 199). Copyright 1987 by Pro-Ed, Inc. Reprinted by permission.

trates the story map. Idol-Maestas and Croll used the procedure for students with learning disabilities (LD), and found significant improvements in comprehension without continuation of the story-mapping procedure, as well as maintenance of comprehension levels after the procedure was discontinued.

In a follow-up study, Idol (1987) implemented the story-map technique with 27 students in a third- and fourth-grade classroom. The strategy employed is a good example of a prereading technique. After showing the set of generic questions that students were to answer after reading the passage (Figure 6.7) and having the students read the story silently, the teacher displayed the story map. Students then completed the story map during a group instruction period led by the teacher. In a subsequent phase, the teacher no longer modeled the use of the story map as students independently completed the map. Students were permitted to fill in the map as they read the story. After the students completed the assignment, the teacher led the group in completing the map by calling on students in the group. Finally, in the last phase, the teacher discontinued completing the maps. A final phase with baseline conditions was then instituted.

Results of the study showed substantial improvements in student comprehension scores once the story-mapping procedure was instituted. This was especially true for the students with LD and low achievement in the classroom. An interesting related finding of the study was that gains in comprehension were observed on a variety of measures of comprehension and general application of reading. Similar positive outcomes for

Name: _____

Date: _____

1. Where did this story take place?
2. When did this story take place?
3. Who were the main characters in the story?
4. Were there any other important characters in the story? Who?
5. What was the problem in the story?
6. How did _____ try to solve the problem?
7. Was it hard to solve the problem? Explain.
8. Was the problem solved? Explain.
9. What did you learn from reading this story? Explain.
10. Can you think of a different ending?

FIGURE 6.7. Questions used to frame the story map. From Idol (1987, p. 197). Copyright 1987 by Pro-Ed, Inc. Reprinted by permission.

story mapping have been reported by several investigators (e.g., Babyak, Koorland, & Mathes, 2000; Baumann & Bergeron, 1993; Billingsley & Ferro-Almeida, 1993; Davis, 1994; Mathes, Fuchs, & Fuchs, 1997; Taylor, Alber, & Walker, 2002; Vallecorsa & deBettencourt, 1997).

Other prereading instructional procedures found useful for teaching comprehension are self-instruction training procedures. Very much like learning strategies, these techniques are designed to have students practice asking themselves a series of questions as they read. Smith and Van Biervliet (1986) described a self-instruction training program used with six comprehension-deficient sixth-grade students. The instruction focused on having students practice

> (a) reading the title of the story; (b) looking at illustrations; (c) reading the story and looking for the main idea; (d) noting the sequence of events; (e) reading through the comprehension questions; (f) rereading the story and answering the questions as they came to the answers in the story; and (g) checking the answers by referring again to the section of the story which provided the answers. (p. 47)

Self-instruction training was provided by using the procedures described by Meichenbaum and Goodman (1971) and involved having the student watch the experimenter model the task aloud; having the child perform the task while the experimenter instructed him or her aloud; having the child perform the task self-instructing aloud, while the experimenter whispered; having the child perform the task, while self-instructing in a whisper; and having the child self-instruct silently. Results of the study showed significant changes in the percentage of comprehension questions answered correctly after training. Three additional students who served as controls showed no change throughout the investigation.

In another study designed to examine self-instruction training, Miller (1986) compared the self-instruction procedure to a control practice technique in which students received equivalent exposure and practice to materials but were not taught the self-verbalization strategy. Results of the study showed that although no differences in performance were evident between conditions when students were exposed to a single self-instruction training session, significant differences were present when three training sessions were employed.

Graham and Wong (1993) compared teaching students a mnemonic strategy and a self-instruction technique to identify relationships in the text that were implicit, explicit, or script implicit. Using a question–answer method, 45 average readers and 45 poor readers were taught a mnemonic strategy called 3H (Here, Hidden, and In My Head) to cue themselves as to how to find answers to comprehension questions. In one of the conditions, a self-instruction procedure was used to teach students how to use the 3H intervention. Results of the study showed that students in both the self-instruction and didactic teaching groups improved their reading comprehension performance. However, self-instruction training was more effective than the didactic teaching technique in maintaining performance over time.

Another prereading strategy that can be used as a previewing technique is the use of a Question Wheel (Elliott et al., 2001). Illustrated in Figure 6.8, the wheel is used to activate background knowledge about the reading that students are starting. The outer and inner circles can be color coded, each containing a question word. Combinations of the words from the two circles form the types of questions students should be asking themselves as they preview material. Although there appears to be a preference in instructional strategies for prereading interventions in teaching comprehension, one postreading procedure may be valuable for improving both fluency and comprehension skills. A problem sometimes faced after conducting an assessment of reading skills is that students are being instructed in texts far beyond their level of effective acquisition. As noted by Lovitt and Hansen (1976a), it becomes difficult for students to achieve academic gains if they are being instructed in materials that clearly exceed their instructional levels. Placing students into lower level materials, however, can present a problem for teachers. For example, it may be unrealistic to expect a teacher to have a single student use curriculum materials that are signifi-

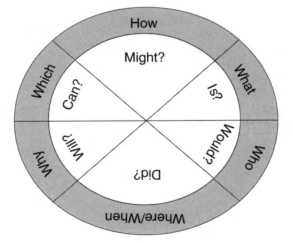

FIGURE 6.8. The Question Wheel for previewing reading passages. From Elliott and DiPerna, with Shapiro (2001, p. 94). Copyright 2001 by The Psychological Corporation. Reprinted by permission.

cantly below the lowest level used by other students in the classroom. In addition, some teachers who are willing to place students into such material may be prevented from doing so by district policy.

Lovitt and Hansen (1976b) described a technique called "contingent skipping and drilling" that may prove useful in these circumstances. After the appropriate level of instruction was determined using CBA, desired performance levels were set for each student, so as to achieve 25% improvement over baseline. During the intervention, students were permitted to skip all the remaining stories in the quarter of the basal reader book if, on the same day, all scores equaled or exceeded the preset criterion score. If a student went 7 days without skipping, a drill procedure was instituted. Drills employed for correct oral reading rate required a student to read the last 100 words from the previous day's assignment until he or she could pass at his or her criterion level. For incorrect rate, the teacher showed the student a list of words he or she had misread. The student was required to rehearse all lists of phrases in which these words were embedded until he or she could read all of them to the teacher. The comprehension drill required the student to rework answers to the questions until they were all correct. Students received drills on those aspects of reading performance that were below the desired scores, and could be drilled on all three components. Drill procedures remained in effect until a student skipped a section. After skipping, another 7 days had to elapse before another drill procedure was implemented.

Results of the study showed improvements across students in oral reading rates, reductions in error rates, and improvements in comprehension questions. Lovitt and Hansen (1976b) pointed out that although the measure of skipping in their procedure was a quarter of the text, teachers concerned about the amount of basal material not read could design the skipping procedure so that students could skip the following story rather than the entire quarter of the book.

Over the last several years, the emphasis in teaching reading comprehension skills has been on metacognition. Defined as conscious control of the skills by which one thinks and reasons, "metacognitive techniques" are designed to provide a framework for acquiring information from text. For example, as a student is reading, he/she may be taught to access prior knowledge, to ask a set of questions to him-/herself, to attempt to predict outcomes, to examine relationships among characters, or other such strategies. The idea is to teach the student strategies to approach the information so that the text becomes meaningful as he/she reads it. The literature exploring the many metacognitive strategies is voluminous. For example, a computerized literature search on the terms "reading comprehension and metacognition" within PSYCHLIT between January 1995 and December

2003 resulted in 105 citations. Any attempt to describe the many possible strategies here is beyond the scope of this book. Strategies offered here are but a small set of examples of the many types of metacognitive techniques that one could use.

Bos and Vaughn (2002) describe what is called the "Click and Clunk" strategy. Students are taught to self-monitor as they read, thinking about what they know and do not know. Throughout the reading process, students practice key words and principles as they grapple with text. "Clicks" are defined as those elements of the reading process that students "get." These are the elements of information, vocabulary, and meaningful understanding that students recognize immediately as they read. "Clunks" are those aspects of the reading process in which students suddenly recognize that they are struggling. Such elements may be words that cannot be decoded, phrases that are not making sense, or aspects of the story that do not seem logical. Students are taught a "declunking" strategy, with the teacher's help, when they reach one of these problems. Such strategies include the mechanisms to attack the problem, such as breaking down words into smaller units, chunking information, and looking back at previous parts of the story that clicked to gain the context of the difficult part. These strategies are written on "declunking cards" and used as reminders when students reach other parts of the story that also create difficulty.

Another set of strategies that can teach students approaches to better understand what they are reading are the "Get the Gist" and "Wrap-Up" strategies. Get the Gist helps students learn the main idea of the passage they are reading by having them identify the most important points through rephrasing. The rephrasing is required to be limited to 10 words or less, which forces students to focus their thinking about the material they are reading. Wrap-Up strategies are excellent for students when they are reading expository types of materials. Here, students are asked to summarize and retell the main points of the story, answering questions with simple stems such as "How do you think _____ could have been prevented?" or "How would you compare and contrast _____?" The Question Wheel, shown in Figure 6.8, could also be applied here to facilitate this process. All of these strategies can be done as part of collaborative processes within classes, in which students assume various roles, such as Leader, Clunk Expert, Gist Expert, Announcer, and so forth.

Ward and Traweek (1993) described another strategy, the think-aloud procedure, as illustrative of metacognitive techniques. Grade-level passages were modified using a cloze technique wherein every fifth word of the passage was left blank. In their procedure, replacement with only the exact word was considered correct. In the think-aloud technique, students were asked to tell the examiner the word that was omitted and why they chose that particular word to fit in the blank. In their study, Ward and Traweek compared the think-aloud condition to another condition in which students were simply told to tell the examiner the word left out in the passage. At the end of the intervention, a series of nine comprehension questions was asked. In addition, a set of questions designed to elicit the metacognitive strategies that students used in completing the cloze technique was asked. Results showed that although both groups of students displayed equivalent performance on word identification and reading tasks, the students who used the think-aloud technique dramatically improved their comprehension scores.

Another metacognitive intervention teaches students to give reasons for responses to questions. In two studies with fifth-grade students, scores on a test of reading comprehension were significantly improved as a result of using the technique. Benito, Foley, Lewis, and Prescott (1993) had students use a question–answer technique in responding to four types of questions usually asked in content-area textbooks. Although the students showed minimal gains on a global measure of reading comprehension, they all showed a substantial increase in the percentage of questions answered correctly in a social studies text.

Reading processes also extend beyond the acquisition of learning basic reading skills. When students are asked to read content materials, such as in science or social studies, even students with developed basic reading skills can struggle. It is at this point that students must use reading to learn, rather than learning to read. Specific strategies to attack the types of materials presented in content-area reading are required.

Two sets of skills necessary to be successful in content-area reading are vocabulary building and comprehension. Strategies for vocabulary development are no different when doing content-area reading then they are in developing basic skills. Previewing, playing word games, pneumonics, word analysis, using synonyms, and other such activities can all be applied when learning content-area material in science, social studies, geography, and other such subjects. Blachowicz and Ogle (2001) is just one of many, many resources available to help readers identify such strategies.

Perhaps even more important than vocabulary building is the ability of students to grasp the complexity of relationships in content-area material they are reading. Two of the best strategies are the use of semantic maps and semantic feature analysis. In semantic mapping, students are asked to make connections between concepts. Brainstorming sessions are used to generate these maps and result in a web that connects one concept to another. Figure 6.9 is an illustration of a semantic map for a reading assignment on seabirds.

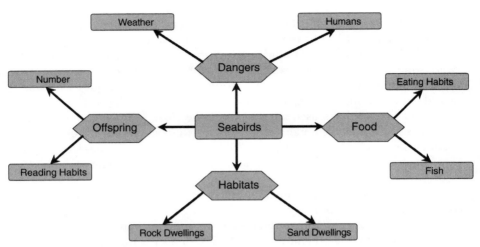

FIGURE 6.9. Example of semantic mapping for reading assignment. Adapted from Bryant, Ugel, Thompson, and Hamff (1999, p. 299). Copyright 1999 by Pro-Ed, Inc. Adapted by permission.

Maps such as these can be useful but bring about the need for the development of new vocabulary as well. Semantic feature analysis can also help students to integrate the concepts with new vocabulary they will need to understand the material. Using a chart, such as the one in Figure 6.10, students can identify through discussions the links between terms.

In general, use of metacognitive and cognitive strategies is the focus of significant interventions to improve reading comprehension skills. Indeed, it appears that the use of these strategies is critical to teaching students with

Features	Causes	Union	Confederacy	Battles
Vocabulary Words				
cannonade	–	+	+	+
slavery	+	+	+	–
cavalry	–	+	+	+
abolitionist	+	+	–	–

FIGURE 6.10. Example of semantic-feature analysis of reading assignment. Adapted from Bryant, Ugel, Thompson, and Hamff (1999, p. 299). Copyright 1999 by Pro-Ed, Inc. Adapted by permission.

academic skills problems in reading. Readers are encouraged to examine the large array of interventions that have appeared in the literature showing the wide range of strategies that can be selected.

MATHEMATICS

Students typically are referred for two types of problems in mathematics. Difficulty in mastering computational skills is the more common problem. These problems can range from failure to learn basic addition, subtraction, and multiplication facts to difficulties learning the correct rules for regrouping. Also, some students who are able to learn basic math facts have difficulty reaching levels of fluency. Mathematics is an area in which speed *and* accuracy are particularly important for success.

The other common type of problem in mathematics involves skills requiring the application of math. This would include such areas as time, money, measurement, and geometry. Word problems also fall into this category.

Although failure in mathematical applications certainly is important. Students who cannot master basic computational skills are very unlikely to succeed at applications. As such, intervention procedures designed as prework activities are focused more on applications and conceptual understanding of operations, whereas postwork activities emphasize acquisition of basic computational skills.

Number Sense

Before students can even begin the process of learning computation, they must develop number sense. As noted by Gersten and Chard (1999), the concept of number sense is the equivalent in mathematics to phonemic awareness in reading. Although difficult to define, number sense is easy to recognize. When young children show a capability to manipulate numbers, one-to-one correspondence, and an understanding of how our number system operates, they are showing number sense. The skills often develop informally through everyday experience. For example, having children count aloud the number of steps as they walk down to breakfast, or asking simple questions in mathematical terms (e.g., "You come home from school at 3:00 P.M. It is now 8:00 A.M. In how many more hours will you be home today?") shows evidence that students have number sense.

Developing number sense serves as a key prerequisite to developing other mathematical skills. The skills are usually taught to very young children using a limited focus for instruction. For example, one would use only addition, subtraction, and equal signs to show relationships between numbers. Another technique would be to use labeling and counting of everyday experiences, such as setting the table and asking a child, "How many forks do we need for dinner tonight?" Using a number line to represent the concepts of "more and less" is another example of how one would teach number sense.

Postwork Activities

Procedures that increase the frequency of accurate responding can provide a built-in mechanism for providing students with reinforcement for their math computation. Some early studies showed that offering students praise and immediate correctness feedback could produce improved performance on math problems (Kirby & Shields, 1972). McLaughlin (1981) described a more extensive token economy program that provided points for many behaviors, including increasing math rates on assigned daily worksheets. Points could be exchanged for a variety of activity reinforcers. Likewise, contingent free time has also been employed in several early investigations to improve math rates (Johnston & McLaughlin, 1982; Luiselli & Downing, 1980; Terry, Deck, Huelecki, & Santogrossi, 1978).

Another simple postwork technique that has been found to improve accuracy and production of math computation is the interspersal of easy material among more difficult material. Skinner and his colleagues first explored this concept with undergraduate college students (Skinner, Fletcher, Wildmon, & Belifore, 1996), but the findings were soon expanded to many other populations with children and adolescents. For example, Logan and Skinner (1998) found that sixth-grade students given a choice between assignments that were more difficult and shorter versus longer but containing problems of both the same and easier difficulty, significantly preferred the longer assignments with items of mixed difficulty. Wildmon, Skinner, McCurdy, and Sims (1999) applied the same principles and obtained the same results with high school students working with word problems. The robustness of this technique has been evident in many other investigations (Cates et al., 1999; Skinner et al., 1999) and has been applied when working with students with LD (Johns, Skinner, & Nail, 2000) and emotional disturbance (Skinner, Hurst, et al., 2002).

Another technique developed by Skinner and his colleagues, which uses corrective feedback to improve student performance in mathematics, is a procedure entitled "cover–copy–compare" (CCC; Skinner, Bamberg, et al., 1993; Skinner, McLaughlin, & Logan, 1997; Skinner et al., 1991, 1992). The procedure involves five steps: (1) Look at the problem; (2) cover the problem with an index card; (3) write the problem and solution on the right side of the page; (4) uncover the problem and solution; and (5) evaluate the response. In Skinner et al. (1992), a comparison was made between feedback in the CCC procedure given by peers or by the student to themselves for six second-grade students. Results showed that student performance was greater for four of the six students when the feedback was self-directed rather than peer-directed. However, across all students, the peer-directed feedback sessions required double the time to complete the intervention. Skinner, Bamberg, et al. (1993) had three third-grade students subvocalize the CCC procedure while working on division problems. Results showed that two of the three students had increased their rate of correct responding to mastery levels. The third student required more directed feedback and goal setting to reach this level of performance. Follow-up data obtained 8 months after the intervention ended showed strong maintenance of division facts.

Clearly, the simple procedure of increased feedback and reward can act as often-needed incentives for improving fluency of basic computational skills. Although this is true, the most straightforward recommendations about increasing fluency in computational skills are hardly novel. Even though students may know their facts, they must be able to perform them at a reasonable pace. Almost all discussions of increasing fluency note that one item is required: practice. Practice through the use of flash cards and oral recitation, practice through writing responses, and practice with and without timing are essential to improving computational skills. This should not be surprising given what we know about increased opportunities to respond and improved academic skills. Practice alone, however, may not be sufficient to increase *accuracy* of responding effectively. When a child's difficulties are not only related to speed or fluency but also show problems in accuracy, the use of prework activities become important.

Prework Activities

Several types of prework activities have been described for math problems. One involves simple reminders and cues for students as they work through problems. These techniques are particularly applicable for students who often struggle with learning aspects of the computational process. Another strategy training method requires students to identify the steps needed to solve a particular task and use self-talk to work through the required tasks as they solve the problem. A third approach uses schematic representations as formats for teaching students how to proceed through tasks and is particularly applicable for students asked to complete complex mathematical problems, such as word problems.

Reminders and Cues

A common computational problem in children stems from their use of incorrect operations. Students may not attend to the operation sign or may perseverate on one sign when asked to perform a set of problems with mixed operations. A simple intervention to assist students is to provide additional visual cues that draw their attention to the operation that the problem asks to be performed. For example, color-coded signs (e.g., green = add, red = subtract) using highlighting pens prior to beginning the assignment can often facilitate student performance.

Computational problems can also occur when students are asked to do more complex problems involving regrouping. Difficulties in both place value, how to "carry," and organization can be evident when students struggle with these types of problems. One of the most effective interventions for this type of computation problem involves providing cues for completing problems that remind students and direct them through the correct sequence. For example, as illustrated in Figure 6.11, problems are structured so that students are unlikely to make common mistakes such as placing two digits under the 1's column (i.e., writing down 13 instead of 3 in the 1's column), or forgetting to add both the regrouped value and the presented value. Other visual cues such as graph paper, charts, color-coded worksheets, and stepwise reminders can all be valuable in improving student performance in computation. It is important that these cues and prompts be faded quickly, so that students do not become dependent on these prompts to accurately complete their computation problems.

1. Add the numbers in the 1's column.

2. Write the first number in the box at the top of the 10's column.

3. Write the second number of the sum in the box below the line of the 1's column.

4. Add the numbers in the 10's column. Be sure to include the number in the box.

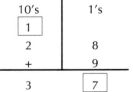

FIGURE 6.11. Reminder cues for addition problem with regrouping to 10's and columns.

Strategy Instruction

Cullinan et al. (1981) provided a detailed explanation of strategy training for arithmetic instruction. Before a strategy can be devised to attack a problem, an analysis of the curriculum must be completed. The specific objectives being taught, such as adding one-digit numbers, writing numerical fractions when given pictures that show fractional relationships, or determining speed when given distance and time, provide the content for which strategies can be developed. Obviously, one can subdivide these objectives into even smaller levels. The optimal size of the task to be taught is often based upon the teacher's preference, the student groups being taught, and the judgment of professionals as to which level of tasks would result in the greatest generalization. In Chapter 5, Figure 5.5 displays an example of a task class for multiplication facts described by Cullinan et al. (1981).

Once the objective is determined, an attack strategy is devised. The strategy employed is based on a rational analysis of the problem (Resnick & Ford, 1978); that is, how does a competent learner solve this problem? Figure 5.5 shows the attack strategy developed for performing multiplication facts. After the strategy has been developed, it is important to task-analyze the strategy to determine whether there are specific skills required to perform the attack strategy that the student has not yet acquired. For example, Figure 5.5 shows the task analysis of the multiplication attack strategy. Obviously, a student who cannot count by 2's, 5's, and so on, will not succeed at the strategy devised to teach multiplication facts.

The attack strategy can be taught using any form of direct instruction. If a student has mastered the preskills, however, simply telling him or her the rule for combining skills may be a successful teaching strategy. One way to teach students these strategies has been through self-instruction. Johnston et al. (1980) and Whitman and Johnston (1983) have provided excellent examples of how self-instruction training can be used to teach addition and subtraction regrouping skills. After the appropriate sequence of steps to solve these problems is defined using a task analysis, students are taught to verbalize these steps as they actually solve problems. Initially, the teacher serves as a model for self-instruction while students observe. Through a series of gradual steps, students begin to self-instruct without teacher prompting. Finally, students are expected to self-instruct "covertly" and talk to themselves. As discussed earlier, these procedures have been widely applied for both academic problems (Van Luit & Naglieri, 1999). In Chapter 5, Figure 5.2 shows an example of the actual self-instruction procedure used by Johnston et al. (1980).

Beyond the acquisition of mathematical operations, strategy training is expected to have additional benefits of teaching students problem solving. One of the important aspects of strategy training is the anticipated generalization of the strategy across related types of tasks. For example, it is expected that by teaching students problem solving for addition problems involving regrouping, acquisition of skills in subtraction or multiplication problems with regrouping should be easier.

Schematic Representation

When students are faced with having to solve word problems, they often fail because they are unable to break down the problem to its essential elements. Jitendra and her colleagues have described a procedure called "schema-based learning," whereby students are taught an organizational framework that serves as a means for depicting the numerical relationships between elements of word problems. Jitendra and Hoff (1996) first described the technique in working with third- and fourth-grade students with LD. For example, as seen in Figure 6.12, a schema is presented for certain types of problems. The teaching process starts with presenting students with story situations rather than problems. These story situations are used to teach students to use the diagram and understand how quantities are changed. An example of a group problem would be, "Over the last month, Bob delivered 100 paperback books per day and Rich delivered 55 hardback books per day. Together, they delivered 155 books per day." Students are taught to identify the relationships among the classifications of objects (i.e., paperback books, hardback books, and books) and to ignore factors irrelevant to the solution (i.e., passage of time, or 1 month). Each of the values is placed into the schema maps. Once students learn the process of using the schema with story situations, story problems are introduced (e.g., "Ken had 37 pins in his collection. He bought 12 more pins at a soccer tournament this weekend. How many pins does he now have in his collection?"). Using modeling, prompting, and feedback, students learn rules for selecting the correct operation (addition or subtraction) and use these in solving the problem by completing the schema diagrams.

Comparisons between students using and not using schema diagrams in math problem solving have shown the procedure to result in significantly more accurate performance among students, especially those with LD (Jitendra, 2002; Jitendra et al., 1998; Jitendra & Hoff, 1996; Jitendra, Hoff, & Beck, 1997, 1999; Xin, Jitendra, Deatline-Buchman, Hickman, & Bentram, 2002). The use of schema diagrams has also been shown to have lasting effects that impact student performance beyond the initial instruction.

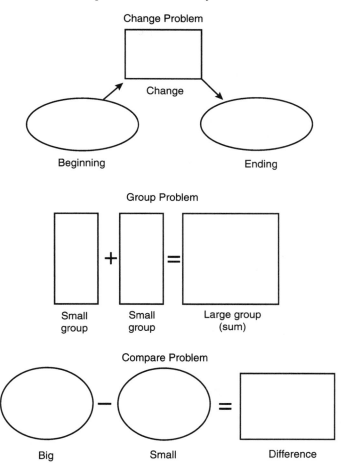

FIGURE 6.12. Schema for change, group, and compare problems. From Jitendra and Griffin (2001). Reprinted by permission from the authors.

SPELLING

At one time, spelling was taught as a separate subject with specific curriculum materials, divorced from other aspects of reading and writing. Today, spelling instruction is usually integrated into the teaching of language arts and is included as part of the curriculum of teaching reading and writing. As a result of the integration, teachers usually select the required spelling words for drill and practice from material that students are expected to read, or from lists of commonly misspelled words. Far fewer teachers today use an explicit curriculum to teach spelling.

Although spelling may not be taught from a prepared curriculum, it is still common for students to have weekly spelling and/or vocabulary tests throughout much of their elementary schooling. These tests do set the stage for mastering word usage and enhancing the vocabulary development needed for reading. Doing well on these tests requires that students engage in repetitive, planned drill and practice. They also need to learn appropriate strategies for enhancing skills development.

Most procedures to improve spelling have involved mostly efforts aimed at postwork activities. In particular, prompting, modeling, feedback, and rehearsal appear to be the most common interventions employed. Instructors have included peer tutors, parents, teachers, and individuals themselves.

Delquadri et al. (1983) investigated the effects of classwide peer tutoring on spelling performance in a regular third-grade classroom. Students were awarded points for correct performance during tutoring. In addition, demonstration and feedback were employed when errors were made during tutoring sessions. Significant reductions in the numbers of errors made on weekly Friday spelling tests were evident when the peer-tutoring procedures were in effect. Others have found that peer tutoring is an excellent way to ensure sufficient practice in spelling (DuPaul et al., 1998; Mortweet et al., 1999). Indeed, Madrid, Terry, Greenwood, Whaley, and Weber (1998) showed that peer-tutored spelling resulted in greater increases in performance when compared to teacher-mediated instruction.

Gettinger (1985) examined the use of imitation to correct spelling errors as a means of increasing spelling performance. Using an alternating treatment design, Gettinger had students engage in one of four conditions: Following a no-instruction control, in which students were told to study and practice, comparison was made between teacher- and student-directed study, with or without cues regarding the incorrect portion of the word. In the teacher-directed condition, students were shown and told the correct spelling of the word. Cues consisted of having the misspelled part of the word circled. Results of the study revealed that the highest performance on posttests occurred when student-directed study with cues was employed. All four conditions, however, were significantly better than the no-instruction control condition.

An interesting procedure used to improve spelling called "Add-a-Word" was described by Pratt-Struthers, Struthers, and Williams (1983). The procedure involves having students copy a list of 10 words, cover each word, and write it a second time, then check each word for correct spelling against the teacher's list. Misspelled words are repeated and remain on the list. If a word is spelled correctly on 2 consecutive days, the word is dropped from the list and replaced with a new word. Results of this study showed that all nine of the fifth- and sixth-grade students with LD increased their percentage of correctly spelled words during a creative writing assignment using this procedure.

McLaughlin, Reiter, Mabee, and Byram (1991) replicated the Add-a-Word program across nine 12- to 14-year-old students with mild handicaps. Comparing the program to the more traditional approach of giving a Monday pretest, followed by an end of the week posttest, students' overall accuracy in spelling was higher during the Add-a-Word program than during any other form of instruction. Similar findings for the Add-a-Word program were reported by several other investigators (McAuley & McLaughlin, 1992; Schermerhorn & McLaughlin, 1997; Struthers, Bartlamay, Bell, & McLaughlin, 1994; Struthers, Bartlamay, Williams, & McLaughlin, 1989).

Although most procedures for academic remediation are based on positive procedures, as is typical in skills acquisition programs, use of a mild aversive technique has also been investigated for improving spelling performance. Foxx and Jones (1978) and Ollendick et al. (1980) examined use of positive-practice overcorrection in improving spelling. In the Foxx and Jones study, 29 students between fourth and eighth grade were assigned to one of four conditions. All students took a pretest on Wednesday and a graded spelling test on Friday. In the control condition, no other manipulation was employed. In the second condition, students took only the Friday test, followed by positive practice on Monday. The positive practice procedure involved having students write out for each misspelled word (1) correct spelling, (2) phonetic spelling, (3) part of speech, (4) dictionary definition, and (5) correct usage in five sentences. In the third condition, students took the pretest, did positive practice on those words, and then took the Friday test. Finally, in the fourth condition, students performed positive practice after both pretest and posttest conditions. Results of their study found that all conditions in which positive practice was employed resulted in improved spelling performance over the control condition. Similar findings were observed in the Ollendick et al. (1980) study in two single-case design experiments, in which positive practice paired with contingent reinforcement resulted in better performance than did traditional teaching procedures. Others have also reported positive outcomes in using overcorrection techniques for improving spelling performance (Stewart & Singh, 1986).

A drill procedure for students that can be very effective in improving spelling performance is self-management spelling (SMS; Shapiro & Cole, 1994). The procedure requires that the list of spelling words be recorded on a standard cassette audiotape, and that the student practice their spelling during some independent work time. The tape provides the word to be spelled, a sentence using the word, if needed, pauses for about 7 seconds, and then says and spells the word. Students are instructed to listen to the word and sentence, pause the tape, write their response, write the correct spelling when they hear the word, and then immediately compare the word they have written to the correct spelling. Students then move through the list of words until completion. After they complete their practice, students chart their performance. This technique is repeated until students are able to achieve success at over 90% of the words presented spelled correctly, at which time they inform the teacher they are ready to take their test. The test itself can be placed on an audiotape, with the correct spelling of the word removed, and students are not permitted to stop the tape. The advantages of SMS are that students can work on the activity independently, manage their own time, receive immediate corrective feedback, and see the outcomes of their work.

Finally, simply providing contingent reward for meeting preset criteria for performance can result in improved spelling performance. We (Goldberg & Shapiro, 1995; Shapiro & Goldberg, 1986, 1990) compared the effects of types of group contingencies on spelling performance of regular sixth-grade students. Students were awarded points that were equivalent to a penny each if they met the preset criterion for performance. Although the findings related to the effectiveness of group contingencies were complex, they strongly suggested that even the poorest spellers significantly improved their performance as a result of contingent reward.

The procedures employed to teach spelling in these studies are typical of how most spelling is usually taught. Students are assigned a list of words that they memorize and recite back when asked on the spelling test. Practice and rehearsal are conducted daily. Although this strategy appears to work, it may not be the best way to teach spelling (Howell & Nolet, 1999). Students who are poor spellers do not have well-developed phonemic awareness or alphabetic principles. However, if these students have good visualization skills, they may be able to learn to memorize the word lists, repeat them during the test, and score high marks for spelling in school. The real test for these individuals, however, is how they spell when they must produce written language. Thus, teaching spelling is usually linked to instruction and remediation for written language.

WRITTEN LANGUAGE

The area of written language involves many interrelated skills. These include grammar, punctuation, handwriting, spelling, creativity, and expressiveness. Over the last two decades, Graham, Harris, and their colleagues have provided extensive descriptions of the best way to teach these skills, especially to children with mild handicaps (e.g., Graham, 1982; Graham & Harris, 2003; Graham, Harris, MacArthur, & Schwartz, 1991; Graham, Harris, & Troia, 2000; Graham, MacArthur, Schwartz, & Page-Voth, 1992; Graham & Miller, 1980; Mason, Harris, & Graham, 2002; Sexton, Harris, & Graham, 1998). Based primarily on a constructivist approach to learning that perceives learning as a series of socially situated events that are functional, meaningful, and authentic (Harris & Graham, 1994), their work has focused primarily on the use of strategy instruction as a mechanism to teach the component skills necessary for effective writing. Entitled, Self-Regulated Strategy Development (SRSD), students are taught to self-regulate to improve the acquisition, maintenance, and generalization of skills required for effective composition. (Interested readers should see Graham et al., 1991, and Harris & Graham, 1996, for a superb description of their program.)

In general, Graham, Harris, and colleagues found that students with LD do not use very effective strategies in conducting writing tasks. For example, in planning an essay, students with LD made the task into a question-answering task, with little consideration given to the relationship of the questions and the material that was to be written. It was also found that students with LD had a difficult time accessing the knowledge they did possess. This is especially true, given the mechanical problems many of these student have in producing written work.

Students with LD are equally ineffective at revising. Graham et al. (1991) noted that students with LD tend to look at revising as an opportunity to improve the appearance of the composition, with little attention to its content. Additionally, students with LD may be unrealistic about the quality of their writing skills.

Based on these deficiencies, writing strategies have been designed to teach students with LD to self-monitor productivity, frame and plan text, generate content, edit, revise, and write sentences. Through a series of empirical studies, the impact of these strategies has been thoroughly tested. For example, in the area of planning, strategies such as brainstorming, framing text, and goal setting can be taught successfully to students with LD.

Harris and Graham (1985) taught two sixth-grade students to brainstorm as part of a larger strategy to improve composition skills. Three objectives of instruction were identified as increasing the number of different action words, action helpers, and describing words. Students were taught the attack strategies (brainstorming) for improving their compositions; each of the three objectives was attacked individually. Results of the study showed substantial increases in performance on the type of words used in the composition, as well as an increase in overall quality of writing.

In another set of studies, students were taught strategies for framing by posing and answering questions, each involving different parts of the story. Using a scale developed by Graham and Harris (1989) that scored each composition for the presence and quality of the inclusion of eight story–grammar elements (main character, locale, time, starter event, goal, action, ending, and reaction), students increased the number of story–grammar parts included significantly. Performance generalized to another writing assignment for a different teacher and was maintained for at least 4 weeks.

Another important part of the planning process in writing is the setting of goals. Graham et al. (1992, p. 325) reported an investigation in which four fifth-grade students with LD were taught a specific prewriting strategy. The strategy included three steps:

1. Do PLANS (Pick goals, List ways to meet goals, And, make Notes, Sequence notes).
2. Write and say more.
3. Test goals.

Both product and process goals were selected by having students choose one goal from three or four listed in each area. For product goals, students chose goals for purpose, structure, and fluency. Under purpose, the student could choose from the following: (1) Write a paper that will convince my friends; (2) write a paper that will be fun to read; or (3) write a paper that will teach something. Under structure, the student's choice of goals was as follows: (1) Write an essay that has all the parts, or (2) write a story that has all the parts. Under fluency, the student chose a goal based on word count, adjusted depending on his/her pretest performance.

The second step of the strategy required students to indicate process goals for accomplishing the product goals previously chosen. The students then self-administered prompts to continue planning once they actually started writing. At the final step, students evaluated whether the goals were met.

The strategy was modeled by the instructor using a self-instruction technique that began with a talk-aloud procedure as an essay was written. Planning worksheets were provided for the students and modeled by the instructor. In a typical self-instruction format, the requirements for students to engage in self-talk were increased. Once the steps of the strategy were memorized, the instructor and the students composed an essay jointly and, finally, the students completed two or three essays independently.

Results of the study showed that the students improved their writing skills in terms of the number of story elements included, as well as the quality of their writing. Prior to learning the strategy, students spent less than 5 seconds of prewriting time on their stories. This increased to approximately 8 minutes following instruction. Total composing time increased from 12 minutes in baseline to 20 minutes after intervention. In addition, when students were asked to write stories in other areas not discussed as part of the intervention, substantial improvements over baseline scores were evident across students. Other studies (Graham & Harris, 1989; Sawyer, Graham, & Harris, 1992) have also shown the potential value of goal setting as a strategy in improving writing skills.

In the area of revising, the use of peers to react and make suggestions has been a commonly applied strategy. Stoddard and MacArthur (1993) and MacArthur, Schwartz, and Graham (1991) reported the use of peer editors by having an assigned student summarize the main points of the essay in a log with suggestions for revisions. Students are provided with a series of questions to help guide their decisions. The editor and student author then discuss the suggestions. Results from these studies showed that students with LD made more mechanical and content revisions compared to baseline.

Finally, the impact of self-monitoring productivity has been examined during the writing process. Harris et al. (1994) compared two procedures for self-monitoring. In one condition, they used the procedure reported by Hallahan, Lloyd, Kauffman, and Loper (1983), whereby students are told to ask themselves, "Was I paying attention?", immediately after hearing a tone played on a tape recorder. Tones occurred at random intervals between 10 and 90 seconds. As each tone was heard, students were instructed to mark their response to the self-directed question on a recording sheet. In the other condition, students were told to simply self-record the number of words in the composition and record it on a graph at the conclusion of their writing. Results showed that both forms of self-monitoring improved the students' on-task and writing quality.

Strategy instruction has also been applied in improving the handwriting of students. Traditional techniques for teaching handwriting usually involve modeling the formation of letters by an instructor, followed by practice. Unfortunately, for many students with LD, these procedures are not always successful. Kosiewicz et al. (1982) used a self-instruction and self-correction procedure to improve the handwriting of a boy with LD. Using the self-instruction procedure in combination with self-correction produced substantially better handwriting. Blandford and Lloyd (1987) used a self-instructional training technique to enhance handwriting of two students with LD. Using a cue card that included self-evaluation questions related to proper handwriting technique, teachers taught the students to covertly ask and answer each question as they completed their handwriting assignment. After the students improved their performance, the cue cards were removed and maintenance data were collected. Results showed that the self-instructional training procedure improved the handwriting of both students, and these effects were maintained after use of cue cards was discontinued.

Despite these two studies, the outcomes of using self-instruction to improve handwriting have been somewhat mixed. Graham (1983) tried using self-instruction training to improve the handwriting skills of three third- and fourth-grade students with LD. After extensive training, however, only modest gains on the letters taught were found. No transfer to untaught letters was evident.

Another prewriting activity that can be a valuable tool in improving the written language skills of students is the use of a web. The web is a nonlinear outline that provides a mechanism for organizing information and linking important concepts together. The web begins with a main idea in the center and then branches to other categories of information. Zipprich (1995) described a study designed to teach webbing as a strategy to improve the written compositions across 13 students with learning and behavior disabilities between ages 9 and 12 years. Prior to the study, students were taught to identify elements of narrative stories using the story map (Idol, 1987). In baseline, students were asked to write their best story during a 30-minute period, based on a picture cue displayed by the teacher. Following baseline, students were shown a prestructured web to help teach them how to clarify components of the story (see Figure 6.13). The teacher then led the students through a brainstorming session, writing their responses on the prestructured web that was displayed on an overhead projector. Next, the students were shown another picture and were told to complete their own individual webs. Students then shared their ideas with the group, and the collective outcomes were recorded by the teacher. Students were then given 30 minutes to write their best story, using either individual ideas or the group ideas from the web. Finally, students were shown another picture and asked to generate a web and a story. Results were scored using a holistic scoring device. Overall, most of the students showed substantial gains in various components of the webbing process. Students were somewhat inconsistent in their improvement across components of the writing process (e.g., number of words, thought units, sentence types), but all showed improvement over baseline in the amount of planning time and quality (holistic score) of their writing.

Another program developed to teach students skills in handwriting is the Process Assessment of the Learner (PAL; Berninger, 1998). The PAL

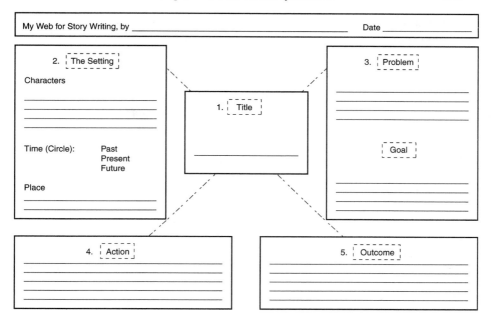

My Web for Story Writing, by _____ Date _____

2. The Setting

Characters

_____
_____
_____

Time (Circle):   Past
                 Present
                 Future

Place

_____
_____

1. Title

_____

3. Problem

_____
_____
_____

Goal

_____
_____
_____

4. Action

_____
_____
_____
_____

5. Outcome

_____
_____
_____
_____

FIGURE 6.13. Prestructured story web form. From Zipprich (1995, p. 6). Copyright 1995 by Pro-Ed, Inc. Reprinted by permission.

was developed to provide strong links between teaching reading and writing to students with difficulties in these areas. The system is based on much of the research on brain development and LD (Berninger, 1994). In particular, Berninger and Amtmann (2003) provide strong research support that teaching handwriting can have significant impact on other skills, such as spelling.

PAL handwriting lessons are designed to develop automaticity in young children as they develop correct letter formation. Using frequent repetition and directed practice, students use numbered arrow cues as models for writing their letters. At the same time as they write, students name letters. Once the letter formation reaches automatic levels, students then are prompted to write short compositions.

CONCLUSIONS AND SUMMARY

Interventions for academic problems can be highly complex. Although studies have been conducted with all skills areas employing postwork activities that do not require extensive intervention development (e.g., reinforcement contingencies, feedback, modeling, and prompting), an emphasis on prework activities requiring strategy training is somewhat involved. These strategies, however, may foster generalization across tasks and can be quite powerful in the instructional process.

Missing, by design, from this review of potential intervention techniques is procedures more commonly viewed as based on information-processing approaches to remediation. For example, no recommendations for examining modality of instruction or altering curriculum materials based on learning approaches of students were made. These types of recommendations, common in the past, are not considered likely to result in improved student performance. Instead, the targets for intervention (i.e., reading, arithmetic, spelling, and writing) become the focus of the interventions. If a student is having problems reading, strategies to improve reading, and not some hypothesized set of underlying skills, should be implemented. If a student is having trouble learning basic math facts, basic math facts should be taught, not just any perceptual process. If a student is having trouble in composition, then designing teaching strategies for effective writing are needed. This approach emphasizes the functional and not structural aspects of academic problems. The approach has worked well and is consistently reinforced through the research.

Given this wide range of intervention procedures, which strategies should we choose? What works? Interestingly, there is a large research literature that supports the types of interventions discussed in this and the previous chapter. In addition, substantial efforts are currently under way to offer a set of empirically tested and validated recommendations to educators as to what procedures work for what types of skills problems. Through a contract with the U.S. Department of Education, the What Works Clearinghouse is expected to gather and disseminate information to educators as to what are effective strategies for academic intervention (*http://www. w-w-c.org*). Other similar efforts have been evident through the work of Swanson, Hoskyn, and Lee (1999), who provided an extensive meta-analysis of interventions for students with LD, covering all areas of academic performance, as well as the work of Swanson, Harris, and Graham (2003), who published the *Handbook of Learning Disabilities*, in which one can find volumes of information on empirically supported interventions for students with LD.

At the same time that we uncover "what works," it is also true that what may work with a particular student may not work with the next student who has a similar problem. Many aspects of the learning environment interact with a student's learning, and it is virtually impossible to predict with certainty when an intervention may be effective and when it may not. This is the point at which we begin the journey into problem solving for effective intervention. We begin where our experience tells us we will have success. Where we go next depends on the research and analysis of our data.

CHAPTER 7

♦♦♦

Step 4: Progress Monitoring

♦

Regardless of which instructional modifications identified in Step 3 of the assessment model are implemented, a key decision for the evaluator is to determine whether the intervention is effective in improving the academic performance of the student. Setting goals for performance is an important element of ensuring student success. Likewise, determining whether a student is making progress toward his or her goal is an essential ingredient in conducting an effective evaluation of academic skills. Failing to evaluate a student's academic progress after starting an intervention program is tantamount to undergoing months of diagnostic tests for a medical condition and being prescribed extensive pharmacotherapy by a physician, but never checking back with the physician to see if the therapy is working. Indeed, progress monitoring is a primary component of any system of problem-solving assessment.

Progress monitoring can be used to determine both short- and long-term outcomes of academic interventions. Monitoring for short-term outcomes is consistent with the subskills mastery model of CBA, whereas monitoring for long-term outcomes follows the general outcomes measurement (GOM) model of CBA (see Chapter 1, this volume, and L. S. Fuchs & Deno, 1991). In either case, the measures must be direct (assess the outcome response), must be repeated (taken frequently throughout the intervention period), and must incorporate a time series analysis (graphed; Marston & Magnusson, 1988; Marston & Tindal, 1995). When subskill mastery monitoring is used, the evaluator is trying to determine whether the specific instructional objective that is being taught is being learned. For example, suppose it is determined during the assessment of instructional placement and instructional modification that a student does not understand the algorithm for regrouping in subtraction. The evaluator constructs a self-instruction procedure to help guide the student through the steps of the process as the intervention. To determine whether the student is learning the strategy, a math probe is constructed, consisting of subtracting two-digit from three-digit numbers with regrouping to the 10's and 100's columns. Repeated twice per week, the percentage of problems correct, as well as the number of digits correct per minute, are calculated. Increases evident in the graphed data would indicate that the student is learning the instructional objective being taught. Once the student reaches mastery level on this objective, the evaluator would repeat the process for any additional objectives that need to be taught. As one can see, this process informs the evaluator that the student has accomplished the short-term goals that were set when the intervention was begun.

Although a student may show consistent acquisition of short-term goals and objectives, the degree to which these accomplishments translate into reaching the yearlong curricular goals set by the teacher is unknown. For example, just because a student increases his or her performance in computational objectives of regrouping in subtraction may or may not impact on the student's overall performance to acquire mastery across all curricular objectives of that grade level. The assessment process for long-term measurement is best described by the type of progress monitoring developed in the curriculum-based measurement (CBM) model and is consistent with other general outcome measurement models of CBA (see Chapter 2).

The process of CBM or GOM uses a standardized, systematic, and repeated process of assessing students directly from material that reflects student outcomes from across all the curricular objectives for that year. For example, to assess a third-grade student in mathematics computation, the evaluator would first identify all computational objectives required for that student during the entire third grade. Drawing randomly from across these objectives, a set of probes consisting of approximately 20–30 problems would be developed. Each probe would then contain problems that reflect the expected performance across the curriculum. A student's score on these probes across time would reflect the degree to which the instructional processes occurring in the classroom were effective.

To illustrate, suppose the third-grade curriculum for mathematics computation indicates that students will be taught up to three-digit addition and subtraction with regrouping. Using CBM or GOM procedures, the evaluator develops a series of 36 probes (36 weeks of school × 1 probe per week) consisting of two- and three-digit addition and subtraction problems with regrouping. These probes are given to the students weekly. During the first few weeks of school, student performance on these probes may not be very high. However, as the teacher begins the process of teaching addition with regrouping, student performance on the probes should improve, if the instruction is effective. After all, the material being taught is appearing on the test, and the student's performance should reflect the learning that is occurring. As the year progresses, the student's performance should steadily increase as the skills are learned. Should the probes begin to show a pattern of no improvement or decline, the teacher would know that the instructional processes that had been working previously were no longer effective. Thus, the progress monitoring data offer a clear message that something in the instructional process needs to change.

Effective progress monitoring requires data collection for the assessment of both short- and long-term objectives. It is impossible to cover the details of all types of progress monitoring in the scope of this book. Readers are directed to several excellent sources that provide superb detail regarding the many forms of progress monitoring (see Howell et al., 1993; Marston & Magnusson, 1988; Shinn, 1989a, 1998). In this chapter, basic principles and examples of short- and long-term progress monitoring in reading, math, spelling, and written language are provided.

READING

General Outcome Measurement: Long-Term Monitoring

Selecting Probes

As with the assessment of instructional placement, the rate of a student's reading aloud of passages is used for long-term progress monitoring. However, unlike the earlier part of the assessment, the passages chosen to monitor the student are taken from goal-level material (i.e., material the student is expected to complete by the end of the assessment period). The determination of the material appropriate for monitoring was made during the assessment for instructional placement. In other words, if a fourth-grade student were found to be instructional at the second-grade level, using fourth-grade material to monitor his or her performance would likely result in little growth, because we are expecting him or her to demonstrate skills at a level that is clearly too difficult (i.e., frustration level). Likewise, monitoring the student in second-grade material may be too easy and result in a ceiling effect, thus showing no sensitivity to instruction. It is also possible that if the student were assessed in material in which he or she was being instructed, practice effects would impact the measurement. Thus, the selection of material for monitoring in this case would be third-grade material. Although this material might be above the student's current instructional level, it represents material that is likely to be sensitive to the instructional process.

In general, the material selected for monitoring should be at a level at which the student's performance is either instructional or just slightly frustrational. Selecting material that is too far from the student's assessed instructional level (as determined in Step 2 of the model) is likely to result in floor effects and show little change over time. Material that is too close to the instructional level may reflect ceiling or practice effects and, again, not be sensitive to student growth.

Questions often arise as to whether one should be using material in which students are currently being instructed, or material with which students are not familiar. A key aspect of using GOM, or long-term monitoring, is that the material being used is well controlled for level of difficulty. If students are supposedly being assessed in third-grade material, it is important that the readability of the material is indeed third grade. Most reading curricula used today in schools are literature-based materials that often do not carefully consider the readability of the material. Reading series are usually anthologies of published literature that are viewed by their developers as meeting the interests and reading levels for most students of the grade at which the particular book of the series is labeled. Although some attempt is made to examine the readability, it is not the only consideration in designating the specific grade level of the material.

When conducting GOM in reading, it is therefore recommended that one use material that is standardized and in which reading levels are carefully controlled. These passages can be used independent of the curriculum of instruction but have been shown to be sensitive to the instructional process. Within grade levels, the passages are controlled for difficulty, and passages increase in difficulty as one moves across different grades. Several commercially available products offer users sets of graded passages that can be used as GOM. Table 7.1 lists these products and where they can be found. In addition to these commercially available products, passages developed by various school districts (e.g., Minneapolis Pubic Schools, Kansas State Department of Education, Louisiana State University Reading Center) have been made available free-of-charge through the Intervention Central website (*http://www.interventioncentral.org*). The degree to which these free-download sites have carefully controlled for grade-level readability is unknown. If one chooses to use any of the available free sets of passages, it is highly recommended that the readability levels of the selected passages be evaluated prior to their use.

There are many formulas used to calculate readability. Popular formulas include the Dale–Chall, Spache, Fry, Flesch Grade, Flesch Reading Ease, FOG, SMOG, FORCAST, and Powers–Somner–Kearl. Each formula brings with it advantages and disadvantages. For example, the Dale–Chall

TABLE 7.1. Commercially Available Reading Passages for General Outcome Measurement

Product	Source
Reading Assessment Passages	AIMSweb (*http://www.aimsweb.com*)
Scholastic Fluency Formula Assessment	Scholastic Fluency (*http://teacher.scholastic.com/products/fluencyformula/*)
Standard Reading Passages	Children's Educational Services (*http://www.readingprogress.com*)
DIBELS (Dynamic Indicators of Basic Early Literacy Skills)	DIBELS Official home page, University of Oregon, College of Education (free download, (*http://dibels.uoregon.edu/*); also from Sopris West (*http://www.sopriswest.com*)
Sequenced Levels	Read Naturally (*http://readnaturally.com*)

and Spache formulas are based on difficulty level of vocabulary; the Dale–Chall is good for assessing upper elementary and secondary level material, and the Spache, for elementary grades up through grade 4. The Flesch Reading Ease formulas is used primarily for adult material, while the Flesch Grade formula is useful primarily with secondary level materials. The Fry formula is used over a wide range of materials from elementary through college levels, while formula such as the FOG are used primarily to obtain readability of materials in the health care and insurance industries. Some formulas, such as the SMOG, are focused on predicting levels of comprehension rather than reading fluency, and others, such as the FORCAST, are aimed at determining levels of functional literacy and used in development of survey instruments. Commercial software is available that offers calculations of all of these readability formula (*http://www.micropowerandlight.com*). Also, through the Intervention Central website, a free tool for building reading passages, as well as assessing readability with the Spache and Dale–Chall formulas, is available (*http://www.interventioncentral.org/htmdocs/tools/okapi/okapi.shtml*).

In addition to these readability formulas, more sophisticated readability formulas have been developed through using a Lexile® framework, which incorporates components of both vocabulary frequency, and sentence length and structure, two key features related to comprehension (see *http://www.lexile.com*). As such, these metrics for calibrating the reading level of passages are far from perfect. However, using the same formula consistently across passages will offer users an opportunity to establish some degree of relative difficulty across reading passages and help identify those passages that stray far from the expected grade level. Among all available formulas for calculating readability when working with reading materials for purposes of GOM, it is recommended that one use either the Fry formula or the Spache formula for materials of fourth grade or less, and the Dale–Chall formula for materials at fifth grade or above.

Developing Probes

Although using free or commercially available passages is highly recommended when conducting GOM monitoring in reading, it is also possible for interested users to develop their own generic passages or even to take passages from the material of instruction. Once the material for assessment is selected, a set of passages is developed from that material in the same way as described in Chapter 3. Each passage is randomly selected and retyped onto a separate page. Given that the readability of published texts can vary widely, it is recommended that the readability level of the passage be checked, so that it remains within ± 1 grade level of the material from which it was selected. As previously discussed, several formulas exist for checking readability, but it is recommended that either the Fry formula be used across all material or that the Spache formula be used for material at fourth grade or less, and the Dale–Chall formula for fifth grade and upward. Enough probes should be developed to assess students twice per week for an entire school year. Usually, this requires between 70 and 80 passages.

Administering and Scoring Probes

Students are asked to read each passage aloud for 1 minute. If students are unable to pronounce or phonetically decode words, they are prompted to continue after 3 seconds. Errors are scored only for omissions and mispronunciations, with self-corrections being scored as correct. The total number of words read correctly and incorrectly per minute are calculated.

Unlike the assessment of instructional placement, GOM monitoring involves only a 1-minute reading sample, with no assessment for comprehension. Studies have shown that this procedure can be conducted under conditions of self-, peer-, or teacher-monitoring with high levels of integrity and reliability (Bentz, Shinn, & Gleason, 1990; McCurdy & Shapiro, 1992).

Selecting Long-Range Goals

In order to provide meaningful interpretation of the data, it is important to select a long-range goal. Several approaches to establishing the goal are available, including the use of local norms, average learning rate, and mastery criteria (Marston & Tindal, 1995).

Use of local norms offers several advantages. First, the data to be used to set goal levels are based on the performance of large numbers of students from the same educational environment. As such, these students are likely to be representative of the performance levels expected of the student being assessed. Several sources are available for readers interested in the procedures to develop and maintain local norms (Canter, 1995; Shinn, 1988, 1989a, 1998). Although establishing local norms can be time-consuming and initially expensive in terms of personnel to collect the data, the results can be quite valuable in selecting appropriate goals for students, as well as establishing expected levels of performance over time.

Given that not all districts will have local norms available, it is possible to use several of the excellent sets of norms reported in the literature. For example, Table 7.2 lists norms reported by Hasbrouck and Tindal (1992), who summarized normative data taken from numerous districts (over 9,000 students) across the country. An important consideration in the selection of which normative data to use when a district does not have its own norms collected is the particular SES represented in the district. An excellent illustration of the degree to which districts of varying SES levels will vary in the normative performance of their students is shown in Chapter 4 (Table 4.1). Using the level of low-income population reported by the districts to determine SES, the performance across types of districts (urban = 59.5% low income, mixed urban–suburban = 33.8%, suburban = 6.3% low income) shows deep discrepancies across and within grades. For exam-

TABLE 7.2. Quartiles for Oral Reading Fluency Averaged across Up to Eight Different School Districts

Grade	Percentile	Fall	Winter	Spring	SD of raw scores
2	25	23	46	65	39
	50	53	78	94	
	75	82	106	124	
3	25	65	70	87	39
	50	79	93	114	
	75	107	123	142	
4	25	72	89	92	37
	50	99	112	118	
	75	125	133	143	
5	25	77	93	100	35
	50	105	118	128	
	75	126	143	151	

Note. From Hasbrouck and Tindal (1992, p. 42). Copyright 1992 by the Council for Exceptional Children. Reprinted by permission.

ple, a student reading at the 50th percentile of the low-income district in the winter of the fourth grade was found to be reading at 59 words correct per minute (WCPM). By comparison, students in the winter of the fourth grade reading at the 50th percentile of the high-income district, were found to be reading at 98 words WCPM, a discrepancy with 50th percentile readers at the same grade reading grade-level material of 39 WCPM. Clearly, districts using the available norms rather than collecting their own need to carefully match socioeconomic levels of their district against those of norms available for use. Failure to do so could easily lead to setting goals that are far too easy or too difficult to achieve.

In selecting goals for students, the evaluator should examine the current level of the student's performance and select a goal that is realistic yet ambitious. Using normative data can help the evaluator make this decision. For example, Figure 7.1, illustrates the performance of students across grades in a moderate-SES district. Each bar represents performance between the 25th and 75th percentiles on grade-based reading passages. A third-grade student is found in the fall to be reading at 38 WCPM in second-grade material, 32 WCPM in third-grade material, and 50 WCPM in first-grade material. Based on an assessment of instructional level, the student is placed in second grade materials for purposes of instruction. For students in this district, in the winter, students scoring at the 25th percen-

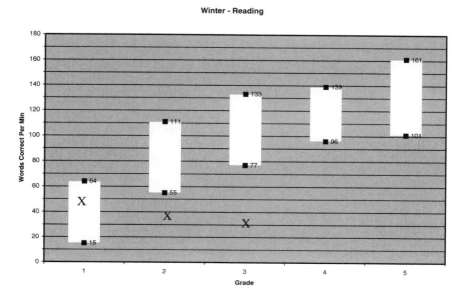

FIGURE 7.1. Goal chart of reading for winter in a moderate-SES school district.

tile in second grade were found to be reading at 55 WCPM. Using the goal chart, the teacher decides to teach the student using second-grade material and to establish a goal for the student to reach the 25th percentile for second-grade readers (i.e., 55 WCPM) by the middle of the winter, which is approximately 15 school weeks from the start of the monitoring process. This would establish an expected rate of growth of 1 word per week.

In establishing a yearlong goal for the target student, one may decide that a reasonable goal would be to move the student to a level equal to at least the 25th percentile of the third grade by the end of the school year. Looking at Figure 7.2, students at the 25th percentile in the spring are reading at 89 WCPM in third-grade material. Thus, a goal of 90 WCPM (rounding upward) is set for the target student once the student is moved to this level of material. This information is then added to the graph on which progress monitoring will be plotted.

A second method for establishing goals is to use an average learning rate for students. Used in combination with local norms, average learning rates establish the amount of gain that students are expected to make over each year of instruction.

L. S. Fuchs et al. (1993) reported progress monitoring data from 2 years in the areas of reading, math, and spelling. Table 7.3 shows the data for reading. These data can be used to establish the average expected levels of gain in oral reading rate across a year for other students. Although using

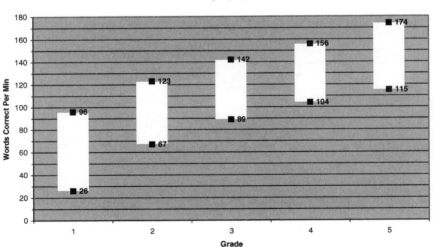

FIGURE 7.2. Goal chart of reading for spring in a moderate-SES school district.

TABLE 7.3. Means and Standard Deviations for Average Gains in Words Read Correct per Minute across 1 Year in Two Midwestern School Districts

Grade	Mean	SD
1	2.10	1.01
2	1.46	0.69
3	1.08	0.52
4	0.84	0.30
5	0.49	0.26
6	0.32	0.33

Note. Adapted from L. S. Fuchs, Fuchs, Hamlett, Walz, and Germann (1993, p. 34). Copyright 1993 by the National Association of School Psychologists. Adapted by permission.

data that come directly from the district where the student is enrolled would be better, the data provided by L. S. Fuchs et al. can be very helpful. For example, in the case of our third-grade student, it can be seen that the average third grader should make a 1.08 WCPM gain per week when instructed in third-grade materials. Since our student will initially be taught in second-grade materials, we may select the second-grade rate of improvement, 1.46 WCPM, as our target for the period of time he or she is instructed in those materials (i.e., 15 weeks). Once moved to third grade materials, and a new baseline is established, one would use the third-grade expected rate of improvement (i.e., 1.08 WCPM) to establish the goal for the remainder of the school year.

The slope of improvement, or average learning rate, can be plotted on the graph by simply multiplying the rate by the number of weeks over which the student will be instructed. In our example using 15 weeks, the expected performance level of our student from fall to winter, using an average rate of gain of 1.08 words per week, would result in a goal of 60 (38 + 22) WCPM at the end of the 15 weeks of monitoring.

A final method for selecting a goal is to use the criteria for instructional levels described in Chapter 4. These data offer general guidelines for expected levels of oral reading rates and can be useful in suggesting appropriate goals for performance. For example, with our fourth-grade student, we note that 70–100 WCPM represents the instructional level for third- and fourth-grade reading material. Given that our student is currently reading 40 WCPM in second-grade material, we might select a level of performance halfway between 70 and 100 (85) as our long-term goal. Although not as precise as using local norms, this procedure will offer a rough guideline for making goal-setting decisions.

Graphing Data

As already mentioned, the graphic depiction of progress monitoring is an essential feature of the procedure. Without graphic displays of the data, decisions about a student's progress are impossible. For most purposes, a simple equal interval graph is used. Time is indicated on the horizontal axis, with performance in oral reading rate scaled along the vertical axis. Marston (1988), in comparing both equal interval and semilogarithmic graphs, found that predictions of goals were more accurate with equal interval graphs. In addition, this type of graph is more understandable by teachers, parents, and students.

Graphs are designed to display student progress across the entire time period during which progress monitoring is being conducted. The graph contains the student's baseline level performance, a goal, an aim line (the line of progress that a student needs to establish to reach his or her goal), and the data collected during each progress monitoring period.

Several computer software programs have been developed to assist the graphing and data display process. For example, AIMSweb has developed a program that facilitates data entry, display, and decision making. The program offered by AIMSweb also provides data storage, as well as many other features to enhance the progress monitoring process. ChartDog, another free graphing service provided through the Intervention Central website (*http://www.interventioncentral.org*), provides graphing capability but does not offer the data monitoring and storage capacity of AIMSweb. Finally, any of the commonly available spreadsheets, such as Microsoft EXCEL, offer graphing capability as well.

Making Instructional Decisions

The most important part of the entire process of academic assessment occurs in this phase. The data collected must be used to make instructional decisions in order for the entire process to be valuable. For example, L. S. Fuchs, Fuchs, Hamlett, and Ferguson (1992) and L. S. Fuchs, Fuchs, Hamlett, and Stecker (1991) found that when a computerized expert system to assist teachers with making instructional decisions based on CBM data was not used, students showed poorer performance than when the expert system was used.

In order to use the data from progress monitoring to make effective instructional decisions, it is important to establish a set of decision-rules that guide the evaluator in determining whether the student is making progress toward the set goal. For example, L. S. Fuchs, Hamlett, and Fuchs (1999a, 1999b, 1999c), in their computerized progress monitoring system, use specific rules for evaluating the appropriateness of goals and determining whether teaching changes are needed. To monitor goal appropriateness, when at least six scores and at least 3 weeks have passed since the last goal was set, the four most recent scores are examined. If all scores are above the aim line, the program recommends that the goal be raised. Increasing the goal is also recommended if, after at least eight assessments and 3 weeks have passed, the program finds that the best line of fit (trend estimate) through the most recent 8–10 data points is steeper than the goal line. Others may simply set initial performance requirements, such as "If four consecutive data points fall below the aim line, a change in instructional intervention should be made."

Trend estimation can also be used. There are several approaches to trend estimation. Two of the more commonly used approaches in the special education literature are the split-middle or quarter-intersect (White & Haring, 1980) methods. Both techniques require that 9–12 data points be collected. In the split-middle technique, the entire data set is divided at the median data point. Next, the median score of each set of data is calculated and the two points are connected. This results in a trend estimation of the entire data set.

A more precise method of trend estimation is to calculate the ordinary least squares (OLS) regression line that fits the data series. This statistic is available with most spreadsheet computer programs used to graph data (e.g., Microsoft Excel®, Quatro-Pro®). In addition, Shinn, Good, and Stein (1989) found that the OLS can result in more accurate predictions than the split-middle technique.

Regardless of which method is used to analyze the data, evaluators need to make instructionally relevant decisions based on their data. Using the data to inform instruction requires that one use some form of data-based problem-solving routine. One such routine would be to divide the process of examining data into four steps using the acronym IDEA. For example, assuming the evaluator is using a decision rule of four data points above or below the aim line, the problem-solving routine would involve the following:

I. Inspect the last four data points.
D. Decide what the scores look like (Are they going up? Down? Variable?).
E. Evaluate why the scores are this way (Motivation? Attendance? Instruction?).
A. Apply a decision to improve achievement (continue instruction without change, increase goal, make a teaching change).

Using this type of problem-solving routine requires those who are collecting the data to use the data to inform instructional decisions.

As illustrated in Figure 7.3, three types of decisions should be considered when looking at the data. First, if the data show that a student is either making progress along his or her expected level of performance (i.e., actual performance closely matches the aim line), then one would conclude that the current instructional processes are successful and should be continued. Likewise, if a student were making progress that was parallel but below the aim line, the decision would also be to "wait and see whether the current instruction will soon improve student performance." Second, should the data show that the student is easily exceeding his or her goal early on in the instructional process, the goal should be increased. Small increments in the goal are appropriate and are decided based on the teacher's best judgment as to what he or she believes students can accomplish. Third, if applying the decision rules shows that the student's performance is not sufficient to make the year-end goal, a change in instructional procedures needs to be implemented. The exact nature of the change is based on an examination of the data that have been collected through the progress monitoring procedure, the informal observation of the instructor, an examination of the data collected during the implementation of the instructional modifications, as

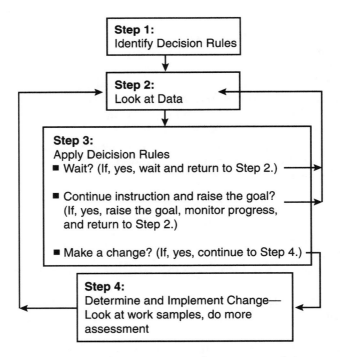

FIGURE 7.3. Flowchart of four-step process for instructional decision making.

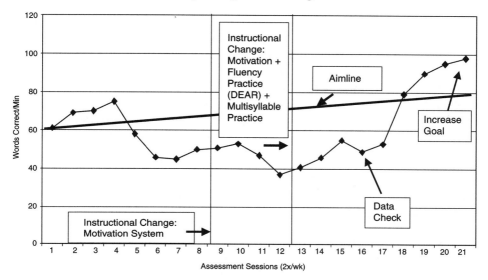

FIGURE 7.4. Progress monitoring of Jay's performance in reading.

well as any "best educational guesses" suggested by the many professionals working with the student. Whatever type of change is suggested, this is noted on the graph (usually by a solid line), and progress monitoring is continued.

Figure 7.4 shows the progress monitoring in reading over 10 weeks (two assessment sessions per week) of a third-grade student, Jay. Following an assessment of the academic environment and instructional placement, and establishing a baseline of 60 WCPM, a goal of 80 WCPM over 10 weeks was set, depicted by the solid line. In the first two weeks, Jay appears to be making good progress and, indeed, almost reaches the goal in only a short time period. Whatever instructional strategies the teacher is using at the time appear to be working. However, after four more data points are collected (2 more weeks), Jay appears to be experiencing difficulties. In using the IDEA problem-solving routine, the teacher and consultant believe that Jay's problem may be motivational. Based on discussions with the teacher, a motivational system is put in place, in which Jay sets daily instructional goals for his performance. Successfully meeting those goals earns Jay points that are redeemable toward homework passes.

After 2 more weeks of data collection, Jay's reading performance had not improved. In consultation with the teacher, it was decided that the motivational system was not sufficient, and additional instructional changes were needed. Specifically, the teacher felt that Jay was not getting enough practice in reading and added a simple intervention called DEAR (Drop Everything and Read). The intervention involved the teacher periodically during the instructional day announcing a "DEAR STOP," during which students were to stop what they were doing, pick up a book, and partner-read for 5 minutes. Also, the teacher noticed that Jay was struggling with multisyllabic words and developed a moderate-level intervention involving minilessons that were supplemental to the regular reading instruction to target this skill. During this intervention, the motivational system also remained in place.

At the next data checkpoint in 2 weeks, Jay's performance appeared to be starting to head in the upward direction. As a result, Jay's teacher decided to wait and see if the instructional program in place would begin showing its anticipated positive effect. In just 2 more weeks, at the next data checkpoint, the teacher found that the intervention plan was highly successful. Jay was now far exceeding his goal. As a result, the teacher decided it was time to raise the goal. After a new baseline was taken and Jay was reading at 85 WCPM, a goal of reading 110 words WCPM was established for the remainder of the school year.

An Alternative to Oral Reading Fluency

Although there is strong and substantial research supporting the use of the oral reading fluency metric as a key indicator of student progress in reading over time, there remains a significant suspicion among many educators that oral reading fluency does not effectively reflect acquisition of comprehension. Indeed, perhaps the greatest criticism of CBM comes from those in the reading field who doubt that a student's reading can be adequately reflected in oral fluency rates alone. Recognizing this problem, L. S. Fuchs and Fuchs (1992) identified an alternative to oral reading fluency that has a stronger comprehension component but is equally sensitive to student growth over time. The technique required students to read a passage in which every seventh word was omitted. Students were provided with three choices to replace the blank, only one of which made any sense in the context of the paragraph. This modified maze technique was implemented, using a computer program that generated graphic displays of student results. In the study, they compared the modified maze technique to a written cloze requiring an exact replacement, written retell using total words written as the score, and a written retell with a matched words written score. Results showed that the retell and cloze techniques were inadequate to reflect ongoing student progress in reading, whereas the criterion validity of the maze technique was very strong. L. S. Fuchs and Fuchs also reported that teachers saw the maze technique as an acceptable measure of decoding, fluency, and comprehension. L. S. Fuchs et al. (1993) provided normative data on the amount of progress students are expected to make over a year on this measure. Specifically, they noted that regardless of grade level, a reasonable level of progress would be at a rate of .39 correct replacements and that .84 correct replacements would be considered a challenging goal. Benchmark performance for students at the 50th percentile were approximately 15 to 17 correct replacements across the task. Modified maze measures that can be used without the assistance of computerized presentation are also available from AIMSweb (*www.aimsweb.com*). Because the maze task in AIMSweb is designed to be completed over a 3 rather than 2.5 minute period, the number of correct replacements at the 50th percentile across grades would be slightly higher than reported by the Fuchs et al. (1993) study and range between 18 and 20 correct replacements across the task.

Subskills Mastery: Short-Term Monitoring

When intervention strategies developed for instructional modification involve specific instructional objectives, the monitoring process for the mastery of those objectives requires the development of a teacher- or evaluator-made test that actually assesses the skill. The primary purpose of this form of assessment is to assist the evaluator in deciding what types of skills need to be taught and to potentially provide information about instructional modifications that may be effective. Howell and Nolet (1999) have identified this type of assessment as a "specific level assessment."

One type of specific level assessment would be a miscue analysis of oral reading fluency. Parker, Hasbrouck, and Tindal (1992) found that this type of analysis could be useful in some forms of progress monitoring. Figure 7.5 provides an example of the type of analysis that might be used when examining a student's performance on an oral reading task. Using these data, the evaluator can design an instructionally relevant program to impact the skills that are weak. Repeated use of this type of measure can be effective in determining whether the student is making progress in mastering these goals.

Another method for conducting short-term monitoring of reading progress is the repeated use of a teacher rating scale. This may be a particularly useful technique when the instructional objective focuses on improving reading comprehension. These measures, again, tend to be teacher- or evaluator-made and are tailored specifically to the instructional lessons being taught.

For example, a sixth-grade student, Ray, was found to have oral reading fluency commensurate with a sixth-grade level. However, an evaluation of his comprehension skills showed that he had great difficulty comprehending what he had read. Specifically, the evaluation showed that he had

ERROR PATTERN ANALYSIS

Student's name <u>Kara</u>   **Date** _____

Content Categories _____   **No. of Errors** _____

Words: errors involving whole words

polysyllabic words	<u>monito</u> (monitor, monshur, morish), also (always)
compound words	
sight words	the (th<u>a</u>t), were (w<u>as</u>), those (th<u>e</u>se), I'd (I'<u>ll</u>d)
silent letters	

Units: errors involving combined letter units

endings (suffixes)	
r-controlled vowels	person (<u>pre</u>son)
vowel teams	thought (that)
consonant digraphs (th, sh, ch, etc.)	thought (that)
consonant clusters (bi, br, ld, etc.)	
CVC words	

Conversions: errors involving sound modification

double consonant words	pepper (pe<u>tt</u>er)
vowel plus e conversions	

Sounds: errors involving individual letters and sounds

vowels	those (th<u>e</u>se), the (th<u>a</u>t), Mrs. (m<u>i</u>ss)
consonants	
sequence	
sounds	
symbols	

FIGURE 7.5. Error pattern analysis for decoding. From Howell, Zucker, and Morehead (1982). Copyright 1982 by The Psychological Corporation. Reprinted by permission.

great problems recognizing main ideas, discriminating relevant from irrelevant details, and making inferences beyond the factual information provided in the story read. After the assessment of the academic environment and instructional placement, the evaluator recommended that Ray be taught a webbing technique (see Chapter 6) to increase his comprehension skills. To assess the acquisition of his comprehension skills, a brief five-item checklist was created (see Figure 7.6). Twice each week, Ray was given a new passage to read. After completing his web, Ray was asked to discuss the story with his teacher, who then completed the checklist. Scores across 5 weeks on each item are shown in Table 7.4. These data reflect the impact of the webbing strategy on Ray's performance.

Another technique that can be useful for short-term monitoring in reading is the use of an oral retell technique. This is particular valuable for narrative text. In the technique, students are asked to read a passage of 200–300 words. Immediately following the reading, students are asked to tell what they read in their own words. The retell can be scored for the presence or absence of elements of the story, such as theme, problem, goal, setting, and so forth. If the retell is aided by the examiner, this can also be indicated. Figure 6.5 illustrates such a scoring technique. Although the retell technique has not fared well in terms of being sensitive to growth across curriculum objectives (L. S. Fuchs & Fuchs, 1992), it may be useful as an indicator of improvement when specific comprehension skills are being taught.

It is important to remember that the use of short-term monitoring is primarily focused on diagnosing the instructional process. As such, it does not meet the psychometric standards of typical progress-monitoring measures. Consistent with a specific subskills mastery model, these methods of monitoring student progress will vary each time a new instructional objective is developed. However, the measures can be very helpful in assisting an

TEACHER RATING MEASURE FOR COMPREHENSION

	Poor			Excellent	
1. Ability to recognize main ideas	1	2	3	4	5
2. Recognition of relevant details	1	2	3	4	5
3. Discriminates relevant from irrelevant detail	1	2	3	4	5
4. Inferences beyond story detail	1	2	3	4	5
5. Overall comprehension skill rating	1	2	3	4	5

FIGURE 7.6. Example of teacher rating measure for assessment of reading comprehension.

TABLE 7.4. Scores on Biweekly Comprehension Probes by Ray's Teachers

Probe no.	Ray's scores on Teacher Comprehension Rating Form				
	MI	DET	D/I	INF	OVR
1	2	3	1	1	2
2	2	3	1	1	2
3	3	3	2	1	2
4	3	3	2	1	2
5	3	3	1	2	2
6	4	4	2	1	3
7	4	4	2	2	3
8	4	4	3	1	3
9	3	4	3	2	3
10	4	4	3	1	3

Note. MI, main idea; DET, relevant detail; D/I, discriminates relevant–irrelevant detail; INF, inferences beyond story; OVR, overall comprehension rating.

evaluator in making effective and relevant recommendations for whether the recommended changes in instruction have been effective in teaching the student the specific skill that the instructional method was designed to teach.

MATHEMATICS

General Outcome Measurement: Long-Term Monitoring

Selecting Probes

As noted in Chapter 3, CBA of math focuses on the acquisition of computational skills as well as concepts–applications of mathematical principles. In choosing the material for assessment, it is important to understand how curricula in math are structured. An examination of the scope and sequence for any published math curriculum shows that the curriculum is recursive. Skills are often introduced and practiced in one grade and then reappear over the next several grades. Mastery of the skill is not expected until several grades after the skill is first taught.

Given that math objectives are repeated over several grades makes selection of material for monitoring important. If the examiner selects the content of the assessment from the objectives being taught at the grade level of instruction, the student is likely to have some problems where mastery is expected, and other problems in the acquisition (instructional) stage of the learning process. Such information would be valuable in informing the evaluator as to the level of student performance within grade-level material. On the other hand, if the material chosen for assessment comes only from instructional objectives where mastery is expected, the outcomes provide the evaluator with information about the student's long-term mastery of computation.

In most CBA long-term progress monitoring, the material selected for assessment involves multiple-skill probes taken from across grade-level computational objectives. Material selected for assessment is usually taken from the grade level or one grade level below the level at which the student is being instructed. This is determined through the teacher interview conducted as part of the assessment of the academic environment, as well as initial assessment that results in performance levels that do not represent either highly frustrational or mastery-level material. It is important to realize that if a student is found during the assessment of instructional placement to have significant deficiencies in computational objectives occurring far below his or her grade level, conducting the progress-monitoring process at grade level may result in a potential floor effect. As such, it may be necessary to select material a year or two below current grade-level functioning, if progress monitoring is to be effective. For example, suppose a fourth-grade student is found to be frustrational in addition with regrouping, a skill initially introduced in the third grade of the curriculum. Using fourth-grade level material for progress monitoring that contains many computational objectives for which addition with regrouping is a prerequisite skill is likely to result in a lack of sensitivity to instruction; thus, the student shows little growth over time. In such a case, using third-grade level computational probes would be recommended.

Developing Probes

Probes for the long-term monitoring in mathematics are developed by randomly selecting problems from across the grade-level curricular objectives chosen for assessment. A total of 35–70 probes, each containing 20–30 problems, is usually developed to allow monitoring to occur approximately once or twice per week for a full academic year. Because each probe contains items selected from across grade-level curriculum objectives, the administered CBM test should reflect student gains in the curriculum over time.

Obviously, it would be somewhat time-consuming to develop a set of 35–70 math probes per grade level, each containing a set of problems that represents the entire curriculum. There are several available computer programs, however, that can be used to generate these problems.

L. S. Fuchs et al. (1999a) in their program, Monitoring Basic Skills Progress: Basic Math Computation, provide a set of black-line masters consisting of grade-level problems that have already been developed. These can be scored by the teacher or student using the computer program. L. S. Fuchs et al. (1999c) have developed a set of black-line masters for assessing concepts–applications in math as well.

Another computer program for generating math worksheets is found at *www.edhelper.com*. This website offers a very wide range of math probes, including both computation and concepts–applications, available for no charge and on a subscriber basis. Included in the website are numerous single and multiple-skills worksheets that can be generated for use in progress monitoring. Schoolhouse Technologies, Inc., also offers a downloadable set of programs called the Mathematics Worksheet Factory (*www.schoolhousetech.com*), which provides an easy-to-use program that allows users to create their own worksheets in all areas of mathematics (as well as other subjects). The program has a free demonstration version available for educators, as well as a commercially available project. A similar set of materials can be found at the aplusmath website (*www. aplusmath.com*). Finally, *www.interventioncentral.org* offers a free worksheet generator for assessing computation that is tied closely to specific computational objectives, as well as an available program that provides mixed operation worksheets.

Administering and Scoring Probes

Probes are administered in much the same way as the assessment of instructional placement described in Chapter 3. Students are given specific time limits to complete as many problems as they can. As the grade level of the students increases, so does the complexity of the problems; thus, the amount of time permitted to complete the probe increases. Table 7.5 lists the recommended time limits for students being monitored within computation and concepts–application probes. Students are instructed to work on the problems in sequence, doing problems they can do quickly right away

TABLE 7.5. Recommended Time Limits
for Students Monitored in Math
Computation and Concepts/Applications

Grade	Computation	Concepts
1	2 min	N/A
2	2 min	8 min
3	3 min	6 min
4	3 min	6 min
5	5 min	7 min
6	6 min	7 min

and skipping those that are difficult, then returning to those difficult problems when they have gone through the entire set. Students are stopped when the time expires, or when they have completed all the problems on the sheet.

Students are given the probes once or twice per week, although it has been found that once-a-week assessment of math is usually sufficient to show sensitivity to student growth. Given time constraints, it is also possible to conduct an assessment of computation one week and concepts–applications the next. Our own research with this process has shown that data collected this way over an entire academic year are quite sensitive to instruction and instructional changes (Shapiro et al., in press). The one disadvantage of collecting data at this pace is that several weeks must elapse before sufficient data are collected to allow for an accurate assessment of trend. Those conducting progress monitoring in math need to make collaborative decisions with teachers as to the feasibility of weekly or biweekly data collection.

The probes for computation are scored for digits correct and incorrect per minute, as described in Chapter 3. (Detailed descriptions of the use of this metric, along with several practice exercises, can be found in the workbook accompanying this text.) An error analysis can also be performed by looking at results of individual items to examine which of the computational objectives the student has mastered, partially mastered, or not mastered. The computer program by L. S. Fuchs et al. (1999a) conducts such an analysis automatically. Results of this analysis can be useful in planning future instructional objectives.

It is also possible to score math computation data used for purposes of progress monitoring by only counting the digits correct (and incorrect) within the answer. Although excluding some digits below the answer line (i.e., in multidigit multiplication, not counting digits except in the final answer) does reduce some of the sensitivity of the digits-per-minute metric, substantial research has shown that the measures can still be quite sensitive to change over time if only the answers are examined for accuracy (e.g., L. S. Fuchs at al., 1999a, 1999c; Shapiro et al., in press).

Although the digits-per-minute metric can be used in progress monitoring for computation, much of the CBM math literature has used the *total* digits metrics instead of digits per minute. Use of total digits results in data that are simple to score (i.e., no need to divide by the number of minutes of the assessment) and have been found to be more interpretable by teachers. For example, a student completing a 3-minute probe found to have 10 total digits correct at baseline would be reported as 3.3 digits correct per minute. If the student improves by one total digit following a week of instruction, the student will have grown by 0.3 digits correct per minute. Despite the mathematical equivalence of a change from 10 to 11 total digits and from 3.3 to 3.6 digits correct per minute, it has been my experience that teachers have difficulty recognizing that a change of 0.3 digits correct per minute in a week is a meaningful unit of improvement. They have less difficulty seeing the change in total digit units. As such, it is recommended that progress monitoring for computation be done in total digits correct rather than digits correct per minute.

Probes for concepts–applications are scored based on the number of problems that students do correct rather than on the number of digits produced for each problem. For example, using the concepts–application probes developed by L. S. Fuchs et al. (1999c), problems are divided into several parts. Each part of a problem is regarded as a point, and the number of points is totaled. Because each grade level has a somewhat different level of possible points, the number of points can also be divided by total points to determine the percentage of possible points scored. However, similar to the use of total digits correct for progress monitoring of computation, *total points* is also an easy metric for teachers to score and interpret. Shapiro et al. (in press) found that use of total points was able to reflect yearlong gains in progress monitoring of concepts–applications and is the metric most often used in studies where concepts–applications were monitored.

Setting Long-Term Goals

Long-term goals in math are determined in the same ways as in reading. Local normative data collected in fall, winter, and spring can be developed and used to signal the expected performance in terms of digits correct per minute per grade level. Average learning rate normative data can also be collected. L. S. Fuchs et al. (1993, 1999c) provided such data for a large number of students monitored once per week in computation (total digits) and concepts–applications (total points) (see Table 7.6). Shapiro (2003b) also reported outcomes of normative data collection for computation (total digits) conducted in a high- and moderate-level SES school districts when data were collected at both grade and instructional levels (i.e., one level below grade level) (see Table 7.7).

These data raise questions about the appropriate goal to set for students once the instructional level of progress monitoring is decided. A good recommendation based on these data is to set goals for students that are at least between the lowest and highest levels found in the research. For example, as seen in Table 7.6 for fourth graders, a level of gain equal to 0.69 digits per week, or 28 digits per year (based on a 40-week school year), would be an expected level of growth for these students. The norms offered in Table 7.7 for a moderate-level SES district, suggest a gain of 24 total digits per year at grade level (i.e., 14 digits in fall, 38 in spring). Thus, setting a

TABLE 7.6. Computation (Total Digits) and Concepts–Applications (Total Points) Findings from Two Studies on Gain Rates per Week and per Year (Based on a 40-Week School Year)

Grade	Computation (1993)		Computation (1999)		Concepts (1999)	
	Gain/wk	Gain/yr	Gain/wk	Gain/yr	Gain/wk	Gain/yr
1	0.34	13.6	—	—	—	—
2	0.28	11.2	0.25	10.0	0.40	16
3	0.30	12.0	0.63	25.2	0.58	23.2
4	0.69	27.6	0.70	28.0	0.69	27.6
5	0.74	29.6	0.38	15.2	0.19	7.6
6	0.42	16.8	0.26	10.4	0.12	4.8

Note. Data from studies of L. S. Fuchs, Fuchs, Hamlett, Walz, and Germann (1993) and L. S. Fuchs, Hamlett, and Fuchs (1999c).

goal level initially at a point halfway between these two points (i.e., 26 total digits per year), would be a reasonable and logical guess. It is still recommended that evaluators use good judgment working with the data, because goal levels are set to avoid levels that are far too challenging or too easy for students.

Graphing

Graphic display of the data remains an essential feature of the progress monitoring process. These graphs can be either hand-drawn or computer generated. For example, the L. S. Fuchs et al. (1999a, 1999c) computer program automatically draws and updates student graphs as the data are collected. These graphs offer opportunities for feedback to students and can be very useful for student motivation, as well as helping teachers make instructional recommendations. In addition, as described previously, any spreadsheet program with graphing capability can be used.

Making Instructional Decisions

The data obtained from progress monitoring in math are interpreted in much the same way as in reading, using the same IDEA acronym presented previously. Using a priori decision rules, outcomes generated by the data tell the evaluator whether the current instructional procedures are having their desired impact. When the data series suggests that the goal needs to be altered or an instructional change needs to be made, the graphic display of the progress monitoring data is used to verify that the new procedures are indeed effective.

TABLE 7.7. Math Computation Normative Data from a Moderate- and High-SES District

	Moderate-SES district					High-SES district			
Grade	Grade level	SD	Below grade level	SD	Grade	Grade level	SD	Below grade level	SD
				Fall					
1	3	3			1	8	4		
2	9	7	16	9	2	11	5	15	8
3	8	5	25	12	3	21	12	45	16
4	14	12	18	16	4	38	16	52	18
5	33	6	61	29	5	38	21	70	26
				Winter					
1	6	7			1	14	8		
2	15	10	23	11	2	15	8	24	12
3	17	10	29	12	3	29	16	41	18
4	32	16	37	17	4	62	23	67	24
5	38	24	64	28	5	53	23	85	32
				Spring					
1	14	7			1	16	9		
2	19	11	31	13	2	22	11	29	14
3	28	18	36	16	3	39	20	46	17
4	38	16	50	28	4	62	23	67	24
5	46	22	83	31	5	53	23	85	32

Note. Data reported in total digits correct for both grade level and instructional grade level (one level below grade level).

Progress monitoring data in math can also be used to identify what potential skills may need specific instruction. The evaluator can examine each probe produced by the student for an analysis of the types of problems with which the student is experiencing difficulties. This would help the instructor plan the teaching necessary for the student to learn this skill. As noted previously, the computer program developed by L. S. Fuchs et al. (1999a, 1999c) does this automatically as the data are entered. Using this program, L. S. Fuchs, Fuchs, Phillips, Hamlett, and Karns (1995) combined a classwide peer-tutoring program in mathematics with progress monitoring. Using the results of weekly CBM tests, computerized feedback was provided to select the instructional objectives to be taught through a peer-tutoring format. Results of the study showed that the combination of these two procedures was very powerful in producing substantial improvements in the mathematics performance of students. Numerous replications of this program have found the combination of GOM and classwide peer tutoring to be a powerful combination in improving student outcomes in mathematics (e.g., Calhoun & Fuchs, 2003; L. S. Fuchs, Fuchs, & Karns, 2001).

Short-Term Monitoring

As noted previously for reading, the primary objective of short-term monitoring is to assess whether a student has achieved the specific curriculum objective that has been instructed. In addition, through short-term monitoring, an error analysis can be performed to reveal the patterns of mistakes that a student is making. This assessment involves the use of single-skill probes.

Single-skill math probes, as described in Chapter 3, are used. The same computer-based resources described previously for conducting long-term monitoring contain opportunities to generate single-skill probes as well. Performance on these probes, before and after instruction on a particular objective, provides the data for determining whether the student is reaching mastery. For example, if the assessment of instructional placement shows a student to be deficient in knowing the algorithm for 2-digit by 2-digit multiplication, the repeated administration of a probe after the strategy was developed to teach this skill would demonstrate the short-term monitoring procedure for acquiring this skill. Although it is possible to obtain such data from the long-term monitoring process as well, because the probes will contain some problems derived from all grade-level curricular objectives, it is important to recognize that the long-term monitoring probes may have only one or two problems that are representative of the skill being taught. As such, there may be limited opportunities to carefully assess exactly the types of errors that students are making. Use of single-skill probes, often given under untimed conditions, permits the evaluator to get a more detailed picture of how a student attacks a particular type of computational problem.

Math probes are analyzed to determine whether students are demonstrating difficulties with knowledge of facts, operations, place value, algorithms, or problem solving. Problems with math facts are seen when students consistently add, subtract, multiply, or divide incorrectly. These problems are due to the lack of mastery of basic math facts, such as multiplying 9×7 and getting 56. Errors in operations occur when students add instead of subtract, or add instead of multiply. For example, Figure 7.7 shows the performance of a student with problems in operation. This student understands the concept of subtraction but consistently performs subtraction rather than attend to the sign indicated for each problem.

Errors in place value usually occur if students are having difficulty with the concept of regrouping. Here, students fail to align numerals prop-

```
   8          3          5          3
 - 5        + 3        - 2        + 1
 ───        ───        ───        ───
   3          0          3          2


   7          4          7          4
 - 5        + 2        - 2        + 1
 ───        ───        ───        ───
   2          2          5          3
```

FIGURE 7.7. Example of errors in operation.

erly and do not recognize the properties of placing numbers into their respective columns (1's, 10's, 100's, etc.). Algorithm problems are a common source of error in math computation. Students who have problems in this area do not understand the correct sequence of steps in completing the problem. For example, as seen in Figure 7.8, although Bill knows his addition math facts, he does not understand the algorithm for adding 2-digit numbers. In fact, Bill's approach to the problem is simply to add everything. An interesting point that might be raised about Bill's behavior is that the algorithm he is apparently using to add is similar to one used in the process of multiplying 2-digit numbers. It might be useful to examine whether multiplication is a skill currently being taught in the classroom, and whether this is partially causing some of Bill's confusion.

A final area of error analysis in math computation is the examination of a student's problem-solving skills. In particular, it is possible to see whether a student uses or understands the process of estimation. For example, Bill's responses to the addition problem show clear signs that he does not use any form of estimation in determining whether his answers are correct. This may point to another area that is ripe for possible intervention.

Readers interested in more detailed examples and exercises to analyze common sources of errors in math should see the workbook accompanying this text, as well as excellent texts by Howell and Nolet (1999), Salvia and Hughes (1990), and Rosenfield and Gravois (1995).

```
     7           11           15           12
 +   8        +   7        + 33         + 26
 ─────        ─────        ─────        ─────
    15           18         4848         3478


     4           15           26           11
 +   8        +   5        + 32         + 67
 ─────        ─────        ─────        ─────
    12           20         5948         7788
```

FIGURE 7.8. Example of errors in algorithm for Bill.

SPELLING

Long-Term Monitoring

Selecting Probes

The decisions that guide the selection of material for long-term progress monitoring of spelling are similar to those used in reading. Using the information from the assessment of the academic environment and the assessment of instructional placement, the grade level at which the student is instructional was identified. In choosing material for monitoring, it is typical that the evaluator uses this level of material for monitoring. Rather than selecting material somewhat beyond the current instructional level, as was recommended for reading, it is more common to use the level at which the student is actually being instructed in spelling. Although this may present some problems in terms of practice effects, using the instructional level material will assure the evaluator of good sensitivity in the data to the instructional process.

Developing Probes

When spelling is being taught from a published spelling series, finding the material to select for developing probes is relatively simple. Once the level in the series at which the student is instructional has been identified (in Step 2, Assessing Instructional Placement), the evaluator will find at the end of each level of the series a list of new spelling words taught from that level. The probes are developed by randomly selecting a list of between 12 and 17 words (12 for grades 1 and 2, 17 for grade 3 and up) from the entire pool of words that the student will be taught across the school year. Approximately 70- to 80-word lists are developed to permit up to two assessments per week.

In recent years, the frequency of spelling instruction delivered from published spelling curricula has steadily diminished. More and more, spelling is being taught as a subject integrated within language arts, reading, and other content areas. When spelling lists are generated for the typical Friday spelling test found in many elementary schools, the words on the list are coming from various nonstandardized sources. Given that long-term progress monitoring requires a systematic, standardized methodology, using such material for progress monitoring would be difficult and is not recommended.

An alternative to long-term progress monitoring, when the instruction is not from a published spelling curriculum, is to use already prepared graded word lists. L. S. Fuchs, Hamlett, and Fuchs (1990) in their computerized program, Monitoring Basic Skills Progress: Spelling, provide a set of such word lists for grades 1–6. Derived from the Harris–Jacobson (Harris & Jacobson, 1972) word lists, the evaluator can use these lists to assess a student's progress in spelling, even if spelling is being taught from nonstandard material. A similar set of materials for grades 1–8 is available from AIMSweb (*www.aimsweb.com*), where lists of spelling words from across various curricula were assembled and tested to be sure that the words assigned to a particular grade level were likely to be words that would be taught at that specific grade level.

Administering and Scoring Probes

Spelling probes are administered and scored in the same way as the probes used in the assessment of instructional placement (Chapter 3). Words are dictated at a rate of one word every 7 seconds for grades 3 and up, and one word every 10 seconds for grades 1 and 2, until the list is exhausted. Scoring is done using letters in a sequence (see Chapter 3) and the percentage of words spelled correctly. (More detailed explanation of letters in a sequence and practice exercises for learning how to score spelling this way are provided in the workbook accompanying this text.) In both the L. S. Fuchs et al. (1990) computerized spelling program and the available progress monitoring module of AIMSweb, the results of the spelling probes are entered and automatically scored for both metrics.

Setting Long-Term Goals

The procedures for selecting long-term goals in spelling are no different than they were for reading or math. Use of local norms, learning-rate norms, and the criteria for the assessment of instructional placement can all be applied. Table 7.8 provides normative data from L. S. Fuchs et al. (1993), indicating the average learning rates across over 3,000 students from grades 1–5.

Graphing

As with all other areas of long-term progress monitoring, data from the assessment of spelling are graphed. Although spelling can be graphed and scored for percentage of words correct, the letters-in-a-sequence data are more often used, because these data tend to be more sensitive to small changes in performance than percentage of words spelled correctly. The L. S. Fuchs et al. (1990) and the AIMSweb computer programs automatically provide this graph.

TABLE 7.8. Means and Standard Deviations for Average Gains (Slope) on Letter Sequences and Words Correct in Spelling across 1 Year for Students in Five Midwestern School Districts

Grade	Letter sequences		Words correct	
	Mean	SD	Mean	SD
2	.92	.48	.17	.10
3	.57	.34	.11	.09
4	.48	.50	.09	.07
5	.41	.41	.06	.07
6	.46	.31	.09	.09

Note. Adapted from L. S. Fuchs, Fuchs, Hamlett, Walz, and Germann (1993 p. 38). Copyright 1993 by the National Association of School Psychologists. Adapted by permission.

Making Instructional Decisions

The data from long-term progress monitoring in spelling indicate the degree to which student performance is being affected by the instructional process. The same types of decision rules applied for reading and math are used to determine whether a change in goals or instructional methods is warranted.

Short-Term Monitoring

Like other areas of instruction, the short-term progress monitoring of spelling is designed to assist the evaluator in identifying the specific skills that the student may be having difficulty learning and involves the use of primarily teacher-made tests. The primary purpose of the monitoring process, however, is to diagnose the student's performance and to identify clear targets for instruction. Unlike the areas of reading and math, however, short-term monitoring of spelling can be ascertained directly from the long-term progress monitoring probes.

By conducting an analysis of error types, the evaluator is able to determine the kinds of skills a student may need to be taught. This is accomplished most easily if a computerized program is used, such as the one developed by L. S. Fuchs et al. (1990). As seen in Figure 7.9, the computer program examines the last 50 words of the student's progress monitoring tests and provides a list of the error types and their frequency. From this information, evaluators can design instructional methods that will emphasize the teaching of these skills. The repeated assessment process used in

```
--------------------------------------------------------------------------------
NAME: Charles Landrum          Spelling 4              Date:  4/10        Page 1
--------------------------------------------------------------------------------


Corrects      (100% LS)              14 word(s)
Near Misses   (60-99%  LS)           19 word(s)
Moderate Misses (10-59% LS)          16 word(s)
Far Misses    (0-19% LS)              1 word(s)
```

Type	Correct	Possible	Pct	Type	Correct	Possible	Pct
Sing cons	48	50	96	Final vow	3	7	42
Blend	7	10	70	Double	3	4	75
FSLZ	0	0	100	c/s	0	1	0
Single vow	21	31	67	c/ck	0	2	0
Digraph	6	8	75	-le	4	7	57
Vowel + N	6	8	75	Ch/tch	2	2	100
Dual cons	13	25	52	-dge	0	1	0
Final e	1	5	52	Vowel team	4	12	33
igh/ign	0	0	100	Suffix	5	6	83
ild/old	0	0	100	tion/sion	0	1	0
a+l+cons	0	0	100	ance/ence	0	0	100
Vowel + R	9	14	64	sure/ture	0	0	100

KEY ERRORS

Dual cons	Final e	Final vow
learner—leaner	alone—alon	taste—tast
sample—samble	knife—knif	hero—hearow
chart—chard	rare—rar	lazy—lazz
mumble—mobble	cube—cub	unlucky—unluke
tractor—trater		
apart—apeot		

FIGURE 7.9. Example of skills analysis in spelling from Monitoring Basic Skills Progress. From L. S. Fuchs, Fuchs, Hamlett, and Allinder (1991, p. 56). Copyright 1991 by the National Association of School Psychologists. Reprinted by permission.

long-term progress monitoring allows the evaluator to see whether the student reduces the frequency of a specific type of error over time.

WRITTEN LANGUAGE

Long-Term Monitoring

The long-term monitoring of performance in written language is identical to the technique for monitoring described in Chapter 3 for assessing instructional placement. Students are asked to write for 3 minutes using a story starter provided by the evaluator collected once per week. Outcomes are scored for total words written but can also be scored for the presence or absence of specific skills. Performance is graphed, and decision rules are applied to determine whether the goals or instructional methods need to be altered.

Short-Term Monitoring

More attention in progress monitoring of written language is devoted to short-term monitoring than to many other areas. Because written language involves the integration of multiple skills, all of which are needed for producing good written products (i.e., grammar, handwriting, planning, punctuation, creativity, thought, etc.), the short-term monitoring process is usually designed to evaluate whether the instructional methods are resulting in the acquisition of these skills.

Scoring of written language samples usually relies on the use of both quantitative and qualitative (subjective judgment) measurement. For example, Table 7.9 shows a list of 12 measures developed by Zipprich (1995) to score narrative written essays of children ages 9–12 years. She also developed a holistic scoring checklist and a scale for evaluating the student's performance for scoring these essays (see Figure 7.10). The repeated administration, along with graphing of these data, can be used to determine whether specific instructional techniques developed to improve the student's skills are evident. Zipprich found that teaching webbing techniques was successful at improving over baseline the number of words for 9 of 13 students, the number of thought units for 7 students, the density factor (ideas in thought units) for 7 students, and the planning time for all students. Holistic scores for all students improved over baseline. Although beyond the study reported by Zipprich, the data from the individual students across these skills could be used to design instructional programs aimed to improve the specific skills not impacted by the webbing technique.

Graham and Harris (1989) described a similar scale to assess writing skills. In their scale, the presence or absence of eight elements of story grammar were assessed: main character, locale, time, starter event, goal, action, ending, and reaction. For each element, scores from 0 to 4 were assigned. Likewise, a holistic scale using a 1 (lowest quality) to 7 (highest quality) rating was employed. These measures were used to assess change in student writing performance over time, following a self-instruction training procedure.

SUMMARY

The final step in the assessment of academic skills involves the assessment of student progress over time. Goals are set for short- and long-term objectives, and progress toward these goals is measured. Progress monitoring in all four areas of basic skills instruction contains both long- and short-term objectives. The primary purpose of GOM long-term monitoring is to determine the impact of the instructional process on the accomplishment of

TABLE 7.9. Target Behaviors Used to Score Narrative Essay Exams

Behavior	Definition	Measurement
1. Planning time	Length of time, measured in minutes, a student requires to complete "My Web for Story Writing."	Teacher records minutes on blackboard.
2. Words produced	Individual words produced by a student within a story.	Evaluator count.
3. Thought unit	A group of words that cannot be further divided without the disappearance of its essential meaning.	Evaluator count.
Sentence types		
4. Fragment	An incomplete thought.	Evaluator count.
5. Simple	A sentence expressing a complete thought that contains a subject and predicate.	Evaluator count.
6. Compound	A sentence containing two or more simple sentences but no subordinate clauses.	Evaluator count.
7. Compound/ complex	A sentence containing two or more simple sentences and one or more subordinate clauses.	Evaluator count.
8. Holistic score	A quality-of-writing factor developed by this researcher.	A 14-item criteria checklist used to render a score that converts to a Likert scale score of 1.0–3.0.
Mechanics		
9. Spelling	A subjective evaluation of overall spelling accuracy.	Scale developed by researcher.
10. Capitals	A subjective evaluation of correct use of capitalization as taught through standard English language text.	
11. Punctuation	A subjective evaluation of correct use of punctuation as taught through standard English language text.	Scale developed by researcher.
12. Density factor	A quality factor developed by researcher to measure amount of information contained in each thought unit.	A criteria checklist used to render a score for number of ideas included in a thought unit.

Note. From Zipprich (1995, p. 7). Copyright 1995 by Pro-Ed, Inc. Reprinted by permission.

	Evaluator		Checker		Comparison
	Yes	No	Yes	No	
1. Did the student include a title?	___	___	___	___	___
2. Did the student have a clear introduction to the story (i.e., a statement of the problem or beginning of the story line?)	___	___	___	___	___
3. Did the student identify characters?	___	___	___	___	___
4. Did the student state the goal of the story?	___	___	___	___	___
5. Did the student add action to the story?	___	___	___	___	___
6. Did the student state an outcome?	___	___	___	___	___
7. Did the student write more than one paragraph?	___	___	___	___	___
8. Did each paragraph deal with only one topic?	___	___	___	___	___
9. Are the major points in each paragraph presented in a correct sequence?	___	___	___	___	___
10. Do the paragraphs have a beginning sentence that adequately introduces the idea discussed?	___	___	___	___	___
11. Is each paragraph started on a new line?	___	___	___	___	___
12. Did the student sequence the story appropriately?	___	___	___	___	___
13. Did the student include only relevant information?	___	___	___	___	___
Total "YES"	___	___	___	___	___
Conversion Score*	___	___	___	___	___

*Holistic Score Conversion Scale

Total =	Score =	Status
0–3	1.0	Unacceptable
4–7	1.5	Unacceptable/some improvement
8–10	2.0	Acceptable with errors/needs improvement
11–12	2.5	Acceptable with errors/showing improvement
13–14	3.0	Acceptable/meets criteria

FIGURE 7.10. Holistic scoring device used for evaluating written language skills. From Zipprich (1995, p. 8). Copyright 1995 by Pro-Ed, Inc. Reprinted by permission.

long-range curriculum goals set by the instructor. Typically, these are year-long goals.

Long-term data are always graphed. Viewed as an essential element of progress monitoring, the graphic display of the data offers continual feedback to the evaluator and student about progress toward these goals. Using decision rules established before the monitoring begins, decisions to change goals or alter instructional methods are made. In most cases, however, the long-term monitoring data do not tell the evaluator about the specific skills areas that need to be targeted, nor the possible instructional techniques that may be useful to improve student performance.

To determine the specific skills that may have to be targeted for improvement, short-term progress monitoring is used. The primary objective of these data is to guide the evaluator in developing effective intervention techniques. By knowing the specific skills that a student needs to master, strategies aimed at teaching those skills can be developed.

It is critical to recognize that both types of progress monitoring are needed to provide a clear picture of a student's progress. The evaluator usually starts with long-term progress monitoring, because a student maintaining performance along the designated aim line under long-term monitoring conditions suggests to the evaluator that the current instructional methods are working fine, and there is no need to change. However, when the instructional methods are no longer successful, short-term monitoring offers the evaluator a methodology for better determining the targets for intervention, as well as assisting in development of better strategies for instruction.

CHAPTER 8

◆ ◆ ◆

Case Illustrations

◆

In this chapter, a number of examples illustrating the use of the assessment procedures and some of the interventions described in the text are presented. Obviously, it would be impossible to offer examples of all of the intervention procedures described in Chapters 5 and 6. Interested readers are directed to texts by Howell and Nolet (1999), Mayer (2002), Rathvon (1999), Rosenfield (1987), and Shinn et al. (1999) for a wider variety of examples of CBA and behavioral interventions for academic problems.

CASE EXAMPLES FOR ACADEMIC ASSESSMENT

Two cases are presented that illustrate the use of curriculum-based assessment (CBA) in assessing the instructional environment and instructional placement. The first case is that of George, a fourth-grade boy referred by his teacher because of academic problems in the areas of reading and writing, as well as a high degree of distractibility. The case illustrates the assessment of all four areas of basic skills development—reading, mathematics, written language, and spelling, particularly for someone whose first language was not English.

The second case, that of Brittany, illustrates the evaluation of a first-grade girl referred because of poor performance in reading and math. The case illustrates the use of the direct assessment of early literacy skills that becomes necessary when a student does not reach first-grade instructional reading levels.

Each assessment case is presented in the form of a psychological report. Completed teacher interview, observation, and assessment forms for the cases are also included, along with narrative material describing the forms.

Case 1: George[1]

Name: George
Birth date: July 3, 1992
Chronological age: 10 years,
                3 months

Grade: 4
Teacher: Mrs. Pickney, Mrs. Bartram (ESL)
School: Hiram
Report date: May 9, 2002

Background Information

George, a fourth-grade student, comes from both Chinese and Cambodian backgrounds. Although he has lived in the United States his entire life, his first language remains Chinese, the language predominately spoken in his home. Over the past 5 years, he has attended six different elementary schools. Due to academic difficulties, he was retained in second grade and was also referred to the instructional support team (IST) while he was in second grade. His grades reflect failures in reading and English.

On the referral request, the teacher reported that although George does not know the definition of words, he is often able to decode the words fluently. Currently, he works with the instructional support teacher twice per week, as well as with an English as Second Language (ESL) teacher (Mrs. Bartram) 5 days per week. Specific effort is made by these teachers to focus on George's writing, reading, and responses to literature. George continues to struggle with development of the English language, and has a limited knowledge of many English words and sayings. In addition, George's teachers report that he is distracted easily and has difficulty concentrating.

Assessment Methods

- Structured teacher interview and Academic Performance Rating Scale (APRS)
- Direct classroom observation—Behavioral Observation of Students in Schools (BOSS)
- Student interview

---

[1]Many thanks to Clarissa Henry, doctoral student in School Psychology at Lehigh University, whose case report is the basis for this material.

- Review of student permanent products
- Direct assessment of reading, mathematics, and spelling

Assessment Results: Reading

Teacher Interview and APRS. Prior to interviewing Mrs. Pickney, George's primary teacher, the APRS was completed. Outcomes on this measure showed that, compared to other fourth-grade boys, George had significantly lower scores in Academic Productivity, Academic Success, and Impulse Control. According to his teacher, compared to his classmates, George was rated as completing 80—89% of his math assignments but only 50–69% of language arts assignments. Although his completion rate in math is acceptable, the accuracy of his work in both math and language arts is poor, rated as between 0% and 64%. The quality of his written work was also reported as poor and often completed in a hasty fashion.

Reading is primarily instructed in work done with the ESL and IST teachers. When interviewed (see Figure 8.1), Mrs. Pickney reported that in the general education class, reading is instructed primarily from novels for which grade levels have been established. George is currently place in the level "N" books, which represent material that is at the third- and fourth-grade levels. Although Mrs. Pickney divides her class into three reading groups, George's performance is so much below that of his peers that he receives directed reading instruction primarily from the ESL teacher every day and is not part of any of the classroom reading groups. The reading period within the class is divided between individual seatwork, small-group reading, and whole-group instruction. However, George's instruction occurs mostly in one-to-one and small-group activities during ESL periods that are provided within the general education classroom while reading instruction is being delivered to the entire class. Some contingencies (receiving a "star") for homework completion and other academic tasks are used regularly by Mrs. Pickney, with those children earning 15 stars by the end of the week being permitted to select a treat from a grab bag. George participates in these activities along with his classmates.

According to Mrs. Bartram, his ESL teacher, George's oral reading skills and sight-word comprehension are somewhat better than those of his peers. Comprehension, however, is much worse than that of others in his group. On a brief behavior rating scale, Mrs. Pickney indicates that George is above satisfactory for oral reading ability, attending to others when reading aloud, and knowing the place in the book. However, he does an unsatisfactory job of volunteering and often gives responses that are inappropriate and unrelated to the topic.

TEACHER INTERVIEW FORM FOR ACADEMIC PROBLEMS

Student: _George_   Teacher: _Mrs. Pickney, Mrs. Bartram_

Birth date: _7/3/93_   Date: _7/9/02_

Grade: _4_   School: _Hiram_

                                           Interviewer: _C. Henry_

GENERAL

Why was this student referred? _Academic problems_

What type of academic problem(s) does this student have?

Reading comprehension, writing

READING

Primary type of reading series used   Secondary type of reading materials used

☐ Basal reader   ☐ Basal reader

☐ Literature-based   ☒ Literature-based

☒ Trade books   ☐ Trade books

                                                ☐ None

Reading series title (if applicable) _Novels/grade level_

    Grade level of series currently placed _Level N—3rd–4th grade_

    Title of book in series currently placed _Native Americans_

How many groups do you teach? _1 group_

Which group is this student assigned to? _ESL reading group_

At this point in the school year, where is the average student in your class reading?

    Level and book _All students in one group, at same point, Levels R–U, 4th–5th grade_

    Place in book (beg., mid., end, specific page) _N/A_

    Time allotted/day for reading _90 minutes/day_

How is time divided? (Independent seatwork? Small group? Cooperative groups? Large groups?)

Independent work, paired work, small groups (6 children), then work in whole group.

George gets lost in whole group, does better in small and one-to-one

FIGURE 8.1. Completed Teacher Interview Form in reading for George.

How is placement in reading program determined? _Reading specialist initial year_
placement test

How are changes made in the program? _Teacher made changes based on student progress_

Does this student participate in remedial reading programs? How much?
Not applicable

Typical daily instructional procedures _Round robin, read aloud, assigned reading roles_
for cooperative groups, discuss passages

Contingencies for accuracy? _No specific contingencies_

Contingencies for completion? _Sometimes coupons for children to reward good work_

Types of interventions already attempted:

   Simple (e.g., reminders, cues, self-monitoring, motivation, feedback, instructions):

   Moderate (e.g., increasing time of existing instruction, extra tutoring sessions):

   Intensive (e.g., changed curriculum, changed instructional modality,
   changed instructional grouping, added intensive one-to-one):
   Changed instructional grouping, say words/sentences by writing

Frequency and duration of interventions used:
Works with IST teacher 2 days/week, small-group ESL students and teacher on responding
to literature

Extent to which interventions were successful:
Improvements on spoken language but no real success on written language.

Daily scores (if available) for past 2 weeks _Not available_

Group standardized test results (if available) _Not available_

FIGURE 8.1. *(continued)*

ORAL READING

How does he/she read orally compared to others in his/her reading group?

____ Much worse   ____ Somewhat worse   ____ About the same

____ Somewhat better   _X_ Much better

In the class?

____ Much worse   _X_ Somewhat worse   ____ About the same

____ Somewhat better   ____ Much better

WORD ATTACK

Does he/she attempt unknown words? _Yes_

WORD KNOWLEDGE/SIGHT VOCABULARY

How does the student's word knowledge (vocabulary) compare to others in his/her reading group?

____ Much worse   ____ Somewhat worse   _X_ About the same

____ Somewhat better   ____ Much better

In the class?

____ Much worse   _X_ Somewhat worse   ____ About the same

____ Somewhat better   ____ Much better

How does the student's sight-word vocabulary compare to others in his/her reading group?

____ Much worse   ____ Somewhat worse   _X_ About the same

____ Somewhat better   ____ Much better

In the class?

____ Much worse   _X_ Somewhat worse   ____ About the same

____ Somewhat better   ____ Much better

COMPREHENSION

How well does the student seem to understand what he/she reads compared to others in his/her reading group?

____ Much worse   _X_ Somewhat worse   ____ About the same

____ Somewhat better   ____ Much better

FIGURE 8.1. *(continued)*

In the class?

__X__ Much worse   ____ Somewhat worse   ____ About the same

____ Somewhat better   ____ Much better

Areas of comprehension where student has success (+)/difficulty (–):

__–__ Main ideas

__–__ Prediction

__+__ Recollection of facts

__–__ Identifying plot

__–__ Identifying main characters

__–__ Synthesizing the story

__–__ Other (describe):

  Peers in ESL group use strategies for comprehension. George does not.

BEHAVIOR DURING READING

Rate the following areas from 1 to 5 (1 = very unsatisfactory, 3 = satisfactory, 5 = superior).

Reading Group

a. Oral reading ability (as evidenced in reading group) __4__
b. Volunteers answers __2__
c. When called upon, gives correct answer __2__
d. Attends to other students when they read aloud __4__
e. Knows the appropriate place in book __4__

Independent Seatwork

a. Stays on task __3__
b. Completes assigned work in required time __2__
c. Work is accurate __2__
d. Works quietly __5__
e. Remains in seat when required __5__

Homework (if any)

a. Handed in on time __3__
b. Is complete __2__
c. Is accurate __2__

Comments:

Does not know how to ask for help when stuck. Says "I don't know" a lot. Sometimes difficulty getting started with independent work.

FIGURE 8.1. *(continued)*

Direct Observation. Data were collected during observations in the regular classroom and in the remedial reading program using the Behavioral Observation of Students in Schools (BOSS; see Table 8.1). Observations were conducted for a total of 20 minutes in the general education classroom, while George was engaged in small-group guided reading and independent seatwork at his desk or a computer. He was also observed for 18 minutes during his ESL reading group, when he was working individually on a report based on the group reading a book on Native Americans. Comparison data were obtained by using a randomly selected peer once every minute.

During the whole-group guided reading lesson in Mrs. Pickney's class, children were expected to pay attention to the teacher, listen to others read, follow along in their books, and read aloud during their turn. Outcomes of the observation revealed that George's peers were far more actively engaged then he was. For much of the time, George was off-task, primarily during the computer time where he played with the mouse, rubbed his face, and put his head down rather than work on the assigned activity.

In contrast to George's behavior during the whole-group activity, he showed substantially higher active engagement than peers when he was working within the ESL, small-group setting. Throughout the activity, Mrs.

TABLE 8.1. Direct Observation Data from the BOSS Collected during Reading for George

		Percentage of intervals	
Behavior	George (total intervals = 64)	Peers (total intervals = 16)	Teacher (total intervals = 16)
	Classroom		
Active Engagement	23.0	56.0	
Passive Engagement	37.5	25.0	
Off-Task Motor	28.0	6.3	
Off-Task Verbal	0	6.3	
Off-Task Passive	6.3	0	
Teacher-Directed Instruction			18.8
	ESL reading group		
Active Engagement	47.3	6.4	
Passive Engagement	26.3	7.1	
Off-Task Motor	5.2	7.1	
Off-Task Verbal	0	14.2	
Off-Task Passive	0	14.2	
Teacher-Directed Instruction			50

Bartram paid high levels of attention to George, as reflected in the percentage of teacher-directed instruction, and was consistently checking with him to see that he was completing the assigned independent work. George showed minimal levels of off-task behavior, levels that were far lower than those of his peers.

Overall, the observational data in reading support the teacher reports during the interview that George does much better in small-group and one-to-one instructional settings compared to whole-class instruction.

Student Interview. George was interviewed after the observations were conducted and was asked questions about his assignment. Results of the interview revealed that George understood the assignment and recognized the expectations of the teacher. However, George believed that he could not do the assignment when it was distributed. Although he really found the work interesting, he reported that he really did not understand the importance of the assignment. When asked to rate how much time he got to complete his assignments on a scale from 1 (not enough) to 3 (too much), George reported that the amount of time given was usually too much. He did feel that his teacher tended to call on him about as much as other students in class. George also reported that he understood what to do if he was confused and how to seek help if he could not answer parts of the assignment.

In general, the interview with George suggested that he understood well his difficulties in completing reading tasks. George also seemed to have a good understanding of the classroom rules and knew the means to access help when it is required.

Direct Assessment. Administration of oral reading probes from books at the fourth- (starting point), third-, second-, and first-grade levels (see Figure 8.2) showed that George was at an instructional level for fluency within the third-grade book, where he was currently placed using instructional levels based on local normative data collection from the school district. Although George attained acceptable oral fluency within third-grade material, his comprehension levels were below instructional levels with second-, third-, and fourth-grade material. Throughout the reading, George would stop and ask for the meaning of words that he was able to successfully read. He showed some difficulties with vowel sounds, particularly final *e*.

George read at a steady pace but tended to focus on individual words rather than read phrases. He attempted to decode unfamiliar words, using effective strategies for blending and synthesizing syllables. Throughout the reading, George read with minimal expression. He often also lost his place while reading and began to use his pencil as a pointer. When answering

DATA SUMMARY FORM FOR ACADEMIC ASSESSMENT

Child's name: _George_

Teacher: _Mrs. Pickney, Mrs. Bartram_

Grade: _4_

School: _Hiram_

School district: _Bethel_

Date: _5/13/02_

READING—SKILLS

Primary type of reading series used

☐ Basal reader
☐ Literature-based
☒ Trade books

Secondary type of reading materials used

☐ Basal reader
☒ Literature-based
☐ Trade books
☐ None

Title of curriculum series: _Novels (Primary), HBJ (Secondary)_

Level/book—target student: _Level N—(3rd–4th grade) - Native Americans_

Level/book—average student: _Level R–U (class), N–Q (ESL students)_

Results of passages administered:

Grade level/ book	Location in book	WC/ min	Words incorrect/ min	% correct	Median scores for level			Learning level (M, I, F)
					WC	ER	%C	
1	Beginning	44	3	80	52	2	80	Mastery
	Middle	72	2					
	End	65	0					
2	Beginning	71	0		71	0	70	Instructional
	Middle	42	0	79				
	End	76	0					
3	Beginning	51	2	50	51	2	50	Instructional
	Middle	51	1					
	End	61	3					
4	Beginning	56	4		64	2	12.5	Frustrational
	Middle	69	2					
	End	64	1	12.5				

FIGURE 8.2. Data summary form and reading probe data for George. WC, words correct. Starting level for assessment was fourth-grade level.

STUDENT-REPORTED BEHAVIOR

_____ None completed for this area

Understands expectations of teacher	☒ Yes	☐ No	☐ Not sure
Understands assignments	☒ Yes	☐ No	☐ Not sure
Feels he/she can do the assignments	☐ Yes	☒ No	☐ Not sure
Likes the subject	☒ Yes	☐ No	☐ Not sure
Feels he/she is given enough time to complete assignments	☒ Yes	☐ No	☐ Not sure
Feels like he/she is called upon to participate in discussions	☐ Yes	☒ No	☐ Not sure

FIGURE 8.2. *(continued)*

questions, George had substantial difficulty with inferential questions. For those questions requiring factual responses, George did not use any strategies to retrieve the information, although he had access to the passage when questions were asked.

Review of Work Samples. George's performance on worksheets linked to the state standards was consistent with teacher reports and the direct assessment. In the area of reading comprehension, George was unable to use ideas presented in stories to make predictions. He also struggled with vocabulary and had difficulty understanding the concepts of action verbs and contractions. Examination of these worksheets did show that George could distinguish between different types of literature.

Assessment Results: Mathematics

Teacher Interview. In the teacher interview for mathematics (see Figure 8.3), Mrs. Pickney indicates that she focuses instruction based on the state curriculum standards but uses the Scott Foresman/Addison-Wesley curriculum as well. All students in the class, including George, are instructed at the same fourth-grade level and taught as a large group. Approximately 1 hour per day is allotted for math. Daily lessons include direct instruction, individual seatwork, and, occasionally, small-group work. No specific contingencies are used for completion of work but students do receive stars for completing homework. Student progress is assessed about once per week using the district standards assessment.

According to George's teacher, the class does not have a large focus on basic computational skills, but instead focuses instruction in areas of mathematical problem solving, such as fractions, positive and negative numbers, decimals, probability, and geometry. Mrs. Pickney did indicate that although she is unsure about George's current knowledge of basic computational skills, his performance in math instruction is quite variable.

TEACHER INTERVIEW FORM FOR ACADEMIC PROBLEMS

Student: _George_   Teacher: _Mrs. Pickney, Mrs. Bartram_

Birth date: _7/3/93_   Date: _7/9/02_

Grade: _4_   School: _Hiram_

                                       Interviewer: _C. Henry_

MATHEMATICS

Curriculum series _Standards based instruction; Scott-Foresman/Addison-Wesley_

What are the specific problems in math? _Fractions_

Time allotted/day for math _1 hour_

How is time divided? (Independent seatwork? Small group? Large group?
Cooperative groups?) _Whole group, independent work, occasional small group_

Are your students grouped in math? _No_

If so, how many groups do you have, and in which group is this student placed? _N/A_

For an **average** performing student in your class, at what point in the planned course
format would you consider this student at mastery?

   (See computational mastery form.) _Unknown_

For an **average** performing student in your class, at what point in the planned course
format would you consider this student instructional?

   (See computational mastery form.) _Unknown_

For an **average** performing student in your class, at what point in the planned course
format would you consider this student frustrational?

   (See computational mastery form.) _Unknown_

For the **targeted** student in your class, at what point in the planned course format would
you consider this student at mastery?

   (See computational mastery form.) _Unknown_

FIGURE 8.3. Completed teacher interview form in mathematics for George.

For the **targeted** student in your class, at what point in the planned course format would you consider this student instructional?

(See computational mastery form.) _Unknown_

For the **targeted** student in your class, at what point in the planned course format would you consider this student frustrational?

(See computational mastery form.) _Unknown_

How is mastery assessed? _Weekly standards tests_

Describe any difficulties this student has in applying math skills in these areas:

Numeration _____

Estimation _____

Time _____

Money _____

Measurement _____

Geometry _____

Graphic display _____

Interpretation of graph _Embedded word problems_____

Word problems _Multiplication operations_____

Other _Fractions_____

How are changes made in the student's math program? _Teacher-based decisions_

_____

Does this student participate in remedial math programs? _N/A_

Typical daily instructional procedures _Direct instruction, review of homework_

_____

_____

Contingencies for accuracy? _Start charts for homework, can pick treat if he gets 15 stars_
by Friday

FIGURE 8.3. *(continued)*

281

BEHAVIOR DURING MATH

Rate the following areas from 1 to 5 (1 = very unsatisfactory, 3 = satisfactory, 5 = superior)

Math Group (large)

a. Volunteers answers   3
b. When called upon, gives correct answer   3
c. Attends to other students when they give answers   3
d. Knows the appropriate place in math book   2

Math Group (small)

a. Volunteers answers   ____
b. When called upon, gives correct answer   ____
c. Attends to other students when they give answers   ____
d. Knows the appropriate place in math book   ____

Math Group (cooperative)

a. Volunteers answers   ____
b. Contributes to group objectives   ____
c. Attends to other students when they give answers   ____
d. Facilitates others in group to participate   ____
e. Shows appropriate social skills in group   ____

Independent Seatwork

a. Stays on task   1
b. Completes assigned work in required time   1
c. Work is accurate   2
d. Works from initial directions   2
e. Works quietly   4
f. Remains in seat when required   4

Homework (if any)

a. Handed in on time   3
b. Is complete   4
c. Is accurate   3

FIGURE 8.3. *(continued)*

Mrs. Pickney rated George's behavior in math as mixed. Although he has satisfactory performance in areas such as volunteering answers, giving correct answers, attending to others, and handing homework in on time, he is below satisfactory in many other areas related to attention, such as knowing his place, staying on task, and completing assignments on time.

Direct Observation. Data were collected through direct observation in one 43 minute period of math instruction in the classroom (see Table 8.2). During the observation, the teacher reviewed the previous night's homework, using a game-like activity of matching answer cards to their own problems, and provided direct instruction on fractions. Peer-comparison data were again collected by random selection of peers on every fifth observation interval.

These data suggest that George had levels of active and passive engagement similar to those of his peers. However, he had much higher levels of off-task motor and passive behavior. His off-task motor behavior consisted of playing with his face, hands, clothes, and pencils. During the lesson, he continually placed his head on the table and gazed around the room. Mrs. Pickney had to tell him on several occasions to sit up straight and pay attention. When he prematurely put his work away, the teacher instructed a peer sitting close by to help George through the activity. In addition, George is somewhat more distractible during math than reading. Mrs. Pickney noted that George's behavior during this observation was typical of the type of behavior she has observed during most lessons.

Student Interview. When interviewed about math following completion of the lesson in which he was observed, George indicated that he was

TABLE 8.2. Direct Observation Data from the BOSS Collected during Math for George

Behavior	George (total intervals = 64)	Percentage of intervals	
		Peers (total intervals = 16)	Teacher (total intervals = 16)
	Percentage of intervals		
Active Engagement	10.0	8.8	
Passive Engagement	47.0	55.9	
Off-Task Motor	21.6	5.9	
Off-Task Verbal	2.9	14.7	
Off-Task Passive	23.7	8.8	
Teacher-Directed Instruction			70.6

unsure whether he understood what was expected of him. In particular, George indicated that he had difficulty with division, and while he understood the specific assignment given and liked math, he sometimes felt rushed in getting his work done. George did appreciate help and was willing to ask for it from a peer if he struggled with problems.

Direct Assessment. Computation skills were assessed in all four basic operations. Given that his teacher could not speculate on the computational skills that George did or did not know, the examiner began assessment at levels commensurate with those probes likely to be instructional for students at a fourth-grade level. In addition to computation, assessment of George's skills at third- and fourth-grade levels for concepts–applications of mathematics were also administered. Results of the assessment are provided in Figure 8.4.

Results of the assessment indicated that George has mastered or was instructional in a number of fourth- and fifth-grade objectives involving multiplication and division. However, subtraction and division involving regrouping proved difficult. Watching George complete subtraction problems suggested that while he understood the process, he lacked fluency. In an examination of the probes given in concepts and applications, there appeared to be a number of areas where George had some difficulty. He was unable to successfully complete any of the word problems, even when matched with graphic representations. He also did not correctly answer problems involving fractions as whole numbers, writing cents using a "$" sign, and had problems with sequencing and questions related to graphs that required computation.

Review of Work Samples. Examination of worksheets from standard curricular tests revealed that George could write and represent decimals. He also appeared to understand the basic concepts of parallel and perpendicular lines, as well as shapes. He was found to struggle in areas involving fractions, two-and three-dimensional shapes, and concepts of symmetry. On fractions and decimal worksheets, George did not know how to turn fractions to decimals.

Assessment Results: Writing

Teacher Interview. Writing assignments are made periodically and include sentences and creative writing. According to his teacher, George has difficulty with written and oral forms, and tends to use fragmented sentences. His teacher also reports that he has difficulties with writing mechanics, punctuation, grammar, spelling, handwriting, and capitalization. Mrs. Pickney also noted that George often works very slowly compared to other children in his class.

DATA SUMMARY FORM FOR ACADEMIC ASSESSMENT

Child's name: _George_

Teacher: _Mrs. Pickney, Mrs. Bartram_

Grade: _4_

School: _Hiram_

School district: _Bethel_

Date: _5/13/02_

MATH—SKILLS

Curriculum series used: _Standards curriculum and SF/AW_

Specific problems in math: _Fractions, word problems, geometry_

Mastery skill of target student: _Unknown_

Mastery skill of average student: _Unknown_

Instructional skill of target student: _Unknown_

Instructional skill of average student: _Unknown_

Problems in math applications: _Fractions, word problems, embedded word problems_

Results of math probes:

Probe type	No.	Digits correct/min	Digits incorrect/min	% problems correct	Learning level (M, I, F)
Addition: 2 addends of 4-digit numbers with regrouping		19.5	0.9	80	Mastery
Subtraction: 2 digits from 2 digits, no regrouping		26.0	0	100	Mastery
Subtraction: 2 digits from 2 digits, with regrouping		9.5	0	100	Instructional
Subtraction: 3 digits from 3 digits, with regrouping		8.5	0.5	86	Frustrational

FIGURE 8.4. Math probe and interview data for George.

Multiplication: Facts 0–9	53.0	2.4	96	Mastery
Multiplication: 2 digits ×1 digit, with regrouping	23.0	0.3	96	Mastery
Multiplication: 2 digits ×2 digit, with regrouping	14.25	1.2	67	Instructional
Division: 2 digits/1 digit, no regrouping	11.0	5.8	68	Instructional
Division: 2 digits/1 digit, with regrouping	2.5	24	0	Frustrational

Concepts–Applications	Number of correct responses	Percentage of problems correct
Applications—3rd grade	15	66
Applications—4th grade	12	61

STUDENT-REPORTED BEHAVIOR _____ None completed for this area

Understands expectations of teacher	☐ Yes	☐ No	☒ Not sure
Understands assignments	☒ Yes	☐ No	☐ Not sure
Feels he/she can do the assignments	☒ Yes	☐ No	☐ Not sure
Likes the subject	☐ Yes	☒ No	☐ Not sure
Feels he/she is given enough time to complete assignments	☐ Yes	☒ No	☐ Not sure
Feels like he/she is called upon to participate in discussions	☐ Yes	☒ No	☐ Not sure

FIGURE 8.4. *(continued)*

Student Interview. When asked, George indicated that he actually enjoys writing. Although he understands assignments and feels he can do them, George indicated that he really did not know what his teacher expected of him in writing.

Direct Assessment. A total of three story starters were administered to George (see Figure 8.5). His stories all fell below instructional levels for a fourth grader. For the first story starter, which was about Chinese basketball player Yao Ming, George wrote 33 words per 3 minutes, which is instructional for a second grader. However, instead of a story, George provided descriptive information only and did not have much creativity. Although his capitalization and spelling were mostly correct, the words he used were fairly simple. His punctuation was inconsistent and the grammar immature. To examine whether George was able to express his ideas without writing, he was asked to tell the evaluator a story after a story prompt. George's response, again, was not to tell a story but simply to give factual information. When asked to write a second story, George wrote 36 words per 3 minutes, again placing him at the instructional level for second graders.

Review of Work Samples. A review of work samples supported Mrs. Pickney's observations that George's writing was quite immature and lacked depth. He had a difficult time formulating ideas into paragraphs and instead made a list of ideas. He also had problems using correct tenses, as well as articles. Words that were not spelled correctly were written phonetically, consistent with George's skills in decoding. George's printing was leg-

Child Name: George
Date: 5/8/03

Writing Probe

Yesterday I met the famous basketball player Yao Ming ...

He is In the rocket he is 22 year old
he a good Player then the he was funny.
He had black hair, black eye his my
Friend. Then he doge in Micle Jackcn.

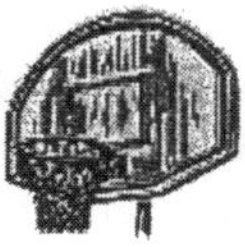

FIGURE 8.5. Writing probe for George.

ible and showed good spacing. There was no evidence that George was able to use cursive writing.

Assessment Results: Spelling

Teacher Interview. Mrs. Pickney uses a list of the 500 most commonly used words for the purpose of teaching spelling. Although time is not specifically set aside for spelling instruction, students are given spelling packets and work independently to complete them within the week. A pretest is given on Wednesday and a final spelling test on Friday. Students are awarded stickers for accurate spelling assignments. Mrs. Pickney indicated that George does not complete his spelling packets and is behind by approximately three packets.

Student Interview. Although George stated that he is a good speller, he reports that he does not always understand the assignments. Often, he does not know how to do the spelling packets, which accounts for the fact that many are not completed.

Direct Observation. No observations of student behavior was conducted for this skills area.

Direct Assessment. The evaluator assessed George in spelling by asking him to spell words presented from fourth-, third-, and second-grade levels. Table 8.3 reports the outcomes of the assessment process.

George appeared to be instructional at a second-grade level based on letter sequences per minute. However, at third- and fourth-grade levels, he averaged only 29% of the words spelled correctly. George was noted to be making a number of consistent errors, including lack of ability to differentiate *c* and *s*, *k* and *c*, *b* and *f*, and *t* and *d*. He also tended to spell words as he said them. Medial vowels were often omitted, and double consonants were not used correctly.

TABLE 8.3. Spelling Probe Data for George

Grade level of probe	LSC/min	% words correct	Level (M, I, F)
2	43	47	Instructional
3	33	29	Frustrational
4	31	24	Frustrational

Review of Work Samples. Weekly spelling tests were examined. Although George tended to get many of these words correct, the words were rather simple, involving mostly three- and four-letter words. Given George's strong decoding skills, it is not surprising that he was successful in many of these weekly spelling tests. Spelling words assessed for this evaluation were more complex and showed substantial deficiencies in George's spelling performance.

Conclusions

George, a student identified as having needs in ESL, was referred because of difficulties primarily in reading and writing. Assessments suggested that George is currently at a third-grade instructional level in reading fluency; however, his comprehension lags much further behind. He appears to be appropriately placed in curricular materials, although he remains primarily a word-by-word reader, which certainly impedes his comprehension development. A review of work samples show that George's comprehension problems are mainly with inferential questions, where he has difficulty making story predictions, and understanding meaning of key vocabulary and action verbs.

In math, George has mastered most computational objectives at a fourth-grade level but still has some difficulty with regrouping skills across all operations. In applications, he shows some problems in the areas of geometry, word problems, and fractions.

Writing remains a significant problem for George. His work lacks creativity, length, and depth. His writing pattern is immature, and mechanics such as punctuation are inconsistent. In spelling, he was noted to be instructional at the second-grade level. Although he is successful in his spelling instruction in class, his work indicates that he has not mastered material expected of fourth-grade students.

George was noted to be somewhat less attentive in reading and language-related activities when taught in large groups. In contrast, his attentive skills, when instructed in one-to-one situations, appeared to be equivalent to that of his peers. These findings were fairly consistent across different subject areas.

Recommendations

Specific recommendations related to reading, writing, and spelling are made given that these areas appear to be the most problematic for George. In addition, a general concern about George is for teachers to have better insight into his current level of language development.

1. *Language development.* It is recommended that a determination of George's level of Cognitive Academic Language Proficiency (CALP) be obtained. CALP is the measure that reflects the level that second language learners need to do well on academic tasks in English. It is possible that George may have developed Basic Interpersonal Communication Skills (BICS) in the English language, but that his CALP is not sufficiently developed to allow him to benefit from language instruction. It is also recommended that an assessment be completed to see whether Chinese remains his dominant language and to determine whether he is proficient in any language.

2. *Reading.* Several strategies are recommended to enhance George's sight-vocabulary development.

- *Folding-in technique.* This is a flashcard drill in which George practices needed sight vocabulary to improve reading performance.
- *Repeated readings.* This technique involves having a student read a passage repeatedly until a specified criterion of fluency is attained. This technique, when paired with modeling of correct phrase reading and reading for meaning, can improve George's word-by-word reading style.
- *Pre-, during-, and postcomprehension strategies.* George needs to be provided with a set of strategies for approaching reading material. Use of self-talk and prompting, story maps, and other activities designed to elicit previous knowledge, is crucial if George is to improve his understanding of material. It is recommended that George be frequently stopped and asked to summarize material he has read, as well as to develop a strategy in which he constantly develops questions and answers about material he is reading.

3. *Writing.* Efforts to improve George's writing need to concentrate on both mechanics and conceptual development in the writing process.

- George needs some direct instruction in the rules of grammar within his ESL instruction.
- Daily opportunities to practice writing skills are needed. Prior to writing, George should develop a story web to organize his ideas. Because interviews with George suggest that he can be highly motivated by some topics (e.g., his excitement when writing about the basketball player Yao Ming), an inventory of his interests should be developed.
- Direct instruction in the editing and revision process are needed. Mrs. Pickney may want to teach George specifically about important aspects of revision, such as locating and diagnosing a problem,

determining the type of changes needed in writing, and using an editing or proofreading checklist to monitor his work.

- Use of a self-monitoring checklist to evaluate his own writing may allow George to better recognize the problems with his work.

4. *Spelling.* Recommendations in spelling involve trying to increase George's vocabulary and capitalizing on his already established skills in decoding.

- The folding-in technique recommended for developing sight words in reading may also be useful in developing spelling words.
- Specific instruction on long- and short-vowel sounds, differences between hard consonants such as *c* and *k*, and the use of rules such as silent *e* should be taught.
- Use of the spelling self-monitoring intervention (described in Chapter 6) may be helpful.

CLARISSA HENRY
School Psychologist

Comments about George's Case

This case illustrates several excellent issues related to academic assessment. It demonstrates the first two steps of the four-step model of academic assessment: Assessing the Academic Environment and Instructional Placement.

George was referred by the teacher due primarily to academic failure in reading and written language. Interview data with the teacher suggested that the psychologist would find a child who was mostly on-task but had poor academic skills in reading and writing. Results of the direct observations also revealed some level of inattention, predominantly in language-related activities involving whole-group instruction. In George's case, the data did not suggest that his inattention was the cause of his academic skills problems; rather, his poor academic skills in certain areas, especially language arts, caused his inattention, particularly because English was not his primary language. It is likely that he had great difficulty when being instructed in the typical large-group, whole-group methods through which most reading and language arts were being instructed.

Regarding academic skills, results of the administration of skill probes showed that George was being instructed at the level at which he should have been reading. However, his performance in oral reading fluency was viewed as potentially not indicative of his much poorer level of comprehension. Recommendations to focus George on comprehension skills and to capitalize on his good skills in decoding were made. Importantly, it was suggested that even George's oral reading fluency, while strong, required some effort to reduce word-by-word reading and increase phrase reading. Improved fluency of reading material in this way would likely increase his reading comprehension as well.

In the area of writing, again, George was found to have substantial difficulties in language usage. His writing required specific and direct attention to use strategies likely to improve his overall conceptualization of written communication.

Finally, George's identification as a student with ESL needs suggested the need for a more thorough examination of his CALP and BICS levels. These concepts are important, since many children who demonstrate adequate BICS levels have CALP levels that lag far behind. Such a situation would easily account for students who are able to communicate and be understood by teachers but cannot yet use their second language development to work adequately on required academic and cognitive tasks.

Case 2: Brittany[2]

Name: Brittany	*Grade*: 1
Birth date: June 18, 1996	*Teacher*: Mrs. Schatz
Chronological age: 6 years,	*School*: Fels Elementary
11 months	*Report date*: May 24, 2003

Background Information

Brittany is a first-grade student who recently moved to the school district at the end of March. Her teacher reported that Brittany has been struggling in all academic areas. In addition, she has difficulty following directions. She is receiving additional support from a reading specialist three times per week, along with math tutoring from an instructional aide twice per week. The purpose of this evaluation is to determine Brittany's strengths and weaknesses, and to make recommendations for appropriate objectives and goals.

Assessment Methods

- Review of records
- Teacher interview
- Student interview
- Direct classroom observation
- Direct assessment of reading, math

---

[2]Many thanks to Kate Tresco, doctoral student in School Psychology at Lehigh University, whose case report is the basis for this material.

Assessment Results: Reading

Teacher Interview. The reading portion of the completed teacher interview (see Figure 8.6) shows that Brittany is currently placed in the Houghton Mifflin series, level E (grade level 1.1). By contrast, the average student in her class is placed at level I (grade 1.4) of the series. Mrs. Butz reported that Brittany has difficulty reading orally and does not work independently. She has limited sight vocabulary and fails to use appropriate decoding strategies to sound out unknown words or to aid comprehension. Reading is allotted 90 minutes each day, with most instruction involving the whole class. In addition, Brittany is part of a small guided reading group led by Mrs. Butz at least three times per week. Currently, there are six different levels of groups in the class, and Brittany is assigned to the lowest level.

In comparison to her peers, Brittany's oral reading, sight vocabulary, and comprehension are far worse. Mrs. Butz reported that when compared to others in her small guided reading group, Brittany reads orally about the same but has much worse sight vocabulary and comprehension. In addition, Mrs. Butz noted that Brittany has difficulty staying on task, does not complete assigned work on time, and rarely hands in any complete homework.

Direct Observation. Reading was observed for 15 minutes using the BOSS during a period of large-group instruction. Students were asked to follow along in their books while Mrs. Butz read aloud. Periodically, Mrs. Butz stopped to discuss the story. Data were also collected on randomly selected peers who were observed every fifth interval (once every 60 seconds). Results of the observations are provided in Table 8.4. During these observations, Brittany's levels of active and passive engagement were fairly equivalent to levels of her peers. She did show somewhat more off-task motor behavior. While other students were following the story with their finger or looking at their book, Brittany was observed to be flipping pages inappropriately or fidgeting with articles of clothing.

Student Interview. Brittany was interviewed following the direct observations. During the interview, Brittany was quite distracted and wanted to discuss topics other then her work assignment. When questioned about her work, Brittany indicated that she did not know what was expected of her or why she needed to do the assignment. Although she indicated she liked to read, Brittany indicated that when asked to read a passage, she "only reads the words she knows" and would "just skip the hard ones."

Direct Assessment. Brittany's reading skills were assessed first by the administration of a set of passages at the first-grade level. Her median oral reading fluency on those passages was 33 WCPM with eight errors, which places her within a frustrational level based on district norms for reading.

TEACHER INTERVIEW FORM FOR ACADEMIC PROBLEMS

Student: _Brittany_____   Teacher: _Mrs. Butz_____

Birth date: _6/18/96_____   Date: _4/30/03_____

Grade: _1___   School: _Fels_____

Interviewer: _K. T._____

GENERAL

Why was this student referred? _Very far behind academically_____

What type of academic problem(s) does this student have?

_Reading, math_____

READING

Primary type of reading series used   Secondary type of reading materials used

☐ Basal reader   ☒ Basal reader

☒ Literature-based   ☐ Literature-based

☐ Trade books   ☐ Trade books

☐ None

Reading series title (if applicable) _Houghton Mifflin—treasures_____

    Grade level of series currently placed _Grade level 1.1—theme 3_____

    Title of book in series currently placed _Guided Reading—Level E, Grumpy Elephants_____

How many groups do you teach? _6_____

Which group is this student assigned to? _lowest_____

At this point in the school year, where is the average student in your class reading?

    Level and book _Grade level 1.4_____

    Place in book (beg., mid., end, specific page) _theme 8_____

    Time allotted/day for reading _90 minutes/day_____

How is time divided? (Independent seatwork? Small group? Cooperative groups? Large groups?)

Varies by group, typically large group reading, followed by shared reading and activities

FIGURE 8.6. Completed teacher interview form in reading for Brittany.

How is placement in reading program determined? _Tested by reading specialist_

How are changes made in the program? _Consultation with reading specialist_

Does this student participate in remedial reading programs? How much?
Yes

Typical daily instructional procedures _Review story themes, read aloud, share ideas,_
review assigned work

Contingencies for accuracy? _None noted_

Contingencies for completion? _None noted_

Types of interventions already attempted:

    Simple (e.g., reminders, cues, self-monitoring, motivation, feedback, instructions):

    Moderate (e.g., increasing time of existing instruction, extra tutoring sessions):
    Has received guided reading 3x per week, adult volunteer tutoring 2x/week, works with
    student intern 3x/week.

    Intensive (e.g., changed curriculum, changed instructional modality,
    changed instructional grouping, added intensive one-to-one):

Frequency and duration of interventions used:

Extent to which interventions were successful:
No significant improvement

Daily scores (if available) for past 2 weeks _Not available_

Group standardized test results (if available) _Not available_

FIGURE 8.6. *(continued)*

ORAL READING

How does he/she read orally compared to others in his/her reading group?

____ Much worse   ____ Somewhat worse   _X_ About the same

____ Somewhat better   ____ Much better

In the class?

_X_ Much worse   ____ Somewhat worse   ____ About the same

____ Somewhat better   ____ Much better

WORD ATTACK

Does he/she attempt unknown words? <u>No</u>

WORD KNOWLEDGE/SIGHT VOCABULARY

How does the student's word knowledge (vocabulary) compare to others in his/her reading group?

_X_ Much worse   ____ Somewhat worse   ____ About the same

____ Somewhat better   ____ Much better

In the class?

_X_ Much worse   ____ Somewhat worse   ____ About the same

____ Somewhat better   ____ Much better

How does the student's sight-word vocabulary compare to others in his/her reading group?

_X_ Much worse   ____ Somewhat worse   ____ About the same

____ Somewhat better   ____ Much better

In the class?

_X_ Much worse   ____ Somewhat worse   ____ About the same

____ Somewhat better   ____ Much better

COMPREHENSION

How well does the student seem to understand what he/she reads compared to others in his/her reading group?

_X_ Much worse   ____ Somewhat worse   ____ About the same

____ Somewhat better   ____ Much better

FIGURE 8.6. *(continued)*

In the class?

__X__ Much worse   _____ Somewhat worse   _____ About the same

_____ Somewhat better   _____ Much better

Areas of comprehension where student has success (+)/difficulty (–):

__–__ Main ideas

__–__ Prediction

__–__ Recollection of facts

__–__ Identifying plot

__–__ Identifying main characters

__–__ Synthesizing the story

_____ Other (describe):

_____

_____

BEHAVIOR DURING READING

Rate the following areas from 1 to 5 (1 = very unsatisfactory, 3 = satisfactory, 5 = superior).

Reading Group

a. Oral reading ability (as evidenced in reading group)   __2__
b. Volunteers answers   __3__
c. When called upon, gives correct answer   __1__
d. Attends to other students when they read aloud   __3__
e. Knows the appropriate place in book   __2__

Independent Seatwork

a. Stays on task   __1__
b. Completes assigned work in required time   __1__
c. Work is accurate   __1__
d. Works quietly   __3__
e. Remains in seat when required   __3__

Homework (if any)

a. Handed in on time   __1__
b. Is complete   __1__
c. Is accurate   __1__

FIGURE 8.6. *(continued)*

TABLE 8.4. Direct Classroom Observation Data from the BOSS Collected during Reading for Brittany

Behavior	Percentage of intervals		
	Brittany (total intervals = 60)	Peers (total intervals = 16)	Teacher (total intervals = 16)
Active Engagement	35.4	41.7	
Passive Engagement	35.4	33.3	
Off-Task Motor	8.3	0	
Off-Task Verbal	0	0	
Off-Task Passive	18.8	16.7	
Teacher-Directed Instruction			83.3

She was unable to answer any comprehension questions correctly. In addition, Brittany's high error rate was a reflection of her skipping many words that she did not feel she could read.

Due to Brittany's below-grade-level performance on first-grade materials, an assessment of prereading skills was conducted. The Dynamic Indicators of Early Literacy Skills, sixth edition (DIBELS), was administered. Measures of Initial Sound Fluency, Letter Naming Fluency, Phonemic Segmentation Fluency, and Nonsense Word Fluency were administered. Results are shown in Table 8.5, which also compares Brittany's attained scores against the national established benchmarks.

Results of the assessment of prereading skills showed that Brittany reached appropriate benchmarks for a first grade student in letter-naming. Her skills in Initial Sound Fluency, identifying and producing the initial sound of a given word, were considered as emerging for a student in the middle of kindergarten. Her skills in Phonemic Segmentation Fluency and Nonsense Word Fluency were within the emerging area of first grade. In particular, her performance on Nonsense Word Fluency, a skill that is one of the later prereading benchmarks, was nearly established.

Review of Work Products. No work products were available for reading.

TABLE 8.5. DIBELS Measures for Brittany

Measure	Score	Level
Initial Sound Fluency	21.7	Middle-kindergarten emerging benchmark
Letter Naming fluency	60.0	Above first-grade benchmark
Phonemic Segmentation Fluency	25.0	First-grade emerging benchmark
Nonsense Word Fluency	44.0	First-grade emerging benchmark

Assessment Results: Mathematics

Teacher Interview. Brittany is currently placed in the first-grade book of the Everyday Mathematics curriculum series, the same level at which the entire first-grade class is placed. Instruction occurs for approximately 60 minutes per day. Typically, new material is introduced to the entire class so that students practice problems independently, then review them. Mrs. Butz also uses small-group work and independent seatwork. During the independent seatwork time, Mrs. Butz often works one-to-one with Brittany.

Brittany's skills were reported as below expected levels. Mrs. Butz indicated that Brittany struggles with number concepts, can only count to 50, has trouble identifying the value of coins, can only tell time to the hour and half-hour, and has little skill in completing subtraction problems. She was reported as successful at some simple addition problems.

Student Interview. No opportunity to conduct a student interview with Brittany was available.

Direct Observation. Two 15-minute observations of Brittany during math instruction were completed using the BOSS. In one observation of the entire group, Mrs. Butz was presenting a new method to compute double-digit addition problems. Instruction during the second observation asked students to complete two worksheets independently. Mrs. Butz worked directly with Brittany during this time.

Data for each of the observations are presented in Table 8.6. During the large-group setting, Brittany was equally actively engaged in completing her work but had lower levels of passive engagement. Typically, while Brittany would attend to her required problems, she would engage in off-task behaviors, such as looking around the room, fidgeting with articles of clothing, and talking to a peer instead of attending to the teacher as instruction was occurring at the board. During the independent seatwork activity, Brittany showed less active and passive engagement compared to her peers. Often, she would either be gazing around the room or fidgeting with her clothes when she was supposed to be working. In terms of the amount of material actually completed, Brittany completed only one worksheet during the observation, whereas the rest of her class completed both assigned and additional worksheets within the same time period.

Review of Work Samples. A review of the worksheet Brittany completed during the independent seatwork activity showed that she was unsure how to apply the strategy she was instructed to use. The worksheet provided place-value blocks for the 10's and 1's columns in two digit addition problems. Brittany was able to complete the worksheet accurately only for problems in which the number zero was added. Her most common er-

TABLE 8.6. Direct Observation Data from the BOSS Collected during Math Large-Group and Independent Work Periods for Brittany

	Percentage of intervals		
Behavior	Brittany (total intervals = 60)	Peers (total intervals = 16)	Teacher (total intervals = 12)
	Large group		
Active Engagement	37.5	33.3	
Passive Engagement	33.8	66.7	
Off-Task Motor	10.4	0	
Off-Task Verbal	6.3	0	
Off-Task Passive	2.1	0	
Teacher-Directed Instruction			75.0
	Independent seatwork		
Active Engagement	45.2	58.3	
Passive Engagement	3.2	16.7	
Off-Task Motor	22.6	8.3	
Off-Task Verbal	0	8.3	
Off-Task Passive	29.0	0	
Teacher-Directed Instruction			41.7

rors were to add all place-value blocks together in the 1's column, instead of distinguishing between the 1's and 10's columns.

Direct Assessment. Brittany's skills with basic addition and subtraction facts were assessed. Results indicated that she was able to add single-digit problems, sums to 10 at a rate of only 1.6 correct per minute, and that she scored no problems correct on a probe of similar types of subtraction facts. Observation of her behavior while trying to do the problems indicates that she has some basic concepts of addition, using her fingers to count. However, she often started with the wrong number in the problem and had difficulty with counting skills.

Conclusions

Brittany was referred for poor academic performance in reading and math. According to her teacher, she was far behind in both skills areas. During both reading and math activities, Brittany appeared to be somewhat more off-task then her peers. Typically, much of her distractibility appeared to be due to her inability to accurately complete her assigned academic work.

In reading, Brittany scored as frustrational in oral reading fluency when assessed at the first-grade level. As such, she was assessed on prereading skills of phonemic segmentation, knowing initial sounds, decoding nonsense words, and letter naming. She was found to be below the expected benchmarks for first-grade students in all skills except for nonsense word decoding. However, Brittany was unable to apply these same decoding skills when reading in context. In math, Brittany showed skills that suggested she was at frustrational levels at even the most basic addition and subtraction facts.

Recommendations

A series of recommendations focused on intervention strategies to improve Brittany's skills in reading and basic math was made.

1. *Reading.* Word segmentation tasks:

- Instruction should be focused on specific blends, digraphs, or "sounds of the day" paired with building words that include the sounds Brittany practices.

2. *Reading.* Practice of words she does not know:

- Use a rereading activity in which Brittany reads a short passage aloud, while monitoring for errors. Omitted or mispronounced words should be identified and reviewed. She should be required to reread the passage a specified number of times, until she reads the passage correctly.
- Use a summarizing strategy after reading the passage to improve comprehension skills.
- Use her passage reading to develop word lists on which concentrated and focused work is conducted using the "folding-in" technique (see Chapter 6).

3. *Math.* Repeated practice:

- Use a single strategy to teach addition and subtraction skills, and repeatedly practice that single strategy until Brittany shows mastery of the skill.
- Use the cover–copy–compare technique to improve Brittany's recall of basic facts.
- Use flashcard drill activity with mixed facts as Brittany acquires new addition and subtraction facts.

KATE TRESCO
School Psychologist

Comments on Brittany's Case

This case represents an example of how direct assessment of academic skills can be used for a student whose reading skills are not instructional at the first-grade level. In Brittany's case, an interesting finding was that although she did not have well-developed reading skills, she seemed to have a level of decoding of nonsense words that were far better than one would expect. The problem seemed to be that Brittany could not transfer the skills to reading words in context.

In math, Brittany again showed only rudimentary ability to apply any strategies she was being taught. Her failure to have basic addition or subtraction skills really requires immediate and intensive interventions aimed at increasing any automaticity. In addition, she needs to be given more explicit instruction within the teaching process to ensure that she continues to use these skills when applied to other parts of the math curriculum.

Finally, Brittany was more distractible than her peers in many places. However, the outcome of the assessment shows that the distractibility was probably due to her poor academic skills development.

Overall, Brittany's case presents a common problem often seen in referrals for students at first-grade level. Her low levels of reading and math require immediate and intensive intervention; otherwise, she is destined to be a student likely to be referred for retention and possibly for special education services. Indeed, one advantage of the type of assessment illustrated in this case is that if the intensive interventions focused on Brittany's skills fail to result in a positive outcome, a referral for further special education eligibility would be both justified and logical.

CASE EXAMPLES FOR ACADEMIC INTERVENTIONS

The next two cases are designed to illustrate the last two steps of the four-step assessment process: Instructional Modification and Progress Monitoring. It would be impossible to provide case illustrations for even a small portion of the many academic interventions covered in Chapters 5 and 6. Readers are encouraged to examine the publications cited in those chapters for specific examples of the procedures of interest. Two types of intervention cases were chosen for presentation here. The first case illustrates a student whose difficulties focused on improving fluency in reading. In particular, emphasis in the intervention was placed on vocabulary development and word fluency. The second case illustrates how CBA can be employed as a monitoring device for a child whose intervention plans are focused in the areas of both reading comprehension, as well as math interventions, with an emphasis on increasing skills in multiplication facts, division, fractions, and place values. In both cases, examples of both short- and long-term progress monitoring are provided.

Case 3: Shawn[3]

Name: Shawn
Birth date: December 16, 1994
Chronological age: 8 years,
                 6 months

Grade: 3
Teacher: Mrs. Dasche
School: Moore
Report date: May 25, 2003

Background Information

Shawn was referred because of poor academic performance in the area of reading. In particular, a CBA of reading found that Shawn is instructional at the second-grade level, although he is being instructed at the 3.2 level of the reading series. Mrs. Dasche supplements Shawn's instruction with drills from phonics book assigned at the second-grade level. Beyond regular classroom instruction, Shawn receives both Title One services 5 days per week and additional remedial help through a special district-run program for students at risk for reading failure.

Goal Setting

A CBA was administered to determine a baseline rate of Shawn's oral reading rates. Baseline probes taken from the third-grade level found that Shawn read at 42 WCPM, with only a few errors. Short- and long-term goals were set for monitoring Shawn's performance. The short-term goal was to increase Shawn's reading fluency in third-grade material in which he was currently being instructed. Shawn's goal was to read 60 WCPM in the third-grade material used for the intervention. Long-term goals deemed reasonable by the IST were for Shawn to reach instructional level in third-grade material with which he had no familiarity. To accomplish this goal, an increase from a baseline level of 42 WCPM to 70 WCPM was set, across the 7 weeks of intervention. This would be equal to a gain of 28 words across the remaining 7 weeks of the school year, or 4 words correct per week. The goal was approached by setting an initial goal for Shawn to increase from 42 WCPM to 54 WCPM over the first 2 weeks of the intervention.

---

[3]Many thanks to Hillary Rogers, Specialist student in School Psychology at Lehigh University, whose case report is the basis for this material.

Intervention

A fourth-grade student was selected to work with Shawn an average of two to three times per week, across a 4-week period. The tutor was trained for 2 days, until the tutor could implement the intervention independently. Sessions occurred for 15–20 minutes at the start of the school day. Each session consisted of a series of strategies, including the following:

1. First, the tutor would collect from Mrs. Dasche a photocopied passage from Shawn's third-grade reader.
2. The tutor would have Shawn do a "cold" reading of the passage, timing him for 1 minute and marking his errors. Shawn would then graph his pretest score.
3. The passage was read again, but Shawn and the tutor would then alternate reading lines. The reading was untimed, and when Shawn struggled with words, the tutor would provide help.
4. Shawn then read the passage for a third time, while the tutor again timed him for 1 minute and mark his errors as he read.
5. Shawn would graph his own posttest score and compare it to his pretest score.
6. At the end of the session, the tutor recorded the date and Shawn's respective scores for the day on a special data sheet prepared by the evaluator.

Progress Monitoring Procedures

Shawn's pre- and posttest reading scores on each session served as a measure of short-term progress. Long-term progress was measured by assessing Shawn twice per week using unfamiliar passages selected at random from across third-grade level material of the AIMSweb reading passages. Each assessment session, Shawn was asked to read three passages and the median words correct per minute across those passages was recorded.

Results

Figure 8.7 reflects the outcomes of Shawn's short-term progress monitoring. The data show that Shawn consistently read passages at posttest at faster rates compared to the initial "cold reading" at the beginning of each session. In particular, Shawn reached fluency levels on nine of 14 sessions at posttest that exceeded the instructional level of 70 WCPM. An examination of Shawn's performance during the initial "cold" reads prior to each session were examined over time to determine whether Shawn was making

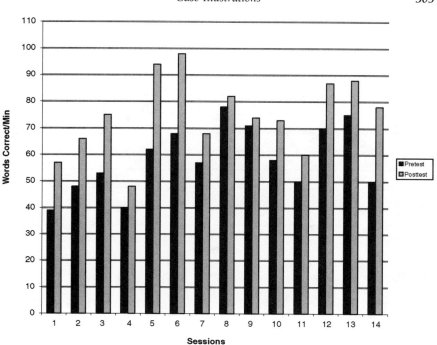

FIGURE 8.7. Results of reading intervention for Shawn.

session-to-session progress in oral reading fluency. As shown in Figure 8.8, Shawn's prereading scores over the first six sessions increased from 39 WCPM to 68 WCPM, which surpassed the initial short-term goal of 60 WCPM. As a result, a new goal to have Shawn increase his fluency to 70 WCPM across the last seven sessions was set. As can be seen from Figure 8.8, Shawn approached and nearly attained the higher goal level set for him.

Using the long-term monitoring, general outcomes measurement (GOM) passages taken from the AIMSweb material with which Shawn was not familiar showed that he made substantial progress toward the desired goal. Based on the goals set for Shawn by the IST, he was expected to reach a level of 54 WCPM across the first 2 weeks of the intervention program, and then reach a level of 70 WCPM across the remaining 5 weeks. Although not quite reaching 70 WCPM, Shawn improved his reading performance from 42 WCPM at baseline to around 60 WCPM across the 7 weeks of intervention. This was a gain of 18 words correct in 7 weeks, or almost 2.6 words correct per week (see Figure 8.9).

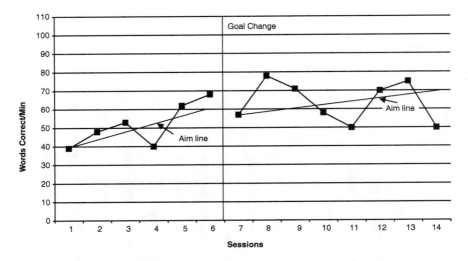

FIGURE 8.8. Presession, short-term progress monitoring of reading intervention for Shawn.

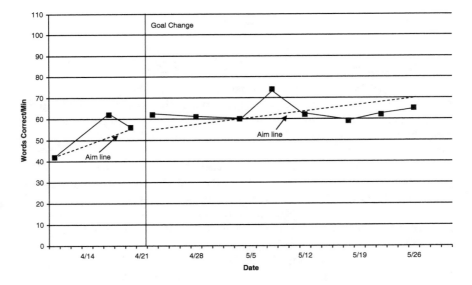

FIGURE 8.9. General outcomes measurement (long-term) progress monitoring for Shawn in reading.

Conclusions and Comments about Shawn's Case

Over the course of 7 weeks, Shawn made considerable progress in his reading fluency. Despite scheduling conflicts and absences that made the intervention less consistent than planned, Shawn increased his fluency in third-grade reading material and approached the goal of reaching third-grade instructional levels. Overall, Shawn was very cooperative and enjoyed the peer-tutoring intervention. During assessment sessions, Shawn also expressed that he really enjoyed graphing his own data.

In this case, the goals set for Shawn were very ambitious. Making progress at a rate of greater than two words per week exceeds the typical performance of most students who do not have any difficulties in reading (see discussion of normative data in Chapter 4). Shawn's case shows the outcomes that can be made when interventions are constructed and implemented with integrity. The nature of the intervention in Shawn's case, use of cross-age peer tutoring, was an excellent and moderately intensive intervention that allowed Shawn the opportunity to practice reading with clear objectives for outcomes. The case illustrates the connections between setting ambitious goals and interventions that are not highly complex to result in significant gains in students who are struggling. In addition, the case shows the links in progress monitoring between short- and long-term assessment methods.

Case 4: Jessi[4]

Name: Jessi
Birth date: November 28, 1991
Chronological age: 11 years,
           3 months

Grade: 5
Teacher: Mrs. Askin
School: Parkway
Report date: March 1, 2003

Background Information

Jessi was referred to the IST of her elementary school for evaluation because of failure to make adequate progress in reading comprehension and math. In particular, her teacher and the team had placed her on a list of students for whom retention was likely. Results of the evaluation revealed that Jessi was being instructed in a fifth-grade reading group for guided reading and read-aloud, and in a fourth-grade group for independent reading. When a CBA for reading was conducted, it was found that Jessi experi-

---

[4]Many thanks to Rebecca Clarkin, graduate student in school psychology at Lehigh University, whose case report is the basis for this material.

enced difficulties in comprehension. She was able to read passages fluently above her grade level but struggled with implicit–inferential comprehension at all levels. In math, Jessi was found to have difficulty with math computation at the third- and fourth-grade levels. In particular, she had her most significant problem with multiplication and division involving two- and three-digit problems. Although her overall accuracy in these skills appeared to be acceptable, her performance rate was extremely slow, suggesting the need for increasing fluency in these areas. Finally, an assessment of Jessi's concepts and applications of math skills revealed that she struggled with many areas, including place value, fractions, and multistep word problems.

Goal Setting

Reading Comprehension. Data obtained through a CBA revealed that Jessi's baseline level for questions answered correctly following the reading of passages was at 63%. A goal of increasing her level to 80% correct or higher was set to be obtained over a 6-week intervention period of instruction designed to focus specifically on improving strategies for reading comprehension.

Mathematics. The initial CBA conducted on Jessi in math identified both aspects of computation and concepts–applications as problematic. In computation, Jessi attained a baseline of 53% of division problems correct and an attained score of six digits correct on an assessment of mixed operations, and only two points correct on an assessment of math applications. Short-term goals set in division problems were for Jessi to achieve a score of 70% or better when presented with 10 division problems. A fluency goal of an 0.5-digit increase per week was established across a 6-week instructional period. In concepts–applications, a similar increase of 0.5 points per week was also established.

Interventions

Reading Comprehension. Based on the finding that Jessi was reading material at fluency rates that exceeded expected grade-level performance, the recommendation was made for Jessi to become more aware of how to read material for meaningful understanding. Specifically, Jessi was found to be reading at a rate of 130 WCPM in fifth-grade reading material but was attaining very low comprehension scores. The initial two sessions of the intervention plan focused on slowing down Jessi's reading rate in order for her to "digest" information and focus on adding emotion to the story by altering voice inflection and volume. A model of good reading was provided by the instructor, who read the material at a rate of approximately 100–110 WCPM and demonstrated the insertion of appropriate inflection.

Subsequent sessions with Jessi focused on reading for a purpose using the fifth-grade reading probes. Strategies such as predicting the outcomes of future events in the story and previewing the comprehension questions to be asked after reading were used. Before each session, the instructor would tell Jessi the title of the story and ask her what she thought the story might be about. Jessi was then asked to tell a story of her own related to the title. The instructor then read the comprehension questions to Jessi, who repeated the question and summarized what was going to be asked when the story was completed. Jessi then read the story and immediately answered the comprehension questions following her reading. The intervention was implemented twice per week for a total of 20 minutes each session.

Mathematics. Interventions were developed to improve Jessi's skills in multiplication facts, division, and fractions. The interventions described below were implemented 3 days per week for the first 2 weeks, and 5 days per week for the remaining 4 weeks. Each lesson lasted approximately 15 minutes.

Interventions for multiplication facts were provided for both school and at home. In school, the drill-sandwich technique (see Chapter 6) was used to help Jessi review her facts. The technique involved first assessing those facts that were known and unknown, then reviewing the facts in a group of 10, where seven facts were known and three were unknown. At home, Jessi was given worksheets to complete, with her mother reviewing multiplication facts as well. Special rewards at school were given for completion of these worksheets, including free time with a friend and lunch with the teacher.

To help Jessi acquire division skills, a set of minilessons was constructed on the steps involved in long division. During these minilessons, Jessi constructed reminder cards (see Figure 8.10) that provided examples of division problems, with and without remainders.

In order to facilitate her response, Jessi was instructed to place boxes over the dividend that corresponded to the correct number of digits she should have in her answer. This technique helped Jessi in sequencing division problems and knowing where to start her answers. The boxes were faded as instruction progressed. Jessi was also taught to prove her answers to division problems by using multiplication. If problems were incorrect, she was instructed to set up and solve the problem again. As instruction progressed and Jessi increased her skill development, proving division problems was reduced to a weekly basis only.

Minilessons in fractions were also constructed. These lessons involved drill and practice taken from Jessi's fractions quiz, on which she had scored 50% correct. Working with Jessi, the instructor, focused the drill on renaming, simplifying, and adding and subtracting fractions. Jessi again constructed a reminder card for each type of problem.

Jessi's Division Reminder

Does McDonald's Sell Cheeseburgers (DMSC)

Divide

Multiply

Subtract

Carry Down

FIGURE 8.10. Jessi's division reminder.

As part of the math intervention, Jessi also graphed her scores on math quizzes. This intervention was used to help Jessi see her progress, as well as to focus on slowing down and increasing the accuracy of her work. She was rewarded for any grade above 80%, earning tickets that could be exchanged for treats or activities.

Progress Monitoring Procedures

Reading Comprehension. Once each week, Jessi was given a fifth-grade passage with which she was not familiar. Following her reading the passage aloud, she was asked a set of eight comprehension questions (five literal, three inferential), and the percentage of questions answered correctly was calculated.

Mathematics. Both long- and short-term assessments of math skills were conducted for Jessi. Once each week, Jessi was assessed on computation or concepts–applications. These two areas were alternated, so that only one of these measures was given each week. Short-term assessment of progress in division was obtained daily, prior to starting each instructional session, by having Jessi complete a probe of division facts (two digits divided by one digit; three digits divided by one digit) similar to those that were being instructed. Long-term assessment involved having Jessi complete fourth-grade mixed-operation probes.

Results

Reading Comprehension. Outcomes for Jessi's performance in reading comprehension are reflected in Figure 8.11. As can be seen, Jessi's performance immediately improved from a baseline of 63% to scores averaging

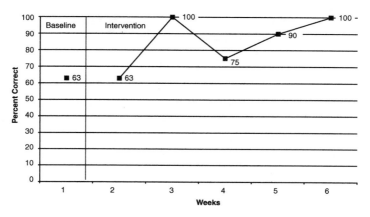

FIGURE 8.11. Short-term progress monitoring of Jessi's performance in reading comprehension.

between 75% and 100% correct after only two instructional sessions. In particular, although slowing Jessi's oral reading fluency contributed to the growth in comprehension, the instructor noted that the greatest gains (sessions 3–6) occurred when Jessi was taught the previewing strategy.

Mathematics. Jessi made tremendous progress in both her multiplication facts and division skills. By the end of the intervention period, Jesse was accurate and fluent in all multiplication facts to 9. She also showed very high accuracy in division skills, increasing from a baseline of 53% correct to 100% for both two-digit by one-digit and three-digit by one-digit division, as reflected in Figure 8.12.

Jessi's short-term gains in division and multiplication were also reflected in long-term progress monitoring. In addition, the instruction in fractions was also evident in the general outcomes measurement assessment collected every other week. These data are shown in Figures 8.13 and 8.14.

Conclusions and Comments about Jessi's Case

Over the course of 6 weeks of intervention, Jessi made considerable progress in all areas of concern that had resulted in her being referred to the IST. She showed considerable success in acquiring skills in multiplication and division, gains in concepts–applications of mathematics, especially fractions, and reading comprehension. These gains occurred as a function of focused and intensive intervention that included multiple strategies. As a result of the intervention program, Jessi was no longer considered at high risk for retention. Instead, the team decided to continue to monitor her progress carefully until the school year ended, and to make recommenda-

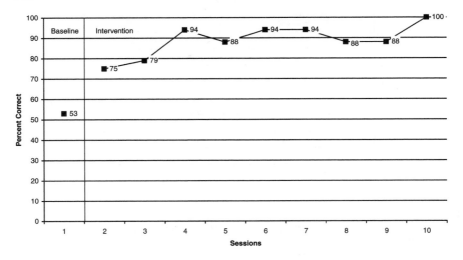

FIGURE 8.12. Short-term progress monitoring of Jessi's accuracy in division facts.

tions for Jessi to obtain ongoing academic support over the upcoming summer months, so that she would start the sixth-grade middle school in the fall with a high degree of success.

The case illustrates several important components of the process of conducting a CBA. First, the assessment data were directly linked to the development of specific intervention strategies. In Jessi's case, these strategies would all be viewed as moderate interventions in which substantial increases in skills were emphasized. Second, the interventions were implemented on a schedule that was reasonable and practical for both Jessi's teacher and the instructor. At the same time, the importance of implementing the intervention with consistency was recognized by everyone on the team. Third, the assessment demonstrates nicely how short- and long-term assessment measures can work together to offer clear determinations of student outcomes. For reading comprehension, Jessi's performance was monitored by only GOM or long-term assessment measures, using Jessi's performance on unknown passages as the mechanism to evaluate outcomes of the intervention. In math, however, short-term assessment was conducted by examining Jessi's performance on the skill being instructed—division of two-digit by one-digit and three-digit by one-digit problems. Jessi's long-term performance on measures involving mixed fourth grade operations showed gains that equaled goal levels set for her. Likewise, her gains from instruction in fractions were evident in her performance on fourth grade concepts/application probes.

Another important aspect of this case was the recognition that although Jessi had strong oral reading fluency that exceeded grade-level

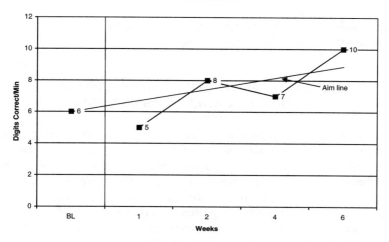

FIGURE 8.13. General outcome measurement (long-term) progress monitoring of Jessi's performance in math computation.

expectations, she lacked success in fully comprehending the material she read. As such, increased fluency was certainly not a goal of the instructional process. Indeed, the opposite was selected as a goal. Jessi's reading rate was purposely decreased to allow her more time to process the information flow and to synthesize what she was reading. Once Jessi slowed down, strategies used to teach comprehension became valuable tools that she was able to use in future reading. Likewise, the fluency rate could be increased

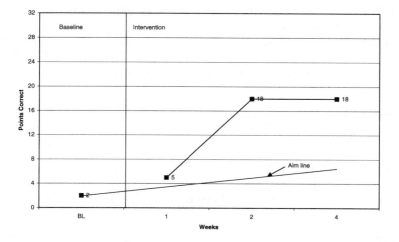

FIGURE 8.14. General outcome measurement (long-term) progress monitoring of Jessi's performance in math concepts–applications.

to levels evident prior to the intervention program, but with Jessi's renewed comprehension of what she was reading.

A CASE EXAMPLE OF THE FOUR-STEP MODEL OF DIRECT ACADEMIC ASSESSMENT

The final case presented here illustrates how all four steps of the model described in this text translate into practice. Although assessment data were collected for the student across academic areas, only the data and intervention technique for reading are presented. During the instructional modification phase, the folding-in procedure, discussed in Chapter 6, for the remediation of problems in reading fluency is presented. Readers interested in an example of the four-step assessment model applied to problems in math computation is provided by Shapiro and Ager (1992).

Case 5: Ace[5]

Name: Ace   *Grade*: 2
Birth date: August 1, 1994   *Teacher*: Mrs. Kregel
Chronological age: 8 years,   *School*: Nyack
                    8 months   *Report date*: April 3, 2003

Background Information

Ace was referred because of his poor reading abilities, as well as other academic skills problems. At the time of referral, his teachers reported that he had often been absent from school.

Currently he attends a general education classroom and is not being considered for special education. However, his teacher reports that Ace is not making the progress expected compared to other second graders.

Step 1: Assessment of the Instructional Environment

Teacher Interview. Mrs. Kregel reported that Ace is currently being instructed in the Houghton-Mifflin reading series, recently finishing the second book of Level 1 (grade 1) and has started in the first book of Level 2 (grade 2). Unfortunately, Ace missed a considerable amount of material as a result of a 6-week absence from school during a family trip abroad. Ac-

---

[5]Many thanks to Amy Kregel, graduate student in School Psychology at Lehigh University, whose case report is the basis for this material.

cording to his teacher, Ace is experiencing difficulties reading. In particular, Mrs. Kregel noted that Ace lacks phonetic analysis skills, has a poor sight vocabulary, and weak oral reading ability.

Although Ace is placed in a book consistent with his grade level, he is instructed in a below-average reading group. He and six other students receive remedial reading with another teacher for 90 minutes per day. During the allotted time, Ace receives a considerable amount of one-to-one instruction attention. Typically, the first 30 minutes of the instructional period are spent in silent reading and reviewing vocabulary. Students than read aloud to the group and complete written assignments. Any tasks not completed during the reading period are assigned as homework. A chart is displayed prominently in front of the classroom, on which accurate assignment completion is noted by stickers.

In terms of behavior, Mrs. Kregel reported that Ace is generally on-task and works quietly to complete his assigned work. Although he volunteers in class, he rarely gives the correct answer when called upon. The teacher's primary concern surrounds the accuracy of Ace's work in reading.

Mrs. Kregel also completed the Academic Performance Rating Scale (DuPaul, Rapport, & Perriello, 1991). She indicated that all aspects of language arts (reading, spelling, and writing) are the most significant problem for Ace. Math was noted as one of Ace's strengths.

Direct Observation. Using the BOSS, Ace was observed during one 20-minute silent reading and one 40-minute oral reading, teacher-directed instruction period. Comparison to peers from Ace's classroom was made during the silent reading period only. As can be seen in Table 8.7, during both sessions, Ace was found to be engaged in schoolwork (combination of

TABLE 8.7. Direct Observation Data from the BOSS Collected during Reading for Ace

	Percentage of intervals		
Behavior	Ace (silent reading, 20 min)	Peers (total intervals = 16)	Ace (oral reading/ teacher-directed instruction)
Active Engagement	31	25	14
Passive Engagement	44	13	56
Off-Task Motor	2	0	2
Off-Task Verbal	0	2	0
Off-Task Passive	20	15	20
Teacher-Directed Instruction	50		90

active and passive engagement) for 70% of the intervals. These levels of engagement were similar to those of his peers. Disruptive behaviors, such as calling out, socializing with peers, or getting out of his or her seat were infrequent for both Ace and his classmates. Ace did show somewhat higher levels of staring-off behavior compared to peers.

During silent reading, Ace received one-to-one instruction from his teacher for most of the intervals. Most of the time, the teacher was trying to teach Ace phonetic analysis. Teacher approval was minimal throughout the observation, despite the high frequency of teacher contact. It was observed during the oral reading that Ace was having great difficulty in identifying basic sight vocabulary and using context cues to answer questions about the material being read. A high degree of on-task behavior was evident, despite Ace's academic problems.

Student Interview. When asked about school, Ace stated that he enjoyed math and felt that it was his strongest area. He thought that most of his problems were in spelling, although he acknowledged having trouble with the reading assignment he had just been asked to complete. Ace noted that he sometimes did not understand the assignments he was given and was not interested in the work, especially if it was related to language arts. Although he thought the time he was given to do his work was fair, he disliked the fact that he often had homework in reading and spelling because he had trouble with class assignments. Ace noted that he often had trouble sounding out words. When asked to explain the procedure he should use if he were confused about his assignments, Ace demonstrated that he knew how to access help from his teacher or peers.

Permanent Product Review. Ace's reading journal and written reading comprehension assignments for the past week were examined. Examination of these materials showed that Ace had good knowledge of beginning consonant sounds. Areas of difficulty appeared to be in consonant blends, punctuation, and medial vowels. Although all assignments were completed, they lacked accuracy.

Summary. The assessment of the academic environment shows that Ace's classroom instruction follows fairly traditional approaches to teaching reading. Students are grouped by ability and much of the instruction is teacher-directed in small groups. Indeed, Ace receives significant teacher attention for his reading problems and is paired with students of similar ability levels. Although Ace is now reading in material consistent with his grade level, he lacks many of the skills needed for success in reading.

The direct observation of Ace's behavior reveals that he is an attentive child, who appears to try hard to overcome his academic problems. He appears to maintain this good level of engaged behavior despite low levels of teacher approval. Examination of Ace's products, as well as the classroom observation is very consistent with the information reported through the teacher interview.

Step 2: Assessing Instructional Placement

Timed passages were administered to Ace across five levels of the reading series. As seen in Table 8.8, Ace was found to be instructional at the Preprimer B level but frustrational at all other levels. Because Ace was found to be frustrational at all levels below the level where he is currently placed (Level 2-1), passages from that level were not administered. During the reading of these passages, Ace was observed to be very dysfluent. He would often lose his place, read a line more than once, and replace unknown words rather than sound them out. However, he was able to answer the comprehension screening questions with at least 80% accuracy for most passages.

In general, the direct assessment of reading showed that Ace is being instructed at a level far beyond his current instructional level. He is likely to experience little success at the 2-1 level at which he is being taught.

Step 3: Instructional Modification

After a review of data from Steps 1 and 2 with the teacher, it was decided to construct an intervention to increase Ace's sight-word recognition and reading fluency in grade-level material. This was considered an essential ingredient for Ace to succeed, especially because his teacher indicated that she was reluctant to move him back to a lower level in the reading series.

The folding-in technique was selected to be implemented three times per week in one-to-one sessions led by an instructional assistant. Baseline data were first collected by the evaluator in the 2-1 level of the reading series in which Ace was being taught. Material selected for instruction dur-

TABLE 8.8. Results of Reading Probe Assessment for Ace

Grade level/ book	Median words correct/min	Median words incorrect/min	% questions correct	Learning level (M, I, F)
B—Preprimer	45	0	100	Instructional
C—Preprimer	38	5	100	Frustrational
D—Preprimer	39	8	80	Frustrational
1.1	31	10	80	Frustrational
1.2	18	6	60	Frustrational

ing the folding-in technique was selected from the story just ahead of where the class was presently reading. This would permit Ace the opportunity to preview and practice reading material prior to his classmates.

Each session began with Ace first being asked to read a passage (usually a paragraph or two consisting of about 100 words) from the upcoming story. The number of words read correctly per minute was calculated and plotted on Ace's bar graph. From the passage, a list of seven words read correctly (identified as "known words") and three words read incorrectly (identified as "unknown words") were selected. The known words selected consisted of words relevant to the content of the story and not simply articles such as *the, and,* and similar types of words. All of the words were written on 3" × 5" index cards.

The unknown words were then interspersed among the known words by folding each unknown word into a review of the seven known words. This was done by having the instructional assistant present the first unknown word to Ace. The instructional assistant taught the word to Ace by saying the word, spelling the word, and using the word in a sentence. Ace was then asked to do the same. After the unknown word was taught, it was presented to Ace, followed by the first known word. Next, the unknown word was presented, followed by the first known word, and then the second known word. This sequence continued until all seven known and the first unknown word had been presented. If at any point in the process Ace hesitated or responded incorrectly, he was asked to again say the word, spell the word, and use it in a sentence.

The second unknown word was then introduced in the same way and folded in among the seven known and one unknown word already presented. The third unknown was then folded in, using the same procedures. The entire procedure took 7–10 minutes.

After the folding-in procedure was completed, Ace was asked to read the same passage he had read at the beginning of the session. His words correct per minute were again calculated and plotted on his bar graph. Ace was also asked to again read the words that were used during the folding-in procedure. If for 2 consecutive days he identified a word that had been classified as an unknown, the word was then considered known. The next session, a previous word from the known pile was discarded and replaced by this previously unknown word. The number of words that moved from unknown to known status was also plotted on a graph by Ace. Each session that Ace learned at least one new word, he was rewarded with an opportunity to select an item from a prize bag.

Step 4: Progress Monitoring

Both long- and short-term progress monitoring of Ace's performance were conducted. In consultation with Ace's teacher, a short-term goal of learning five new words per week was selected. In addition, at the end of the 4-week intervention, Ace would be able to read at least 40 words per minute during the presession reading. A long-term (end-of-year) goal was selected by examining the normative data for students in the 25th percentile of grade 2 in Ace's school district. Those data suggested that Ace should be able to read at least 40 words per minute in the grade 2-1 book.

Short-term monitoring was reflected in Ace's performance on the passage read before and after each folding-in session. In addition, the cumulative number of words learned per week was used to show the acquisition of new words for Ace. Long-term monitoring was obtained through the collection of CBMs taken twice per week by randomly selecting passages from across the second half of the Level 2-1 book.

Results

The results of the four-step process are shown in Figures 8.15, 8.16, and 8.17. Ace demonstrated consistent improvement in his reading fluency from pre- to postsession readings during each time the folding-in intervention was conducted. As seen in Figure 8.15, Ace initially had a reading rate of 10 WCPM in the materials being taught. Following each folding-in session, Ace improved his rate by 10–20 WCPM. An examination of his presession reading rate reflects steady improvement toward the goal of 40 WCPM in presession reading performance over the 4 weeks of intervention. As seen in Figure 8.16, Ace also displayed consistent gains each day in the number of new words learned.

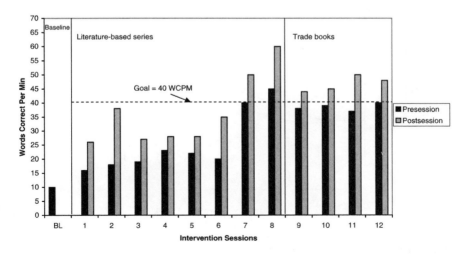

FIGURE 8.15. Results of folding-in intervention sessions for Ace.

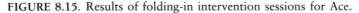

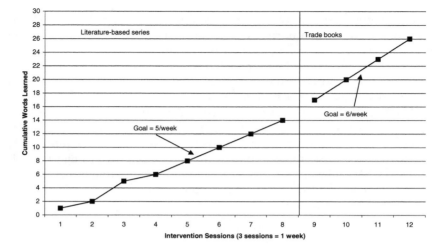

FIGURE 8.16. Results of short-term progress monitoring (cumulative words learned) for Ace during folding-in intervention.

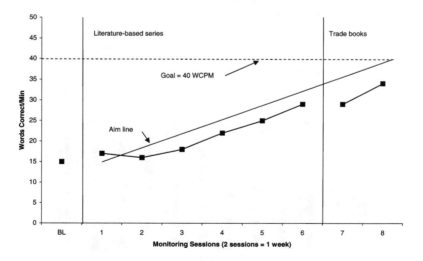

FIGURE 8.17. General outcomes measurement (long-term) progress monitoring for Ace as a result of the folding-in intervention for reading.

Given Ace's strong performance on short-term objectives, an increase from five to six new words per week occurred after the eighth session. As is evident from Figure 8.16, Ace was able to easily achieve this goal throughout the rest of the intervention. Also, at the end of the eighth session, the teacher decided to shift Ace (as well as the rest of the class) from the literature-based reading series to grade-based trade books. Across the last four intervention sessions, the words and passages used for the folding-in technique were taken from the new instructional material. Passages for CBM were still taken from the latter portion of the Level 2-1 basal reading series. Ace maintained his performance across the final week of the intervention using this new material.

An examination of Figure 8.17 shows that Ace was moving toward the long-term goal set for him by his teacher. Despite a change in the instructional material, the data show that Ace was making excellent progress.

Comments about Ace's Case

This case illustrates how the full, four-step model discussed throughout this text can be applied. In this particular example, an assessment of the instructional environment showed that Ace was receiving substantial assistance from the teacher. Indeed, despite high levels of teacher-directed instruction, he was not succeeding. In addition, he had been moved through curriculum materials, even though he clearly lacked mastery with those materials. The teacher was unable or unwilling to move him to material that would be instructional for his fluency level.

Using these data, the evaluator was able to pinpoint what might be keystone behaviors to predict future success. Specifically, the evaluator recognized that increasing sight-word recognition and fluency was likely to result in Ace increasing his effective participation in class, as well as maintaining himself within the present classroom environment. By constructing an intervention that included opportunities to preview upcoming material, the probabilities that Ace would succeed were enhanced.

The case also illustrates the use of the powerful folding-in technique. Because this intervention mixes known and unknown material in a way that guarantees student success, it is likely to result in increased student motivation to learn. Indeed, bar graphs and other visual displays of the data are known to be excellent mechanisms to motivate challenging students.

Finally, the case illustrates how the data can be used to make instructional decisions. In this case, Ace had demonstrated the ability to meet the short-term goals set for him (five new words per week). Seeing this, the evaluator determined that the goal could be increased to six words. When this change was made, Ace's performance improved.

The case also shows the outcomes of an unexpected change, an alteration in the instructional materials. Although the data collection ended as the school year came to a close, the results did show that Ace could maintain his performance when a new set of reading materials were introduced.

CONCLUSIONS

Interventions that may be effective in improving academic performance cannot always be predicted on the basis of assessment data alone. Although the evaluation may provide clues as to the best choices of potentially potent strategies, it is through the ongoing collection of data that one can best determine whether a procedure is working as planned. What works for Jessi may not work for Ace. What works for Ace now may not work for him as well later. These are the realities of academic interventions, and they make the collection of data to assess progress imperative.

The cases provided here are only a brief sampling of the richness of possible examples that could have been selected. These cases represent the performance of actual students and are not hypothetical. Obviously, many other cases could have been chosen.

The future of effective academic interventions most likely will rely on the ability to convince teachers, psychologists, school administrators, and consultants of the importance of data collection to evaluate student progress. Being aware of the range of potential interventions to improve academic skills surely will help the consultant plan effective teaching procedures. However, even those less skilled in developing interventions can greatly facilitate the process of intervention by understanding how to collect data on student progress. Teachers often offer a wealth of experience, knowledge, and training to suggest interventions. It may be unnecessary for those working in a consultative arrangement with these teachers ever to suggest interventions. Data collection, however, appears to be the key to effective intervention. Without the data, we are left to guess the effectiveness of our procedures.

This text has presented a wealth of techniques and strategies for assessing academic problems, as well as potential interventions for solving these complex problems. Reading about them, however, is only the first step. Readers should not be fearful of "trying out" these procedures with one or two representative cases, with teachers who are willing to experiment, and in situations likely to result in success. Such readers will probably find that the procedures are both extremely easy to implement and time-efficient, and will result in successful and rewarding delivery of services.

References

♦

Abt Associates. (1976). *Education as experimentation* (Vol. III). Cambridge, MA: Author.

Abt Associates. (1977). *Education as experimentation* (Vol. IV). Cambridge, MA: Author.

Adams, G., & Carnine, D. (2003). Direct instruction. In H. L. Swanson, K. R. Harris, & S. Graham (Eds.), *Handbook of learning disabilities* (pp. 403–416). New York: Guilford Press.

Adams, M. J., Foorman, B. R., Lundberg, I., & Beeler, T. (1998). The elusive phoneme: Why phonemic awareness is so important and how to help children develop it. *American Educator, 22*(1–2), 18–29.

Ager, C. L., & Shapiro, E. S. (1995). Template matching as a strategy for assessment of and intervention for preschool students with disabilities. *Topics in Early Childhood Special Education, 15,* 187–218.

Alessi, G., & Kaye, J. H. (1983). *Behavior assessment for school psychologists.* Kent, OH: National Association of School Psychologists.

Allen, L. J., Howard, V. F., Sweeney, W. J., & McLaughlin, T. F. (1993). Use of contingency contracting to increase on-task behavior with primary students. *Psychological Reports, 72,* 905–906.

Allsopp, D. H. (1997). Using classwide peer tutoring to teach beginning algebra problem-solving skills in heterogeneous classrooms. *Remedial and Special Education, 18,* 367–379.

Allyn and Bacon. (1978). *Pathfinder—Allyn and Bacon reading program.* Boston: Author.

American Psychiatric Association. (1994). *Diagnostic and statistical manual of mental disorders* (4th ed.). Washington, DC: Author.

Arblaster, G. R., Butler, A. L., Taylor, C. A., Arnold, C., & Pitchford, M. (1991). Same-age tutoring, mastery learning and the mixed ability teaching of reading. *School Psychology International, 12,* 111–118.

Armbruster, B. B., Stevens, R. J., & Rosenshine, B. V. (1977). *Analyzing content coverage and emphasis: A study of three curricula and two tests* (Technical Report No.

26). Urbana–Champaign: Center for the Study of Reading, University of Illinois at Urbana–Champaign.

Arter, J. A., & Jenkins, J. R. (1979). Differential diagnosis–prescriptive teaching: A critical appraisal. *Review of Educational Research, 49,* 517–555.

Axelrod, S., & Greer, R. D. (1994). Cooperative learning revisited. *Journal of Behavioral Education, 4,* 41–48.

Ayres, R. R., & Cooley, E. J. (1986). Sequential and simultaneous processing on the K-ABC: Validity in predicting learning success. *Journal of Psychoeducational Assessment, 4,* 211–220.

Ayres, R. R., Cooley, E. J., & Severson, H. H. (1988). Educational translation of the Kaufman Assessment Battery for Children: A construct validity study. *School Psychology Review, 17,* 113–124.

Babyak, A. E., Koorland, M., & Mathes, P. G. (2000). The effects of story mapping instruction on the reading comprehension of students with behavioral disorders. *Behavioral Disorders, 25,* 239–258.

Bandura, A. (1976). Self-reinforcement: Theoretical and methodological considerations. *Behaviorism, 4,* 135–155.

Barlow, D. H., & Wolfe, B. E. (1981). Behavioral approaches to anxiety disorders: A report of the NIMH-SUNY, Albany, research conference. *Journal of Consulting and Clinical Psychology, 49,* 448–454.

Barsch, R. H. (1965). *A moviegenic curriculum.* Madison, WI: Bureau for Handicapped Children.

Baumann, J. F., & Bergeron, B. S. (1993). Story map instruction using children's literature: Effects on first graders' comprehension of central narrative elements. *Journal of Reading Behavior, 25,* 407–437.

Beck, A. T., Rush, A. J., Shaw, B. F., & Emery, G. (1979). *Cognitive therapy of depression.* New York: Guilford Press.

Becker, W. C., & Carnine, D. W. (1981). Direct instruction: A behavior theory model for comprehensive educational intervention with the disadvantaged. In S. W. Bijou & R. Ruiz (Eds.), *Behavior modification: Contributions to education* (pp. 145–210). Hillsdale, NJ: Erlbaum.

Becker, W. C., & Engelmann, S. (1978). Systems for basic instruction: Theory and applications. In A. C. Cantania & T. A. Brigham (Eds.), *Handbook of applied behavior research* (pp. 325–377). New York: Irvington.

Becker, W. C., & Gersten, R. (1982). A follow-up of Follow-Through: The later effects of the Direct Instruction model on children in the fifth and sixth grades. *American Educational Research Journal, 19,* 75–92.

Beirne-Smith, M. (1991). Peer tutoring in arithmetic for children with learning disabilities. *Exceptional Children, 57,* 330–337.

Bell, P. F., Lentz, F. E., & Graden, J. L. (1992). Effects of curriculum–test overlap on standardized test scores: Identifying systematic confounds in educational decision making. *School Psychology Review, 21,* 644–655.

Benito, Y. M., Foley, C. L., Lewis, C. D., & Prescott, P. (1993). The effect of instruction in question–answer relationships and metacognition on social studies comprehension. *Journal of Research in Reading, 16*(1), 20–29.

Bentz, J., Shinn, M. R., & Gleason, M. M. (1990). Training general education pupils to monitor reading using curriculum-based measurement procedures. *School Psychology Review, 19,* 23–32.

Bergan, J. R. (1977). *Behavioral consultation.* Columbus, OH: Merrill.

Bergan, J. R., & Kratochwill, T. R. (1990). *Behavioral consultation and therapy.* New York: Plenum Press.

Bergan, J. R., & Tombari, M. L. (1975). The analysis of verbal interactions occurring during consultation. *Journal of School Psychology, 13,* 209–226.

Berliner, D. C. (1979). Tempus educare. In P. L. Peterson & H. J. Walberg (Eds.), *Research on teaching* (pp. 120–135). Berkley, CA: McCutchan.

Berliner, D. C. (1988). Effective classroom management and instruction: A knowledge base for consultation. In J. L. Graden, J. E. Zins, & M. J. Curtis (Eds.), *Alternate educational delivery systems: Enhancing instructional options for all students* (pp. 309–326). Washington, DC: National Association of School Psychologists.

Berninger, V. W. (1994). Introduction. In V. Berninger (Ed.), *The varieties of orthographic knowledge: I. Theoretical and developmental issues* (pp. 1–25). Dordrecht, The Netherlands: Kluwer.

Berninger, V. W. (1998). *Process assessment of the learner: Guide for intervention: Reading, writing.* San Antonio, TX: Psychological Corporation.

Berninger, V. W., & Amtmann, D. (2003). Preventing written expression disabilities through early and continuing assessment and intervention for handwriting and/or spelling problems: Research into practice. In H. L. Swanson, K. R. Harris, & S. Graham (Eds.), *Handbook of learning disabilities* (pp. 345–363). New York: Guilford Press.

Berninger, V. W., Vaughn, K., Abbott, R. D., Brooks, A., Abbott, S. P., Rogan, L., et al. (1998). Early intervention for spelling problems: Reaching functional spelling units of varying size with a multiple-connections framework. *Journal of Educational Psychology, 90,* 587–605.

Betts, E. A. (1946). *Foundations of reading instruction,* New York: American Book.

Billingsley, B. S., & Ferro-Almeida, S. C. (1993). Strategies to facilitate reading comprehension in students with learning disabilities. *Reading and Writing Quarterly: Overcoming Learning Difficulties, 9,* 263–278.

Blachman, B. A., Ball, E. W., Vlack, R., & Tangei, D. M. (2000). *Road to the code.* Baltimore, MD: Brookes.

Blachowicz, C., & Ogle, D. (2001). *Reading comprehension: Strategies for independent learners.* New York: Guilford Press.

Blandford, B. J., & Lloyd, J. W. (1987). Effects of a self-instructional procedure on handwriting. *Journal of Learning Disabilities, 20,* 342–346.

Blankenship, C. S. (1985). Using curriculum-based assessment data to make instructional management decisions. *Exceptional Children, 42,* 233–238.

Bornstein, P. H., & Quevillon, R. P. (1976). The effects of a self-instructional package on overactive preschool boys. *Journal of Applied Behavior Analysis, 9,* 179–188.

Bos, C. S., & Vaughn, S. (2002). *Strategies for teaching students with learning and behavior problems* (5th ed). Boston: Allyn & Bacon.

Bourque, P., Dupuis, N., & Van Houten, R. (1986). Public posting in the classroom: Comparison of posting names and coded numbers of individual students. *Psychological Reports, 59,* 295–298.

Braden, J. P. (2002). Best practices for school psychologists in educational accountability: High stakes testing and educational reform. In A. Thomas & J. Grimes (Eds.), *Best practices in school psychology IV* (Vol. 1, pp. 301–320). Bethesda, MD: National Association of School Psychologists.

Bradley-Klug, K. L., Shapiro, E. S., Lutz, J. G., & DuPaul, G. J. (1998). Evaluation of oral reading rate as a curriculum-based measure within literature-based curriculum. *Journal of School Psychology, 36,* 183–197.

Bramlett, R. K., Murphy, J. J., Johnson, J., & Wallingsford, L. (2002). Contemporary practices in school psychology: A national survey of roles and referral problems. *Psychology in the Schools, 39,* 327–335.

Brigance, A. (1981). *Brigance Inventory of Essential Skills.* North Billerica, MA: Curriculum Associates.

Brigance, A. (1999). *Brigance Comprehensive Inventory of Basic Skills—Revised.* North Billerica, MA: Curriculum Associates.

Brigance, A. (2004). *Brigance Inventory of Early Development –II.* North Billerica, MA: Curriculum Associates.

Brigham, T. A. (1980). Self-control revisited: Or why doesn't anyone actually read Skinner (1953). *Behaviorism, 3,* 25–33.

Broussard, C. D., & Northrup, J. (1995). An approach to functional assessment and analysis of disruptive behavior in regular educational classrooms. *School Psychology Quarterly, 10,* 151–164.

Browder, D. M., & Shapiro, E. S. (1985). Applications of self-management to individuals with severe handicaps: A review. *Journal of the Association for Persons with Severe Handicaps, 10,* 200–208.

Bryan, T., Burstein, K., & Bryan, J. (2001). Students with learning disabilities: Homework problems and promising practices. *Educational Psychologist, 36,* 167–180.

Bryant, D., Ugel, N., Thompson, S., & Hamff, A. (1999). Instructional strategies for content-area reading instruction. *Intervention in School and Clinic, 34,* 293–302.

Burns, M. K. (2001). Measuring sight-word acquisition and retention rates with curriculum-based assessment. *Journal of Psychoeducational Assessment, 19,* 148–157.

Burns, M. K., Tucker, J. A., Frame, J., Foley, S., & Hauser, A. (2000). Interscorer, alternate-form, internal consistency, and test–retest reliability of Gickling's model of curriculum-based assessment for reading. *Journal of Psychoeducational Assessment, 18,* 353–360.

Caldwell, J. H., Huitt, W. G., & Graeber, A. O. (1982). Time spent in learning: Implications from research. *Elementary School Journal, 82,* 471–480.

Calhoun, M. B., & Fuchs, L. S. (2003). The effects of peer-assisted learning strategies and curriculum-based measurement on the mathematics performance of secondary students with disabilities. *Remedial and Special Education, 24,* 235–245.

Campbell, J. A., & Willis, J. (1978). Modifying components of creative behavior in the natural environment. *Behavior Modification, 2,* 549–564.

Cancelli, A. A., & Kratochwill, T. R. (1981). Advances in criterion-referenced assessment. In T. R. Kratochwill (Ed.), *Advances in school psychology* (Vol. 1, pp. 213–254). Hillsdale, NJ: Erlbaum.

Canter, A. (1995). Best practices in developing local norms in behavioral assessment. In A. Thomas & J. Grimes (Eds.), *Best practices in school psychology III* (pp. 689–700). Washington, DC: National Association of School Psychologists.

Carnine, D. (1976). Effects of two teacher presentation rates on off-task behavior, answering correctly, and participation. *Journal of Applied Behavior Analysis, 9,* 199–206.

Carr, E. G., Newson, C., & Binkoff, J. (1980). Escape as a factor in the aggressive behavior of two retarded children. *Journal of Applied Behavior Analysis, 13,* 101–117.

Carr, S. C., & Punzo, R. P. (1993). The effects of self-monitoring of academic accuracy and productivity on the performance of students with behavioral disorders. *Behavioral Disorders, 18,* 241–250.

Carroll, J. B. (1963). A model of school learning. *Teachers College Record, 64,* 723–733.

Carta, J. J., Atwater, J. B., Schwartz, I. S., & Miller, P. A. (1990). Applications of ecobehavioral analysis to the study of transitions across early education. *Education and Treatment of Children, 13,* 298–315.

Carta, J. J., Greenwood, C. R., & Atwater, J. (1985). *Ecobehavioral system for complex assessments of preschool environments (ESCAPE).* Kansas City: Juniper Gardens Children's Project, Bureau of Child Research, University of Kansas.

Carta, J. J., Greenwood, C. R., Schulte, D., Arreaga-Mayer, C., & Terry, B. (1987). *The Mainstream Code for Instructional Structure and Student Academic Response (MS-CISSAR): Observer training manual.* Kansas City: Juniper Garden Children's Project, Bureau of Child Research, University of Kansas.

Cartledge, G., & Milburn, J. F. (1983). Social skill assessment and teaching in the schools. In T. R. Kratochwill (Ed.), *Advances in school psychology* (Vol. III, pp. 175–236). Hillsdale, NJ: Erlbaum.

Carver, R. P. (1974). Two dimensions of tests: Psychometric and edumetric. *American Psychologist, 29,* 512–518.

Case, L. P., Harris, K. R., & Graham, S. (1992). Improving the mathematical problem-solving skills of students with learning disabilities: Self-regulated strategy development. *Journal of Special Education, 26,* 1–19.

Cates, G. L., Skinner, C, H., Watkins, C. E., Rhymer, K. N., McNeill, S. L., & McCurdy, M. (1999). Effects of interspersing additional brief math problems on student performance and perception of math assignments: Getting students to prefer to do more work. *Journal of Behavioral Education, 9,* 177–192.

Chadwick, B. A., & Day, R. C. (1971). Systematic reinforcement: Academic performance of underachieving students. *Journal of Applied Behavior Analysis, 4,* 311–319.

Chard, D. J., Vaughn, S., & Tyler, B. J. (2002). A synthesis of research on effective interventions for building reading fluency with elementary students for learning disabilities. *Journal of Learning Disabilities, 35,* 386–406.

Christenson, S. L., & Ysseldyke, J. E. (1989). Assessment student performance: An important change is needed. *Journal of School Psychology, 27,* 409–425.

Clark, F. L., Deshler, D. D., Schumaker, J. B., & Alley, G. R. (1984). Visual imagery and self-questioning: Strategies to improve comprehension of written materials. *Journal of Learning Disabilities, 17,* 145–149.

Clark, L., & Elliott, S. N. (1988). The influence of treatment strength information of knowledgeable teachers' pretreatment evaluation of social skills training methods. *Professional School Psychology, 3,* 241–251.

Clymer, T., & Fenn, T. (1979). *Ginn Reading 720, Rainbow Edition.* Lexington, MA: Ginn.

Cobbs, J. A., & Hopps, H. (1973). Effects of academic survival skill training on low achieving first graders. *Journal of Educational Research, 67,* 108–113.

Cochran, L., Feng, H., Cartledge, G., & Hamilton, S. (1993). The effects of cross-age tutoring on the academic achievement, social behavior, and self-perceptions of low-achieving African-American males with behavior disorders. *Behavioral Disorders, 18,* 292–302.

Combs, M. L., & Lahey, B. B. (1981). A cognitive social skills training program: Evaluation with young children. *Behavior Modification, 5,* 39–60.

Cone, J. D. (1978). The Behavioral Assessment Grid (BAG): A conceptual framework and a taxonomy. *Behavior Therapy, 9,* 882–888.

Cone, J. D. (1981). Psychometric considerations. In M. Hersen & A. S. Bellack (Eds.), *Behavioral assessment: A practical handbook* (2nd ed., pp. 38–68). New York: Pergamon Press.

Cone, J. D. (1988). Psychometric considerations and multiple models of behavioral assessment. In M. Hersen & A. S. Bellack (Eds.), *Behavioral assessment: A practical handbook* (3rd ed., pp. 42–66). New York: Pergamon Press.

Cone, J. D., & Hoier, T. S. (1986). Assessing children: The radical behavioral perspective. In R. Prinz (Ed.), *Advances in behavioral assessment of children and families* (Vol. 2, pp. 1–27). New York: JAI Press.

Connell, M. C., Carta, J. J., & Baer, D. M. (1993). Programming generalization of in-class transition skills; Teaching preschoolers with developmental delays to self-assess and recruit contingent praise. *Journal of Applied Behavior Analysis, 26,* 345–352.

Connoley, A. J. (1997). *KeyMath Revised/Normative Update: A diagnostic inventory of essential mathematics.* Circle Pines, MN: American Guidance Service.

Cooke, N. L., Guzaukas, R., Pressley, J. S., & Kerr, K. (1993). Effects of using a ratio of new items to review items during drill and practice: Three experiments. *Education and Treatment of Children, 16,* 213–234.

Cooper, L. J., Wacker, D. P., Sasso, G. M., Reimers, T. M., & Donn, L. K. (1990). Using parents as therapists to evaluate the appropriate behavior of their children: Applications to a tertiary diagnostic clinic. *Journal of Applied Behavior Analysis, 23,* 285–296.

Cooper, L. J., Wacker, D. P., Thursby, D., Plagmann, L. A., Harding, J., Millard, T., & Derby, M. (1992). Analysis of the effects of task preferences, task demands, and adult attention on child behavior in outpatient and classroom settings. *Journal of Applied Behavior Analysis, 23,* 285–296.

Copeland, S. R., Hughes, C., Agran, M., Wehneyer, M. L., & Fowler, S. E. (2002). An intervention package to support high school students with mental retardation in general education classrooms. *American Journal on Mental Retardation, 107,* 32–45.

Cosden, M. A., & Haring, T. G. (1992). Cooperative learning in the classroom: Contingencies, group interactions, and students with special needs. *Journal of Behavioral Education, 2,* 53–71.

Cossairt, A., Hall, R. V., & Hopkins, B. L. (1973). The effects of experimenter's instruction, feedback, and praise on teacher praise and student attending behavior. *Journal of Applied Behavior Analysis, 6,* 89–100.

Coulter, W. A., & Coulter, E. M. B. (1991). *C. B. A. I. D. : Curriculum-based assessment for instructional design* [Training manual]. New Orleans: Louisiana State University Medical Center.

Crawford, L., Tindal, G., & Stieber, S. (2001). Using oral reading rate to predict student performance on statewide assessment tests. *Educational Assessment, 7,* 303–323.

Cronbach, L. J., & Snow, R. E. (1977). *Aptitudes and instructional methods.* New York: Irvington.

Cullinan, D., Lloyd, J., & Epstein, M. H. (1981). Strategy training: A structured approach to arithmetic instruction. *Exceptional Education Quarterly, 2,* 41–49.

Daly, E. J., III, & Martens, B. K. (1994). A comparison of three interventions for increasing oral reading performance: Application of the instructional hierarchy. *Journal of Applied Behavior Analysis, 27,* 459–469.

Daly, E. J., III, & Martens, B. K. (1999). A brief experimental analysis for identifying instructional components needed to improve oral reading fluency. *Journal of Applied Behavior Analysis, 32,* 83–94.

Daly, E. J., III, & Murdoch, A. (2000). Direct observation in the assessment of academic skills problems. In E. S. Shapiro & T. R. Kratochwill (Eds.), *Behavioral assessment in schools: Theory, research, and clinical foundations* (2nd ed., pp. 46–77). New York: Guilford Press.

Daly, E. J., III, Witt, J. C., Martens, B. K., & Dool, E. J. (1997). A model for conducting a functional analysis of academic performance problems. *School Psychology Review, 26,* 554–574.

Das, J. P., Kirby, J., & Jarman, R. F. (1975). Simultaneous and successive syntheses: An alternative model for cognitive abilities. *Psychological Bulletin, 82,* 87–103.

Das, J. P., Kirby, J. R., & Jarman, R. F. (1979). *Simultaneous and successive cognitive processes.* New York: Academic Press.

Davis, Z. T. (1994). Effects of prereading story mapping on elementary readers' comprehension. *Journal of Educational Research, 87,* 353–360.

de Haas-Warner, S. J. (1991). Effects of self-monitoring on preschoolers' on-task behavior: A pilot study. *Topics in Early Childhood Special Education, 11,* 59–73.

Delquadri, J. C., Greenwood, C. R., Stretton, K., & Hall, R. V. (1983). The peer tutoring spelling game: A classroom procedure for increasing opportunities to respond and spelling performance. *Education and Treatment of Children, 6,* 225–239.

Delquadri, J., Greenwood, C. R., Whorton, D., Carta, J., & Hall, R. V. (1986). Classwide peer tutoring. *Exceptional Children, 52,* 535–542.

Denham, C., & Lieberman, P. (1980). *Time to learn.* Washington, DC: National Institute of Education.

Deno, S. L. (1985). Curriculum-based measurement: The emerging alternative. *Exceptional Children, 52,* 219–232.

Deno, S. L., Fuchs, L. S., Marston, D., & Shin, J. (2001). Using curriculum-based measurement to establish growth standards for students with learning disabilities. *School Psychology Review, 30,* 507–524.

Deno, S. L., King, R., Skiba, R., Sevcik, B., & Wesson, C. (1983). *The structure of instruction rating scale (SIRS): Development and technical characteristics* (Research Report No. 107). Minneapolis: University of Minnesota, Institute for Research on Learning Disabilities.

Deno, S. L., Marston, D., & Mirkin, P. K. (1982). Valid measurement procedures for continuous evaluation of written expression. *Exceptional Children, 48,* 368–371.

Deno, S. L., Marston, D., & Tindal, G. (1985–1986). Direct and frequent curriculum-based measurement: An alternative for educational decision making. *Special Services in the Schools, 2,* 5–27.

Deno, S. L., & Mirkin, P. K. (1977). *Data-based program modification: A manual.* Reston, VA: Council for Exceptional Children.

Deno, S. L., Mirkin, P. K., & Chiang, B. (1982). Identifying valid measures of reading. *Exceptional Children, 49,* 36–47.

Deno, S. L., Mirkin, P. K., Lowry, L., & Kuehnle, K. (1980). *Relationships among simple measures of spelling and performance on standardized achievement tests* (Research Report No. 21). Minneapolis: University of Minnesota, Institute for Research on Learning Disabilities. (ERIC Document Reproduction Service No. ED197508).

Derr, T. F., & Shapiro, E. S. (1989). A behavioral evaluation of curriculum-based assessment of reading. *Journal of Psychoeducational Assessment, 7,* 148–160.

Derr-Minneci, T. F., & Shapiro, E. S. (1992). Validating curriculum-based measurement in reading from a behavioral perspective. *School Psychology Quarterly, 7,* 2–16.

Deshler, D. D., & Schumaker, J. B. (1986). Learning strategies: An instructional alternative for low-achieving adolescents. *Exceptional Children, 52,* 583–590.

Deshler, D. D., & Schumaker, J. B. (1993). Strategy mastery by at-risk students: Not a simple matter. *Elementary School Journal, 94,* 153–167.

Deshler, D. D., Schumaker, J. B., Alley, G. R., Warner, M. M., & Clark, F. L. (1982). Learning disabilities in adolescent and young adult populations: Research implications (Part I). *Focus on Exceptional Children, 15*(1), 1–12.

Deshler, D. D., Schumaker, J. B., Lenz, B. K., & Ellis, E. S. (1984). Academic and cognitive interventions for LD adolescents (Part II). *Journal of Learning Disabilities, 17,* 170–187.

Dineen, J. P., Clark, H. B., & Risley, T. R. (1977). Peer tutoring among elementary students: Educational benefits to the tutor. *Journal of Applied Behavior Analysis, 10,* 231–238.

DiPerna, J. C., & Elliott, S. N. (1999). Development and validation of the Academic Competence Evaluation Scales. *Journal of Psychoeducational Assessment, 17,* 207–225.

DiPerna, J. C., & Elliott, S. N. (2002). Promoting academic enablers to improve student achievement: An introduction to the mini-series. *School Psychology Review, 31,* 293–297.

DiPerna, J. C., Volpe, R. J., & Elliott, S. N. (2002). A model of academic enablers and elementary reading/language arts achievement. *School Psychology Review, 31,* 298–312.

Donovan, M. S., & Cross, C. T. (Eds.). (2002). *Minority students in special and gifted education*. Washington, DC: National Academies Press.

Duarte, A. M. M., & Baer, D. M. (1994). The effects of self-instruction on preschool children's sorting of generalized in-common tasks. *Journal of Experimental Child Psychology, 57*, 1–25.

Dunlap, G., Clarke, S., Jackson, M., & Wright, S. (1995). Self-monitoring of classroom behaviors with students exhibiting emotional and behavioral challenges. *School Psychology Quarterly, 10*, 165–177.

Dunlap, G., Kern, L., & Worcester, J. A. (2001). ABA and academic instruction. *Focus on Autism and Other Developmental Disabilities, 16*, 129–136.

Dunlap, G., Kern-Dunlap, L., Clarke, S., & Robbins, F. R. (1991). Functional assessment, curricular revision, and severe behavior problems. *Journal of Applied Behavior Analysis, 24*, 387–397.

Dunn, L. M., & Markwardt, F. C. (1970). *Peabody Individual Achievement Test*. Circle Pines, MN: American Guidance Services.

DuPaul, G. J., Ervin, R. A., Hook, C. L., & McGoey, K. E. (1998). Peer tutoring for children with attention deficit hyperactivity disorder: Effects on classroom behavior and academic performance. *Journal of Applied Behavior Analysis, 31*, 579–592.

DuPaul, G. J., Guevremont, D. C., & Barkley, R. A. (1991). Attention deficit-hyperactivity disorder in adolescents: Critical assessment parameters. *Clinical Psychology Review, 11*, 231–245.

DuPaul, G. J., & Henningson, P. N. (1993). Peer tutoring effects on the classroom performance of children with attention deficit hyperactivity disorder. *School Psychology Review, 22*, 134–142.

DuPaul, G. J., Rapport, M. D., & Perriello, L. M. (1991). Teacher ratings of academic skills: The development of the Academic Performance Rating Scale. *School Psychology Review, 20*, 284–300.

Durost, W., Bixler, H., Wrightstone, J. W., Prescott, G., & Balow, I. (1970). *Metropolitan Achievement Test: Primary I and II battery*. New York: Harcourt, Brace, Jovanovich.

Eckert, T. L., Hinzte, J. M., & Shapiro, E. S. (1999). Development and refinement of a measure for assessing the acceptability of assessment methods: The Assessment Rating Profile—Revised. *Canadian Journal of School Psychology, 15*, 21–42.

Eckert, T. L., & Shapiro, E. S. (1999). Methodological issues in analog research: Are teachers' acceptability ratings of assessment methods influenced by experimental design? *School Psychology Review, 28*, 5–16.

Eckert, T. L., Shapiro, E. S., & Lutz, J. G. (1995). Teacher's ratings of the acceptability of curriculum-based assessment methods. *School Psychology Review, 24*, 499–510.

Eiserman, W. D. (1988). Three types of peer tutoring: Effects on the attitudes of students with learning disabilities and their regular class peers. *Journal of Learning Disabilities, 21*, 249–252.

Elley, W. N. (1989). Vocabulary acquisition from listening to stories. *Reading Research Quarterly, 14*, 174–187.

Elliott, S. N., Busse, R. T., & Gresham, F. M. (1993). Behavior rating scales: Issues of use and development. *School Psychology Review, 22*, 313–321.

Elliott, S. N., DiPerna, J. C., with Shapiro, E. S. (2001). *AIMS: Academic Intervention Monitoring System guidebook*. San Antonio, TX: Psychological Corporation.

Elliott, S. N., & Fuchs, L. S. (1997). The utility of curriculum-based measurement and performance assessment as alternatives to traditional intelligence and achievement tests. *School Psychology Review, 26*, 224–233.

Elliott, S. N., & Gresham, F. M. (1990). *Social Skills Rating System (SSRS)*. Circle Pines, MN: AGS Publishing.

Elliott, S. N., & Shapiro, E. S. (1990). Intervention techniques and programs for academic performance. In T. Gutkin & C. R. Reynolds (Eds.), *The handbook of school psychology* (2nd ed., pp. 635–660). Oxford, UK: Wiley.

Elliott, S. N., Turco, T. L., & Gresham, F. M. (1987). Consumers' and clients' pretreatment acceptability ratings of classroom group contingencies. *Journal of School Psychology, 25,* 145–153.

Ellis, E. S., & Lenz, B. K. (1987). A component analysis of effective learning strategies for LD students. *Learning Disabilities Focus, 2,* 94–107.

Ellis, E. S., Lenz, B. K., & Sabournie, E. J. (1987a). Generalization and adaptation of learning strategies to natural environments: Part I. Critical agents. *Remedial and Special Education, 8*(1), 6–20.

Ellis, E. S., Lenz, B. K., & Sabournie, E. J. (1987b). Generalization and adaptation of learning strategies to natural environments: Part 2. Research into practice. *Remedial and Special Education, 8*(2), 6–23.

Englemann, S., Becker, W. C., Carnine, D. W., & Gersten, R. (1988). The Direct Instruction Follow Through Model: Design and outcomes. *Education and Treatment of Children, 11,* 303–317.

Englemann, S., & Carnine, D. (1982). *Theory of instruction.* New York: Irvington.

Erchul, W. P., Covington, C. G., Hughes, J. N., & Meyers, J. (1995). Further explorations of request-centered relational communication within school consultation. *School Psychology Review, 24,* 621–632.

Ervin, R. A., DuPaul, G. J., Kern, L., & Friman, P. C. (1998). Classroom-based functional and adjunctive assessments: Proactive approaches to intervention selection for adolescents with attention-deficit hyperactivity disorder. *Journal of Applied Behavior Analysis, 31,* 65–78.

Espin, C. A., Scierka, B. J., Skare, S., & Halverson, N. (1999). Criterion-related validity of curriculum-based measures in writing for secondary school students. *Reading and Writing Quarterly, 15,* 5–27.

Espin, C., Shin, J., Deno, S. L., Skare, S., Robinson S., & Benner, B. (2000). Identifying indicators of written expression proficiency for middle school students. *Journal of Special Education, 34,* 140–153.

Espin, C. A., & Tindal, G. (1998). Curriculum-based measurement for secondary students. In M. R. Shinn (ed,), *Advanced applications of curriculum-based measurement* (pp. 214–253). New York: Guilford Press.

Evans, G. W. (1985). Building systems model as a strategy for target behavior in clinical assessment. *Behavioral Assessment, 7,* 21–32.

Evans, G. W., & Oswaldt, G. L. (1968). Acceleration of academic progress through the manipulation of peer influence. *Behaviour Research and Therapy, 6,* 189–195.

Fantuzzo, J. W., King, J. A., & Heller, L. R. (1992). Effects of reciprocal peer tutoring on mathematics and school adjustment: A component analysis. *Journal of Educational Psychology, 84,* 331–339.

Fantuzzo, J. W., & Polite, K. (1990). School-based, behavioral self-management: A review and analysis. *School Psychology Quarterly, 5,* 180–198.

Fantuzzo, J. W., Polite, K., & Grayson, N. (1990). An evaluation of reciprocal peer tutoring across elementary school settings. *Journal of School Psychology, 28,* 209–224.

Fantuzzo, J. W., Rohrbeck, C. A., & Azar, S. T. (1987). A component analysis of behavioral self-management interventions with elementary school students. *Child and Family Behavior Therapy, 9,* 33–43.

Ferster, C. B. (1965). Classification of behavioral pathology. In L. Krasner & L. P. Ullmann (Eds.), *Research in behavior modification* (pp. 6–26). New York: Holt, Rinehart & Winston.

Fink, W. T., & Carnine, D. W. (1975). Control of arithmetic errors using informational feedback and errors. *Journal of Applied Behavior Analysis, 8,* 461.

Finkel, A. S., Derby, K. M., Weber, K. P., & McLaughlin, T. F. (2003). Use of choice to identify behavioral function following an inconclusive brief functional analysis. *Journal of Positive Behavior Interventions, 5,* 112–121.

Fisher, C., & Berliner, D. C. (1985). *Perspectives on instructional time.* New York: Longman.

Fletcher, J. M., Foorman, B. R., Boudousquie, A., Barnes, M. A., Schatschneider, C., & Francis, D. J. (2002). Assessment of reading and learning disabilities: A research-based intervention-oriented approach. *Journal of School Psychology, 40,* 27–63.

Fletcher, J. M., Francis, D. J., Shaywitz, S. E., Lyon, G. R., Foorman, B. R., Stuebing, K. K., et al. (1998). Intelligent testing and the discrepancy model for children with learning disabilities. *Learning Disabilities Research and Practice, 13,* 186–203.

Fletcher, J. M., Morris, R. D., & Lyon, G. R. (2003). Classification and definition of learning disabilities: An integrative perspective. In H. L. Swanson, K. R. Harris, & S. Graham (Eds.), *Handbook of learning disabilities* (pp. 30–56). New York: Guilford Press.

Foegen, A., & Deno, S. L. (2001). Identifying growth indicators for low-achieving students. *Journal of Special Education, 35,* 4–16.

Foorman, B. R., Francis, D. J., Fletcher, J. M., & Lynn, A. (1996). Relation of phonological and orthographic processing to early reading: Comparing two approaches to regression-based, reading-level-match designs. *Journal of Educational Psychology, 88,* 639–652.

Fowler, S. A. (1984). Introductory comments: The pragmatics of self-management for the developmentally disabled. *Analysis and Intervention in Developmental Disabilities, 4,* 85–90.

Fowler, S. A. (1986). Peer-monitoring and self-monitoring: Alternatives to traditional teacher management. *Exceptional Children, 52,* 573–582.

Fox, D. E. C., & Kendall, P. C. (1983). Thinking through academic problems: Applications of cognitive behavior therapy to learning. In T. R. Kratochwill (Ed.), *Advances in school psychology* (Vol. III, pp. 269–301). Hillsdale, NJ: Erlbaum.

Foxx, R. M., & Jones, J. R. (1978). A remediation program for increasing the spelling achievement of elementary and junior high students. *Behavior Modification, 2,* 211–230.

Franca, V. M., Kerr, M. M., Reitz, A. L., & Lambert, D. (1990). Peer tutoring among behaviorally disordered students: Academic and social benefits to tutor and tutee. *Education and Treatment of Children, 13,* 109–128.

Francis, D. J., Shaywitz, S. E., Stuebing, K. K., Shaywitz, B. A., & Fletcher, J. M. (1996). Developmental lag versus deficit models of reading disability: A longitudinal, individual growth curves analysis. *Journal of Educational Psychology, 88,* 3–17.

Frederick, W. C., Walberg, H. J., & Rasher, S. P. (1979). Time, teacher comments, and achievement in urban high schools. *Journal of Educational Research, 13,* 63–65.

Freeman, T. J., & McLaughlin, T. F. (1984). Effects of a taped-words treatment procedure on learning disabled students' sight-word reading. *Learning Disability Quarterly, 7,* 49–54.

Friedling, C., & O'Leary, S. G. (1979). Effects of self-instruction on second and third grade hyperactive children: A failure to replicate. *Journal of Applied Behavior Analysis, 12,* 211–219.

Friedman, D. L., Cancelli, A. A., & Yoshida, R. K. (1988). Academic engagement of elementary school children with learning disabilities. *Journal of School Psychology, 26,* 327–340.

Frostig, M., & Horne, D. (1964). *The Frostig Program for the Development of Visual Perception: Teachers guide.* Chicago: Follett.

Fuchs, D., Fuchs, L. S., Benowitz, S., & Barringer, K. (1987). Norm-referenced tests: Are they valid for use with handicapped students? *Exceptional Children, 54,* 263–271.

Fuchs, D., Fuchs, L. S., & Burish, P. (2000). Peer-assisted learning strategies: An evidence-based practice to promote reading achievement. *Learning Disabilities Research and Practice, 15,* 85–91.

Fuchs, D., Fuchs, L. S., Thompson, A., Svennson, E., Yen, L., Otaiba, S. A., et al. (2001). Peer-assisted learning strategies in reading: Extensions for kindergarten, first grade, and high school. *Remedial and Special Education, 22,* 15–21.

Fuchs, L. S. (1986). Monitoring progress among mildly handicapped pupils: Review of current practice and research. *Remedial and Special Education, 7*(5), 5–12.

Fuchs, L. S., & Deno, S. L. (1982). *Developing goals and objectives for education programs* [Teaching guide]. U.S. Department of Education Grant, Institute for Research in Learning Disabilities, University of Minnesota, Minneapolis.

Fuchs, L. S., & Deno, S. L. (1991). Paradigmatic distinctions between instructionally relevant measurement models. *Exceptional Children, 57,* 488–500.

Fuchs, L. S., & Deno, S. L. (1992). Effects of curriculum within curriculum-based measurement. *Exceptional Children, 58,* 232–243.

Fuchs, L. S., & Deno, S. L. (1994). Must instructionally useful performance assessment be based in the curriculum? *Exceptional Children, 61,* 15–24.

Fuchs, L. S., Deno, S. L., & Marston, D. (1983). Improving the reliability of curriculum-based measures of academic skills for psychoeducational decision making, *Diagnostique, 8,* 135–149.

Fuchs, L. S., Deno, S. L., & Mirkin, P. K. (1984). The effects of frequent curriculum-based measures and evaluation on pedagogy, student achievement, and student awareness of learning. *American Educational Research Journal, 21,* 449–460.

Fuchs, L. S., & Fuchs, D. (1986a). Curriculum-based assessment of progress toward long-term and short-term goals. *Journal of Special Education, 20,* 69–82.

Fuchs, L. S., & Fuchs, D. (1986b). Effects of systematic formative evaluation: A meta-analysis. *Exceptional Children, 53,* 199–208.

Fuchs, L. S., & Fuchs, D. (1992). Identifying a measure for monitoring student reading progress. *School Psychology Review, 21,* 45–58.

Fuchs, L. S., & Fuchs, D. (1998). Treatment validity: A unifying concept for reconceptualizing the identification of learning disabilities. *Learning Disabilities Research and Practice, 13,* 204–219.

Fuchs, L. S., Fuchs, D., & Bishop, N. (1992). Instructional adaptation for students at risk. *Journal of Educational Research, 86,* 70–84.

Fuchs, L. S., Fuchs, D., Hamlett, C. L., & Allinder, R. M. (1991a). The contribution of skills analysis within curriculum-based measurement in spelling. *Exceptional Children, 57,* 443–452.

Fuchs, L. S., Fuchs, D., Hamlett, C. L., & Allinder, R. M. (1991b). Effects of expert system advice within curriculum-based measurement on teacher planning and student achievement in spelling. *School Psychology Review, 20,* 49–66.

Fuchs, L. S., Fuchs, D., Hamlett, C. L., & Ferguson, C. (1992). Effects of expert system consultation within curriculum-based measurement using a reading maze task. *Exceptional Children, 58,* 436–450.

Fuchs, L. S., Fuchs, D., Hamlett, C. L., Phillips, N. B., & Bentz, J. (1994). Classwide curriculum-based measurement: Helping general educators meet the challenge of student diversity. *Exceptional Children, 60,* 518–537.

Fuchs, L. S., Fuchs, D., Hamlett, C. L., Phillips, N. B., & Karns, K. (1995). General educators' specialized adaptation for students with learning disabilities. *Exceptional Children, 61,* 440–459.

Fuchs, L. S., Fuchs, D., Hamlett, C. L., & Stecker, P. M. (1991). Effects of curriculum-based measurement and consultation on teacher planning and student achievement in mathematics operations. *American Educational Research Journal, 28,* 617–641.

Fuchs, L. S., Fuchs, D., Hamlett, C. L., Walz, L., & Germann, G. (1993). Formative evaluation of academic progress: How much growth can we expect? *School Psychology Review, 22,* 27–48.

Fuchs, L. S., Fuchs, D., Hamlett, C. L., & Whinnery, K. (1991). Effects of goal line feedback on level, slope, and stability of performance within curriculum-based measurement. *Learning Disabilities Research and Practice, 6*(2), 66–74.

Fuchs, L. S., Fuchs, D., & Karns, K. (2001). Enhancing kindergartner's mathematical development: Effects of peer-assisted learning strategies. *Elementary School Journal, 101,* 495–510.

Fuchs, L. S., Fuchs, D., & Kazdan, S. (1999). Effects of peer-assisted learning strategies on high school students with serious reading problems. *Remedial and Special Education, 20,* 309–318.

Fuchs, L. S., Fuchs, D., Phillips, N. B., Hamlett, C. L., & Karns, K. (1995). Acquisition and transfer effects of classwide peer-assisted learning strategies in mathematics for students with varying learning histories. *School Psychology Review, 24,* 604–630.

Fuchs, L. S., Fuchs, D., Prentice, K., Burch, M., Hamlett, C. L., Owen, R., et al. (2003). Enhancing third-grade student mathematical problem solving with self-regulated learning strategies. *Journal of Educational Psychology, 95,* 306–315.

Fuchs, L. S., Fuchs, D., & Speece, D. L. (2002). Treatment validity as a unifying construct for identifying learning disabilities. *Learning Disability Quarterly, 25,* 33–45.

Fuchs, L. S., Fuchs, D., Yazdian, L., & Powell, S. R. (2002). Enhancing first-grade children's mathematical development with peer-assisted learning strategies. *School Psychology Review, 31,* 569–583.

Fuchs, L. S., Hamlett, C. L., & Fuchs, D. (1990). *Monitoring basic skills progress: Basic spelling* [computer program]. Austin, TX: Pro-Ed.

Fuchs, L. S., Hamlett, C. L., & Fuchs, D. (1999a). *Monitoring Basic Skills Progress: Basic Math Computation* (2nd ed.) [computer program]. Austin, TX: Pro-Ed.

Fuchs, L. S., Hamlett, C. L., & Fuchs, D. (1999b). *Monitoring Basic Skills Progress: Basic Reading* (2nd ed.) [computer program]. Austin, TX: Pro-Ed.

Fuchs, L. S., Hamlett, C. L., & Fuchs, D. (1999c). *Monitoring Basic Skills Progress: Basic Math Concepts and Applications* [computer program]. Austin, TX: Pro-Ed.

Fuchs, L. S., Tindal, G., & Deno, S. L. (1984). Methodological issues in curriculum-based reading assessment. *Diagnostique, 9,* 191–207.

Gansle, K. A., Noell, G. H., VanDerHeyden, A. M., Naquin, G. M., & Slider, N. J. (2002). Moving beyond total words written: The reliability, criterion validity, and time cost of alternate measures of curriculum-based measurement in writing. *School Psychology Review, 31,* 477–497.

Garcia, J., & Rothman, R. (2002). *Three paths, one destination: Standards-based reform in Maryland, Massachusetts, and Texas.* Washington, DC: Achieve, Inc.

Gardner, W. I., & Cole, C. L. (1988). Self-monitoring procedures. In E. S. Shapiro, & T. R. Kratochwill (Eds.), *Behavioral assessment in schools: Conceptual foundations and practical applications* (pp. 206–246). New York: Guilford Press.

Germann, G., & Tindal, G. (1985). An application of curriculum-based measurement: The use of direct and repeated measurement. *Exceptional Children, 52,* 244–265.

Gersten, R., & Chard, D. (1999). Number sense: Rethinking arithmetic instruction for students with mathematical disabilities. *Journal of Special Education, 33,* 18–28.

Gersten, R., Keating, T., & Becker, W. (1988). The continued impact of the direct instruction model: Longitudinal studies of follow through students. *Education and Treatment of Children, 11,* 318–327.

Gersten, R., Woodward, J., & Darch, C. (1986). Direct instruction: A research-based approach to curriculum design and teaching. *Exceptional Children, 53,* 17–31.

Gettinger, M. (1984). Achievement as a function of time spent in learning and time needed for learning. *American Educational Research Journal, 21,* 617–628.

Gettinger, M. (1985). Time allocated and time spent relative to time needed for learning as determinants of achievement. *Journal of Educational Psychology, 77,* 3–11.

Gettinger, M. (1986). Issues and trends in academic engaged time of students. *Special Services in the Schools, 2,* 1–17.

Gickling, E., & Havertape, J. (1981). *Curriculum-based assessment.* Minneapolis, MN: National School Psychology Inservice Training Network.

Gickling, E. E., & Rosenfield, S. (1995). Best practices in curriculum-based assessment. In A. Thomas & J. Grimes (Eds.), *Best practices in school psychology III* (pp. 587–595). Washington, DC: National Association of School Psychologists.

Gickling, E. E., & Thompson, V. P. (1985). A personal view of curriculum-based assessment. *Exceptional Children, 52,* 205–218.

Gilberts, G. H., Agran, M., Hughes, C., & Wehmeyer, M. (2001). The effects of peer delivered self-monitoring strategies on the participation of students with severe disabilities in general education classrooms. *Journal of the Association for Persons with Severe Handicaps, 26,* 25–36.

Goh, D. S., Teslow, C. J., & Fuller, G. B. (1981). The practices of psychological assessment among school psychologists. *Professional Psychology, 12,* 699–706.

Goldberg, R. (1998). In vivo rating of treatment acceptability by children: Effects of probability instruction and group size on students' spelling performance under group contingency conditions. *Dissertation Abstracts International Section A: Humanities and Social Sciences, 59*(4-A), 1067.

Goldberg, R., & Shapiro, E. S. (1995). In-vivo rating of treatment acceptability by children: Effects of probability instruction on student's spelling performance under group contingency conditions. *Journal of Behavioral Education, 5,* 415–432.

Good, R. H., III, & Kaminski, R. A. (1996). Assessment for instructional decisions: Toward a proactive/prevention model of decision-making for early literacy skills. *School Psychology Quarterly, 11,* 326–336.

Good, R. H., III, & Kaminski, R. A. (Eds.). (2002). *Dynamic Indicators of Basic Early Literacy Skills* (6th ed.). Eugene, OR: Institute for the Development of Educational Achievement.

Good, R. H., III, & Salvia, J. (1988). Curriculum bias in published, norm-referenced reading tests: Demonstrable effects. *School Psychology Review, 17,* 51–60.

Good, R. H., III, Simmons, D. C., & Kame'enui, E. J. (2001). The importance and decision-making utility of a continuum of fluency-based indicators of foundational reading skills for third-grade high-takes outcomes. *Scientific Studies of Reading, 5,* 257–288.

Good, R. H., III, Vollmer, M., Creek, R. J., Katz, L., & Chowdhri, S. (1993). Treatment utility of the Kaufman Assessment Battery for Children: Effects of matching instruction and student processing strength. *School Psychology Review, 22,* 8–26.

Goodman, L. (1990). *Time and learning in the special education classroom.* Albany: State University of New York Press.

Gordon, E. W., DeStefano, L., & Shipman, S. (1985). Characteristics of learning persons and the adaptation of learning environments. In M. C. Wang, & H. J. Walberg (Eds.), *Adapting instruction to individual differences* (pp. 44–65). Berkeley, CA: McCutchan.

Graden, J. L., Casey, A., & Bonstrom, O. (1985). Implementing a prereferral intervention system: Part II. The Data. *Exceptional Children, 51,* 487–496.

Graden, J. L., Casey, A., & Christensen, S. L. (1985). Implementing a prereferral intervention system: Part I. The model. *Exceptional Children, 51,* 377–384.

Graham, L., & Wong, B. Y. (1993). Comparing two modes of teaching a question-answering strategy for enhancing reading comprehension: Didactic and self-instructional training. *Journal of Learning Disabilities, 26,* 270–279.

Graham, S. (1982). Composition research and practice: A unified approach. *Focus on Exceptional Children, 14*(8).

Graham, S. (1983). The effects of self-instructional procedures on LD students' handwriting performance. *Learning Disability Quarterly, 6,* 231–234.

Graham, S., & Harris, K. R. (1987). Improving composition skills of inefficient learners with self-instructional strategy training. *Topics in Language Disorders, 7*(4), 66–77.

Graham, S., & Harris, K. R. (1989). A components analysis of cognitive strategy instruction: Effects on learning disabled students' compositions and self-efficacy. *Journal of Educational Psychology, 81,* 353–361.

Graham, S., & Harris, K. R. (2003). Students with learning disabilities and the process of writing: A meta-analysis of SRSD studies. In H. Swanson, K. R. Harris, & S. Graham (Eds.), *Handbook of learning disabilities* (pp. 323–344). New York: Guilford Press.

Graham, S., Harris, K. R., MacArthur, C. A., & Schwartz, S. (1991). Writing and writing instruction for students with learning disabilities: Review of a research program. *Learning Disabilities Quarterly, 14,* 89–114.

Graham, S., Harris, K. R., & Troia, GA. (2000). Self-regulated strategy development revisited: Teaching writing strategies to struggling writers. *Topic in Language Disorders, 20,* 1–14.

Graham, S., MacArthur, C. A., Schwartz, S., & Page-Voth, V. (1992). Improving the compositions of students with learning disabilities using a strategy involving product and process goal setting. *Exceptional Children, 58,* 322–334.

Graham, S., & Miller, L. (1980). Handwriting research and practice: A unified approach. *Focus on Exceptional Children, 13*(2).

Gravois, T. A., Knotek, S., & Babinski, L. M. (2002). Educating practitioners as consultants: Development and implementation of the instructional consultation team consortium. *Journal of Educational and Psychological Consultation, 13,* 113–132.

Greenwood, C. R. (1991). Longitudinal analysis of time, engagement, and achievement in at-risk versus non-risk students. *Exceptional Children, 57,* 521–535.

Greenwood, C. R. (1996). The case for performance-based instructional models. *School Psychology Quarterly, 11,* 283–296.

Greenwood, C. R., Arreaga-Mayer, C., Utley, C. A., Gavin, K. M., & Terry, B. J. (2001). Classwide Peer Tutoring Learning Management System: Applications with elementary-level English language learners. *Remedial and Special Education, 22,* 34–47.

Greenwood, C. R., Carta, J. J., & Atwater, J. J. (1991). Ecobehavioral analysis in the classroom: Review and implications. *Journal of Behavioral Education, 1,* 59–77.

Greenwood, C. R., Carta, J. J., & Hall, R. V. (1988). The use of peer tutoring strategies in classroom management and educational instruction. *School Psychology Review, 17,* 258–275.

Greenwood, C. R., Carta, J. J., Hart, B., Kamos, D., Terry, B., & Delquadri, J. C. (1992). Out of the laboratory and into the community: Twenty-six years of applied behavior analysis at the Juniper Gardens Children's Project. *American Psychologist, 47,* 1464–1474.

Greenwood, C. R., Carta, J. J., Kamps, D., & Delquadri, J. (1993). *Ecobehavioral assessment systems software (EBASS): Observational instrumentation for school psychologists.* Kansas City: Juniper Gardens Children's Project, University of Kansas.

Greenwood, C. R., Carta, J. J., Kamps, D., Terry, B., & Delquadri, J. (1994). Development and validation of standard classroom observation systems for school practitioners: Ecobehavioral assessment systems software (EBASS). *Exceptional Children, 61,* 197–210.

Greenwood, C. R., Delquadri, J., & Carta, J. J. (1997). *Together we can!: Classwide peer tutoring to improve basic academic skills.* Longmont, CO: Sopris West.

Greenwood, C. R., Delquadri, J. C., & Hall, R. V. (1984). Opportunity to respond and student academic performance. In U. L. Heward, T. E. Heron, D. S. Hill, & J. Trap-Porter (Eds.), *Focus on behavior analysis in education* (pp. 58–88). Columbus, OH: Merrill.

Greenwood, C. R., Delquadri, J., & Hall, R. V. (1989). Longitudinal effects of classwide peer tutoring. *Journal of Educational Psychology, 81,* 371–383.

Greenwood, C. R., Delquadri, J. C., Stanley, S. O., Terry, B., & Hall, R. V. (1985). Assessment of eco-behavioral interaction in school settings. *Behavioral Assessment, 7,* 331–347.

Greenwood, C. R., Dinwiddie, G., Bailey, V., Carta, J. J., Kohler, F. W., Nelson, C., et al. (1987). Field replication of classwide peer tutoring. *Journal of Applied Behavior Analysis, 20,* 151–160.

Greenwood, C. R., Dinwiddie, G., Terry, B., Wade, L., Stanley, S. O., Thibadeau, S., et al. (1984). Teacher- versus peer-mediated instruction: An ecobehavioral analysis of achievement outcomes. *Journal of Applied Behavior Analysis, 17,* 521–538.

Greenwood, C. R., Hops, H., & Walker, H. M. (1977). Issues in social interaction/withdrawal assessment. *Exceptional Children, 43,* 490–501.

Greenwood, C. R., Hops, H., Walker, H. M., Guild, J. J., Stokes, J., Young, K. R., et al. (1979). Standardized classroom management program: Social validation and replication studies in Utah and Oregon. *Journal of Applied Behavior Analysis, 12,* 235–253.

Greenwood, C. R., Horton, B. T., & Utley, C. A. (2002). Academic engagement: Current perspectives on research and practice. *School Psychology Review, 31,* 326–349.

Greenwood, C. R., Hou, L. S., Delquadri, J., Terry, B., & Arreaga-Mayer, C. (2000). The Class Wide Peer Tutoring Learning Management System (CWPT-LMS). In J. Woodward & L. Cuban (Eds.), *Technology, curriculum, and professional development: Adapting schools to meet the needs of students with disabilities.* Thousand Oaks, CA: Corwin.

Greenwood, C. R., Luze, G. J., Cline, G., Kuntz, S., & Leitschuh, C. (2002). Developing a general outcome measure of growth in movement for infants and toddlers. *Topics in Early Childhood Special Education, 22,* 143–157.

Greenwood, C. R., Terry, B., Arreaga-Mayer, C., & Finney, R. (1992). The Classwide Peer Tutoring Program: Implementation factors moderating students' achievement. *Journal of Applied Behavior Analysis, 25,* 101–116.

Greenwood, C. R., Terry, B., Utley, C. A., Montagna, D., & Walker, D. (1993). Achievement, placement, and services: Middle school benefits of Classwide Peer Tutoring used at the elementary school. *School Psychology Review, 22,* 497–516.

Gresham, F. M. (1984). Behavioral interviews in school psychology: Issues in psychometric adequacy and research. *School Psychology Review, 13,* 17–25.

Gresham, F. M. (2002). Responsiveness to intervention: An alternative approach to the identification of learning disabilities. In R. Bradley, L. Danielson, & D. P. Hallahan (Eds.), *Identification of learning disabilities: Research to practice* (pp. 467–519). Mahwah, NJ: Erlbaum

Gross, A. M., & Shapiro, R. (1981). Public posting of photographs: A new classroom reinforcer. *Child Behavior Therapy, 3,* 81–82.

Gruber, R., DuPaul, G. J., Jitendra, A. K., Volpe, R. J., & Lorah, K. S. (2004). *Classroom observations of students with and without ADHD: Differences across academic subject and types of engagement.* Unpublished manuscript, Lehigh University, Bethlehem, PA.

Gumpel, T. P., & Frank, R. (1999). An expansion of the peer tutoring program: Cross-age peer tutoring of social skills among socially rejected boys. *Journal of Applied Behavior Analysis, 32,* 115–118.

Haile-Griffey, L., Saudargas, R. A., Hulse-Trotter, K., & Zanolli, K. (1993). *The class-*

room behavior of elementary school children during independent seatwork: Establishing local norms. Unpublished manuscript, Department of Psychology, University of Tennessee.

Hall, R. V., Delquadri, J. C., Greenwood, C. R., & Thurston, L. (1982). The importance of opportunity to respond in children's academic success. In E. B. Edgar, N. G. Haring, J. R. Jenkins, & C. G. Pious (Eds.), Mentally handicapped children: Education and training (pp. 107–140). Baltimore: University Park Press.

Hall, R. V., Lund, D. E., & Jackson, D. (1968). Effects of teacher attention on study behavior. Journal of Applied Behavior Analysis, 1, 1–12.

Hallahan, D. P., Lloyd, J. W., Kauffman, J., & Loper, A. V. (1983). Summary of research findings at the University of Virginia Learning Disabilities Institute. Exceptional Education Quarterly, 4(1), 95–114.

Hallahan, D. P., Lloyd, J. W., Kneedler, R. D., & Marshall, K. J. (1982). A comparison of the effects of self- versus teacher-assessment of on-task behavior. Behavior Therapy, 13, 715–723.

Hallahan, D. P., Marshall, K. J., & Lloyd, J. W. (1981). Self-recording during group instruction: Effects on attention to task. Learning Disability Quarterly, 4, 407–413.

Hamilton, C., & Shinn, M. R. (2003). Characteristics of word callers: An investigation of the accuracy of teachers' judgments of reading comprehension and oral reading skills. School Psychology Review, 32, 228–240.

Hammill, D., & Larsen, S. (1978). Test of written language. Austin, TX: Pro-Ed.

Hansen, C. L., & Eaton, M. (1978). Reading. In N. Haring, T. Lovitt, M. Eaton, & C. Hansen (Eds.), The fourth R: Research in the classroom (pp. 41–92). Columbus, OH: Merrill.

Harding, L. R., Howard, V. F., & McLaughlin, T. F. (1993). Using self-recording of on-task behavior by a preschool child with disabilities. Perceptual and Motor Skills, 77(3), 786.

Hargis, C. H., Terhaar-Yonker, M., Williams, P. C., & Reed, M. T. (1988). Repetition requirements for word recognition. Journal of Reading, 31, 320–327.

Harris, A. J., & Jacobson, M. D. (1972). Basic elementary vocabularies. New York: Macmillan.

Harris, K. R., & Graham, S. (1985). Improving learning disabled students' composition skills: Self-control strategy training. Learning Disability Quarterly, 8, 27–36.

Harris, K. R., & Graham, S. (1994). Constructivism: Principles, paradigms, and integration. Journal of Special Education, 28, 233–247.

Harris, K. R., & Graham, S. (1996). Making the writing process work: Strategies for composition and self-regulation (2nd ed.). Cambridge, MA: Brookline.

Harris, K. R., Graham, S., Reid, R., McElroy, K., & Hamby, R. (1994). Self-monitoring of attention versus self-monitoring of performance: Replication and cross-task comparison. Learning Disability Quarterly, 17, 121–139.

Hasazi, J. E., & Hasazi, S. E. (1972). Effects of teacher attention on digit reversal behavior in an elementary school child. Journal of Applied Behavior Analysis, 5, 157–162.

Hasbrouck, J. E., Ihnot, C., & Rogers, G. H. (1999). "Read Naturally": A strategy to increase oral reading fluency. Reading Research and Instruction, 39, 27–38.

Hasbrouck, J. E., & Tindal, G. (1992). Curriculum-based oral reading fluency norms for students in grades 2 through 5. Teaching Exceptional Children, 24(3), 41–44.

Haynes, M. C., & Jenkins, J. R. (1986). Reading instruction in special education resource rooms. American Educational Research Journal, 23, 161–190.

Heller, K. A., Holtzman, W., H., & Messick, S. (Eds.). (1982). Placing children in special education: A strategy for equity. Washington, DC: National Academy Press.

Hendrickson, J. M., Gable, R. A., Novak, C., & Peck, S. (1996). Functional assessment as strategy assessment for teaching academics. Education and Treatment of Children, 19, 257–271.

Hintze, J. M., Callahan, J. E., III, Matthews, W. J., Williams, S. A. S., & Tobin, K. G. (2002). Oral reading fluency and prediction of reading comprehension in African-American and Caucasian elementary schoolchildren. *School Psychology Review, 31*, 540–553.

Hintze, J. M., Christ, T. J., & Keller, L. A. (2002). The generalizability of CBM survey-level mathematics assessments: Just how many samples do we need? *School Psychology Review, 31,* 514–528.

Hinzte, J. M., Owen, S. V., Shapiro, E. S., & Daly, E. J., III. (2000). Generalizability of oral reading fluency measures: Application of G theory to curriculum-based measurement. *School Psychology Quarterly, 15,* 52–68.

Hintze, J. M., & Pelle Petitte, H. A. (2001). The generalizability of CBM oral reading fluency measures across general and special education. *Journal of Psychoeducational Assessment, 19,* 158–170.

Hintze, J. M., & Shapiro, E. S. (1997). Curriculum-based measurement and literature-based reading: Is curriculum-based measurement meeting the needs of changing reading curricula? *Journal of School Psychology, 35,* 351–375.

Hintze, J. M., Shapiro, E. S., & Lutz, J. G. (1994). The effects of curriculum on the sensitivity of curriculum-based measurement in reading. *Journal of Special Education, 28,* 188–202.

Hintze, J. M., Volpe, R. J., & Shapiro, E. S. (2002). Best practices in the systematic direct observation of student behavior. In A. Thomas & J. Grimes (Eds.), *Best practices in school psychology* (Vol. 4, pp. 993–1006). Washington, DC: National Association of School Psychologists.

Hively, W., & Reynolds, M. C. (Eds.). (1975). *Domain-reference testing in special education*. Minneapolis: University of Minnesota, Leadership Training Institute.

Hoge, R. D., & Andrews, D. A. (1987). Enhancing academic performance: Issues in target selection. *School Psychology Review, 16,* 228–238.

Hoier, T. S., & Cone, J. D. (1987). Target selection of social skills for children: The template-matching procedure. *Behavior Modification, 11,* 137–164.

Hoier, T. S., McConnell, S., & Pallay, A. G. (1987). Observational assessment for planning and evaluating educational transitions: An initial analysis of template matching. *Behavioral Assessment, 9,* 6–20.

Holman, J., & Baer, D. M. (1979). Facilitating generalization of on-task behavior through self-monitoring of academic tasks. *Journal of Autism and Developmental Disabilities, 9,* 429–446.

Hopkins, B. L., Schultz, R. C., & Garton, K. L. (1971). The effects of access to a playroom on the rate and quality of printing and writing of first and second grade students. *Journal of Applied Behavior Analysis, 10,* 121–126.

Houghton, S., & Bain, A. (1993). Peer tutoring with ESL and below-average readers. *Journal of Behavioral Education, 3,* 125–142.

Howell, K. W., Fox, S. L., & Morehead, M. K. (1993). *Curriculum-based evaluation: Teaching and decision making* (2nd ed.). Pacific Grove, CA: Brooks/Cole.

Howell, K. W., & Nolet, V. (1999). *Curriculum-based evaluation: Teaching and decision making* (3rd ed.). Belmont, CA: Wadsworth.

Howell, K. W., Zucker, S. H., & Morehead, M. K. (1982). *Multilevel Academic Skills Inventory*. San Antonio, TX: Psychological Corp.

Hughes, C., Copeland, S. R., Agran, M., Wehneyer, M. L., Rodi, M. S., & Presley, J. A. (2002). Using self-monitoring to improve performance in general education high school classes. *Education and Training in Mental Retardation and Developmental Disabilities, 37,* 262–272.

Hughes, C., & Lloyd, J. W. (1993). An analysis of self-management. *Journal of Behavioral Education, 3,* 405–425.

Hughes, C. A., Korinek, L., & Gorman, J. (1991). Self-management for students with mental retardation in public school settings: A research review. *Education and Training in Mental Retardation, 26,* 271–291.

Hultquist, A. M., & Metzke, L. K. (1993). Potential effects of curriculum bias in individual norm-referenced reading and spelling achievement tests. *Journal of Psychoeducational Assessment, 11,* 337–344.

Hutton, J. B., Dubes, R., & Muir, S. (1992). Assessment practices of school psychologists: Ten years later. *School Psychology Review, 21,* 271–284.

Idol, L. (1987). Group story mapping: A comprehension strategy for both skilled and unskilled readers. *Journal of Learning Disabilities, 20,* 196–205.

Idol, L., Nevin, A., & Paolucci-Whitcomb, P. (1996). *Models of curriculum-based assessment: A blueprint for learning* (2nd ed.). Austin, TX: Pro-Ed.

Idol-Maestas, L. (1983). *Special educator's consultation handbook.* Rockville, MD: Aspen Systems Corporation.

Idol-Maestas, L., & Croll, V. J. (1987). The effects of training in story mapping procedures on the reading comprehension of poor readers. *Learning Disability Quarterly, 10,* 214–229.

Iwata, B., Dorsey, M., Slifer, K., Bauman, K., & Richman, G. (1982). Toward a functional analysis of self-injury. *Analysis and Intervention in Developmental Disabilities, 2,* 3–20.

Jastak, J., & Jastak, S. (1978). *Wide Range Achievement Test.* Wilmington, DE: Jastak Associates, Inc.

Jastak, S., & Wilkinson, G. S. (1984). *Wide Range Achievement Test—Revised.* Wilmington, DE: Jastak Associates, Inc.

Jenkins, J. R., Deno, S. L., & Mirkin, P. K. (1979). Measuring progress toward the least restrictive alternative. *Learning Disability Quarterly, 2,* 81–91.

Jenkins, J. R., Larson, K., & Fleisher, L. (1983). Effects of error correction on word recognition and reading comprehension. *Learning Disability Quarterly, 6,* 139–145.

Jenkins, J. R., & Pany, D. (1978). Standardized achievement tests: How useful for special education? *Exceptional Children, 44,* 448–453.

Jenson, W. R., Rhode, G., & Reavis, H. K. (1994). *The tough kid tool box.* Longmont, CO: Sopris West.

Jitendra, A. K. (2002). Teaching students math problem-solving through graphic representations. *Teaching Exceptional Children, 34*(4), 34–38.

Jitendra, A. K., & Griffin, C. C. (2001). *Enhancing mathematical word problem solving performance of students with learning disabilities in general education mathematics classrooms.* Grant No. 84.324D, Office of Special Education, Washington, DC.

Jitendra, A. K., Griffin, C. C., McGoey, K., Gardill, M. C., Bhat, P., & Riley, T. (1998). Effects of mathematical word problem solving by students at risk or with mild disabilities. *Journal of Educational Research, 91,* 345–355.

Jitendra, A. K., & Hoff, K. (1996). The effects of schema-based instruction on the mathematics word-problem solving performance of students with learning disabilities. *Journal of Learning Disabilities, 29,* 422–431.

Jitendra, A. K., Hoff, K., & Beck, M. M. (April, 1997). *The role of schema-based instruction on solving multistep word problems.* Paper presented at the Annual Convention of the Council for Exceptional Children, Salt Lake City, UT.

Jitendra, A. K., Hoff, K., & Beck, M. M. (1999). Teaching middle school students with learning disabilities to solve word problems using a schema-based approach. *Remedial and Special Education, 20,* 50–64.

Johns, G. A., Skinner, C. H., & Nail, G. L. (2000). Effects of interspersing briefer mathematics problems on assignment choice in students with learning disabilities. *Journal of Behavioral Education, 10,* 95–106.

Johnson, D. J., & Myklebust, H. R. (1967). *Learning disabilities: Educational principles and practices*. New York: Grune & Stratton.

Johnson, D. W., & Johnson, R. T. (1985). Cooperative learning and adaptive education. In M. C. Wang & H. J. Walberg (Eds.), *Adapting instruction to individual differences* (pp. 105–134). Berkley, CA: McCutchan.

Johnson, D. W., & Johnson, R. T. (1986). Mainstreaming and cooperative learning strategies. *Exceptional Children, 52,* 553–561.

Johnson, D. W., Maruyama, G., Johnson, R., Nelson, D., & Skon, L. (1981). The effects of cooperative, competitive, and individualistic goal structures on achievement: A meta-analysis. *Psychological Bulletin, 89,* 47–62.

Johnson, L. J., & Idol-Maestes, L. (1986). Peer tutoring as a reinforcer for appropriate tutee behavior. *Journal of Special Education Technology, 7*(4), 14–21.

Johnston, M. B., Whitman, T. L., & Johnson, M. (1980). Teaching addition and subtraction to mentally retarded children: A self-instructional program. *Applied Research in Mental Retardation, 1,* 141–160.

Johnston, R. J., & McLaughlin, T. F. (1982). The effects of free time on assignment completion and accuracy in arithmetic: A case study. *Education and Treatment of Children, 5,* 33–40.

Kame'enui, E. J. (2002). *An analysis of reading instruments for K–3.* Eugene: University of Oregon, Institute for the Development of Educational Achievement [*http://idea.uoregon.edu/assessment*].

Kame'enui, E. J., Carnine, D. W., Dixon, R. C., Simmons, D. C., & Coyne, M. D. (2002). *Effective teaching strategies that accommodate diverse learners* (2nd ed.). Upper Saddle River, NJ: Prentice-Hall.

Kame'enui, E. J., Simmons, D. C., & Coyne, M. D. (2000). Schools as host environments: Toward a school wide reading improvement model. *Annals of Dyslexia, 50,* 33–51.

Kame'enui, E. J., Simmons, D. C., Chard, D., & Dickson, S. (1997). Direct instruction reading. In S. Stahl & D. A. Hayes (Eds.), *Instructional models in reading* (pp. 59–64). Hillsdale, NJ: Erlbaum.

Kaminski, R. A., & Good, R. H., III. (1996). Toward a technology for assessing basic early literacy skills. *School Psychology Review, 25,* 215–227.

Kamps, D. M., Dugan, E., Potucek, J., & Collins, A. (1999). Effects of cross-age peer tutoring networks among students with autism and general education students. *Journal of Behavioral Education, 9,* 97–115.

Kamps, D., Leonard, B. R., Dugan, E. P., & Boland, B. (1991). The use of ecobehavioral assessment to identify naturally occurring effective procedures in classrooms serving students with autism and developmental disabilities. *Journal of Behavioral Education, 4,* 367–397.

Kanfer, F. H. (1971). The maintenance of behavior by self-generated stimuli and reinforcement. In A. Jacobs & L. B. Sachs (Eds.), *The psychology of private events* (pp. 39–58). New York: Academic Press.

Karlsen, B., Madden, R., & Gardner, E. F. (1975). *Stanford Diagnostic Reading Test* (Green level form B). New York: Harcourt Brace Jovanovich.

Karoly, P. (1982). Perspectives on self-management and behavior change. In P. Karoly & F. H. Kanfer (Eds.), *Self-management and behavior change: From theory to practice* (pp. 3–31). New York: Pergamon Press.

Karweit, N. L. (1983). *Time on task: A research review* (Report No. 332). Baltimore: Johns Hopkins University, Center for Social Organization of Schools.

Karweit, N. L., & Slavin, R. E. (1981). Measurement and modeling choices in studies of time and learning. *American Educational Research Journal, 18,* 157–171.

Kastelen, L., Nickel, M., & McLaughlin, T. F. (1984). A performance feedback system:

Generalization of effects across tasks and time with eighth-grade English students. *Education and Treatment of Children, 7,* 141–155.

Kaufman, A. S., & Kaufman, N. L. (1983). *Administration and scoring manual for the Kaufman Assessment Battery for Children.* Circle Pines, MN: American Guidance Service.

Kaufman, A. S., & Kaufman, N. L. (1997). *Kaufman Test of Educational Achievement—Normative Update.* Circle Pines, MN: American Guidance Service.

Kavale, K. A., & Forness, S. R. (1987). Substance over style: Assessing the efficacy of modality testing and teaching. *Exceptional Children, 54,* 228–239.

Kazdin, A. E. (1985). Selection of target behaviors: The relationship of the treatment focus to clinical dysfunction. *Behavioral Assessment, 7,* 33–48.

Keith, T. Z., Kranzler, J. H., & Flanagan, D. P. (2001). What does the Cognitive Assessment System (CAS) measure?: Joint confirmatory factor analysis of the CAS and the Woodcock–Johnson Tests of Cognitive Ability (3rd ed.). *School Psychology Review, 30,* 89–119.

Kelley, M. L., & Stokes, T. F. (1982). Contingency contracting with disadvantaged youths: Improving classroom performance. *Journal of Applied Behavior Analysis, 15,* 447–454.

Kelley, M. L., & Stokes, T. F. (1984). Student–teacher contracting with goal setting for maintenance. *Behavior Modification, 8,* 223–244.

Kephart, N. C. (1971). *The slow learner in the classroom.* Columbus, OH: Merrill.

Kirby, F. D., & Shields, F. (1972). Modification of arithmetic response rate and attending behavior in a seventh grade student. *Journal of Applied Behavior Analysis, 5,* 79–84.

Koegel, L. K., Harrower, J. K., & Koegel, R. L. (1999). Support for children with developmental disabilities in full inclusion classrooms through self-management. *Journal of Positive Behavior Interventions, 1,* 26–34.

Kosiewicz, M. M., Hallahan, D. P., Lloyd, J., & Graves, A. W. (1982). Effects of self-instruction and self-correction procedures on handwriting performance. *Learning Disability Quarterly, 5,* 71–78.

Kranzler, J. H., & Keith, T. Z. (1999). Independent confirmatory factor analysis of the Cognitive Assessment System (CAS): What does the CAS measure? *School Psychology Review, 29,* 117–144.

Kranzler, J. H., Keith, T. Z., & Flanagan, D. P. (2000). Independent examination of the factor structure of the Cognitive Assessment System (CAS): Further evidence challenging the construct validity of the CAS. *Journal of Psychoeducational Assessment, 18,* 143–159.

Kratochwill, T. R. (1985a). Case study research in school psychology. *School Psychology Review, 14,* 204–215.

Kratochwill, T. R. (1985b). Selection of target behaviors in behavioral consultation. *Behavioral Consultation, 7,* 49–62.

Kratochwill, T. R., & Bergan, J. R. (1990). *Behavioral consultation in applied settings: An individual guide.* New York: Plenum Press.

Kraotchwill, T. R., Elliott, S. R., & Busse, R. T. (1995). Behavioral consultation: A five-year evaluation of consultant and client outcomes. *School Psychology Quarterly, 10,* 87–117.

Kunzelmann, H. D. (Ed.). (1970). *Precision teaching.* Seattle: Special Child Publications.

Lahey, B. B., & Drabman, R. S. (1973). Facilitation of the acquisition and retention of sight word vocabulary through token reinforcement. *Journal of Applied Behavior Analysis, 6,* 101–104.

Lahey, B. B., McNees, M. P., & Brown, C. C. (1973). Modification of deficits in reading for comprehension. *Journal of Applied Behavior Analysis, 6,* 475–480.

Lalli, J. S., Browder, D. M., Mace, F. C., & Brown, D. K. (1993). Teacher use of descriptive analysis data to implement interventions to decrease students' problem behaviors. *Journal of Applied Behavior Analysis, 26,* 227–238.

Lam, A., Cole, C. L., Shapiro, E. S., & Bambara, L. M. (1994). Relative effects of self-monitoring on-task behavior, academic accuracy, and disruptive behavior in students with behavior disorders. *School Psychology Review, 23,* 44–58.

Lane, K. L., O'Shaughnessy, T. E., Lambros, K. M., Gresham, F. M., & Bebee-Frankenberger, M. E. (2001). The efficacy of phonological awareness training with first-grade students who have behavior problems and reading difficulties. *Journal of Emotional and Behavioral Disorders, 9,* 219–231.

Larsen, S. C., & Hammill, D. D. (1976). *Test of Written Spelling.* Austin, TX: Empiric Press.

Leach, D. J., & Dolan, N. K. (1985). Helping teacher increase student academic engagement rates: The evaluation of a minimal feedback procedure. *Behavior Modification, 9,* 55–71.

Lee, C., & Tindal, G. A. (1994). Self-recording and goal-setting: Effects on on-task and math productivity with low-achieving Korean elementary school students. *Journal of Behavioral Education, 4,* 459–479.

Lee, L., & Canter, S. M. (1971). Developmental sentence scoring. *Journal of Speech and Hearing Disorders, 36,* 335–340.

Leinhardt, G., Zigmond, N., & Cooley, W. W. (1981). Reading instruction and its effects. *American Educational Research Journal, 18,* 343–361.

Lentz, F. E., Jr. (1988). Direct observation and measurement of academic skills: A conceptual review. In E. S. Shapiro & T. R. Kratochwill (Eds.), *Behavioral assessment in schools: Conceptual foundations and practical applications* (pp. 76–120). New York: Guilford Press.

Lentz, F. E., Jr., & Shapiro, E. S. (1985). Behavioral school psychology: A conceptual model for the delivery of psychological services. In T. R. Kratochwill (Ed.), *Advances in school psychology* (Vol. 4, pp. 191–232). Hillsdale, NJ: Erlbaum.

Lentz, F. E., Jr., & Shapiro, E. S. (1986). Functional assessment of the academic environment. *School Psychology Review, 15,* 346–357.

Lentz, F. E., Jr., & Wehmann, B. A. (1995). Interviewing. In A. Thomas & J. Grimes (Eds.), *Best practices in school psychology* (Vol. 3, pp. 637–650). Washington, DC: National Association of School Psychologists.

Lenz, B. K., Ehren, B. J., & Smiley, L. R. (1991). A goal attainment approach to improve completion of project-type assignments by adolescents with learning disabilities. *Learning Disabilities Research and Practice, 6*(3), 166–176.

Lenz, B. K., Schumaker, J. B., Deshler, D. D., & Beals, V. L. (1984). *Learning strategies curriculum: The word identification strategy.* Lawrence: University of Kansas.

Lenz, B. K., Singh, N. N., & Hewett, A. E. (1991). Overcorrection as an academic remediation procedure: A review and reappraisal. *Behavior Modification, 15,* 64–73.

Levendowski, L. S., & Cartledge, G. (2000). Self-monitoring for elementary school children with serious emotional disturbances: Classroom applications for increased academic responding. *Behavioral Disorders, 25,* 211–224.

Lindsley, O. R. (1971). Precision teaching in perspective: An interview with Ogden R. Lindsley. *Teaching Exceptional Children, 3,* 114–119.

Linn, R. L. (2000). Assessments and accountability. *Educational Researcher, 29*(2), 4–16.

Litow, L., & Pumroy, D. K. (1975). A brief review of classroom group-oriented contingencies. *Journal of Applied Behavior Analysis, 8,* 341–347.

Lloyd, J. (1980). Academic instruction and cognitive behavior modification: The need for attack strategy training. *Exceptional Education Quarterly, 1,* 53–63.

Lloyd, J. W., Hallahan, D. P., Kosciewicz, M. M., & Kneedler, R. D. (1982). Reactive effects of self-assessment and self-recording on attention to task and academic productivity. *Learning Disability Quarterly, 5,* 216–227.

Lloyd, J. W., Kneedler, R. D., & Cameron, N. A. (1982). Effects of verbal self-guidance on word reading accuracy. *Reading Improvement, 19*, 84–89.

Lochman, J. E., & Curry, J. F. (1986). Effects of social problem-solving training and self-instruction training with aggressive boys. *Journal of Clinical Child Psychology, 15*, 159–164.

Logan, P., & Skinner, C. H. (1998). Improving students' perceptions of a mathematics assignment by increasing problem completion rates: Is problem completion a reinforcing event? *School Psychology Quarterly, 13*, 322–331.

Lovaas, O. I. (1977). *The autistic child: Language development through behavior modification*. New York: Irvington.

Lovaas, O. I., Koegel, R., Simmons, J. Q., & Long, J. S. (1973). Some generalization and follow-up measures on autistic children in behavior therapy. *Journal of Applied Behavior Analysis, 6*, 131–166.

Lovitt, T. C. (1978). Arithmetic. In N. Haring, M. Eaton, & C. Hansen (Eds.), *The fourth R: Research in the classroom* (pp. 127–167). New York: Merrill.

Lovitt, T. C., Eaton, M., Kirkwood, M. E., & Perlander, A. (1971). Effects of various reinforcement contingencies on oral reading rate. In E. Ramp & B. L. Hopkins (Eds.), *A new direction for education: Behavior analysis* (pp. 54–71). Lawrence: University of Kansas Press.

Lovitt, T. C., & Hansen, C. C. (1976a). The use of contingent skipping and drilling to improve oral reading and comprehension. *Journal of Learning Disabilities, 9*, 481–487.

Lovitt, T. C., & Hansen, C. C. (1976b). Round one—placing the child in the right reader. *Journal of Learning Disabilities, 9*, 347–353.

Luiselli, J. K., & Downing, J. N. (1980). Improving a student's arithmetic performance using feedback and reinforcement procedures. *Education and Treatment of Children, 3*, 45–49.

Lysynchuk, L. M., Pressley, M., & Vye, N. J. (1990). Reciprocal instruction improves standardized reading comprehension performance in poor grade-school comprehenders. *Elementary School Journal, 90*, 469–484.

Maag, J. W. (1990). Social skills training in schools. *Special Services in the Schools, 6*, 1–19.

Maag, J. W., Reid, R., & DiGangi, S. A. (1993). Differential effects of self-monitoring attention, accuracy, and productivity. *Journal of Applied Behavior Analysis, 26*, 329–344.

MacArthur, C. A., Schwartz, S. S., & Graham, S. (1991). Effects of a reciprocal peer revision strategy in special education classrooms. *Learning Disabilities Research and Practice, 6*, 201–210.

Mace, F. C., Browder, D. M., & Lin, Y. (1987). Analysis of demand conditions associated with stereotypy. *Journal of Behavior Therapy and Experimental Psychiatry, 18*, 25–31.

Mace, F. C., & Knight, D. (1986). Functional analysis and treatment of severe pica. *Journal of Applied Behavior Analysis, 19*, 411–416.

Mace, F. C., & Kratochwill, T. R. (1985). Theories of reactivity in self-monitoring: A comparison of cognitive-behavioral and operant models. *Behavior Modification, 9*, 323–343.

Mace, F. C., & West, B. J. (1986). Unresolved theoretical issues in self-management: Implications for research and practice. *Professional School Psychology, 1*, 149–163.

Mace, F. C., Yankanich, M. A., & West, B. (1988). Toward a methodology of experimental analysis and treatment of aberrant classroom behaviors. *Special Services in the Schools, 4*(3/4), 71–88.

MacQuarrie, L. L., Tucker, J. A., Burns, M. L., & Hartman, B. (2002). Comparison of retention rates using traditional, drill sandwich, and incremental rehearsal flash card methods. *School Psychology Review, 31,* 584–595.

Madden, R., Gardener, E. R., Rudman, H. C., Karlsen, B., & Merwin, J. C. (1973). *Stanford Achievement Test.* New York: Harcourt Brace Jovanovich.

Madrid, D., Terry, B., Greenwood, C., Whaley, M., & Webber, N. (1998). Active vs. passive peer tutoring: Teaching spelling to at-risk students. *Journal of Research and Development in Education, 31,* 236–244.

Maheady, L., Harper, G., Mallette, B., & Winstanley, N. (1991). Training and implementation requirements associated with the use of a classwide peer tutoring system. *Education and Treatment of Children, 14,* 177–198.

Mahn, C., & Greenwood, G. E. (1990). Cognitive behavior modification: Use of self-instruction strategies by first graders on academic tasks. *Journal of Educational Research, 83,* 158–161.

Malecki, C. K., & Jewell, J. (2003). Developmental, gender, and practical considerations in scoring curriculum-based measurement writing probes. *Psychology in the Schools, 40,* 379–390.

Manning, B. H. (1990). Cognitive self-instruction for an off-task fourth grader during independent academic tasks: A case study. *Contemporary Educational Psychology, 15,* 46–46.

March, R. E., & Horner, R. H. (2002). Feasibility and contributions of functional behavioral assessment in schools. *Journal of Emotional and Behavioral Disorders, 10,* 158–170.

Markwardt, F. C. (1997). *Peabody Individual Achievement Test—Revised/NU.* Circle Pines, MN: American Guidance Service.

Marston, D. (1988). Measuring progress on IEP's: A comparison of graphing approaches. *Exceptional Children, 55,* 38–44.

Marston, D., Fuchs, L. S., & Deno, S. L. (1986). Measuring pupil progress: A comparison of standardized achievement tests and curriculum-related measures. *Diagnostique, 11,* 77–90.

Marston, D., & Magnusson, D. (1985). Implementing curriculum-based measurement in special and regular settings. *Exceptional Children, 52,* 266–276.

Marston, D., & Magnusson, D. (1988). Curriculum-based measurement: District level implementation. In J. L. Graden, J. E. Zins, & M. J. Curtis (Eds.), *Alternative educational delivery systems: Enhancing instructional options for all students* (pp. 137–177). Washington, DC: National Association of School Psychologists.

Marston, D., & Tindal, G. (1995). Best practices in performance monitoring. In A. Thomas & J. Grimes (Eds.), *Best practices in school psychology* (Vol. 3, pp. 597–607). Washington, DC: National Association of School Psychologists.

Martens, B. K., Steele, E. S., Massie, D. R., & Diskin, M. T. (1995). Curriculum bias in standardized tests of reading decoding. *Journal of School Psychology, 33,* 287–296.

Mash, E., & Terdal, L. (1997). *Assessment of childhood disorders* (3rd ed.). New York: Guilford Press.

Mason, L. H., Harris, K. R., & Graham, S. (2002). Every child has a story to tell: Self-regulated strategy development for story writing. *Education and Treatment of Children, 25,* 496–506.

Mathes, P. G., Fuchs, D., & Fuchs, L. S. (1997). Cooperative story mapping. *Remedial and Special Education, 18,* 20–27.

Mathes, P. G., Grek, M. L., Howard, J. K., Babyak, A. E., & Allen, S. H. (1999). Peer-assisted learning strategies for first-grade readers: A tool for preventing early reading failure. *Learning Disabilities Research and Practice, 14,* 50–60.

Mayer, R. (2002). *Learning and instruction.* Upper Saddle River, NJ: Prentice-Hall.

McAuley, S. M., & McLaughlin, T. F. (1992). Comparison of Add-a-Word and Compu

Spell programs with low-achieving students. *Journal of Educational Research, 85,* 362–369.

McCandliss, B., Beck, I. L., Sandak, R., & Perfetti, C. (2003). Focusing attention on decoding for children with poor reading skills: Design and preliminary tests of the word building intervention. *Scientific Studies of Reading, 7,* 75–104.

McComas, J. J., Hoch, H., & Mace, F. C. (2000). Functional analysis. In E. S. Shapiro & T. R. Kratochwill (Eds.), *Conducting school-based assessment of child and adolescent behavior* (pp. 78–120). New York: Guilford Press.

McComas, J. J., & Mace, F. C. (2000). Theory and practice in conducting functional analysis. In E. S. Shapiro & T. R. Kratochwill (Eds.), *Behavioral assessment in schools: Theory, research, and clinical foundations* (2nd ed., pp. 78–103). New York: Guilford Press.

McConaughy, S. H., & Achenbach, T. M. (1989). Empirically-based assessment of serious emotional disturbances. *Journal of School Psychology, 27,* 91–117.

McConaughy, S. H., & Achenbach, T. M. (1996). Contributions of a child interview to mutltimethod assessment of children with EBD and LD. *School Psychology Review, 25,* 24–39.

McCurdy, B. L., & Shapiro, E. S. (1992). A comparison of teacher-, peer-, and self-monitoring with curriculum-based measurement in reading among students with learning disabilities. *Journal of Special Education, 26,* 162–180.

McGlinchey, & M. T., Hixson, M. D. (in press). Using curriculum-based measurement to predict performance on state assessments in reading. *School Psychology Review.*

McKenzie, M. L., & Budd, K. S. (1981). A peer tutoring package to increase mathematics performance: Examination of generalized changes in classroom behavior. *Education and Treatment of Children, 4,* 1–15.

McKinney, J. D., Mason, J., Perkersen, K., & Clifford, M. (1975). Relationship between classroom behavior and academic achievement. *Journal of Educational Psychology, 67,* 198–203.

McKnight, D. L., Nelson, R. O., Hayes, S. C., & Jarrett, R. B. (1984). Importance of treating individually-assessed response classes in the amelioration of depression. *Behavior Therapy, 15,* 315–335.

McLaughlin, T. F. (1981). The effects of a classroom token economy on math performance in an intermediate grade class. *Education and Treatment of Children, 4,* 139–147.

McLaughlin, T. F., Burgess, N., & Sackville-West, L. (1982). Effects of self-recording and self-recording + matching on academic performance. *Child Behavior Therapy, 3(2/3),* 17–27.

McLaughlin, T. F., & Helm, J. L. (1993). Use of contingent music to increase academic performance of middle-school students. *Psychological Reports, 72, 658.*

McLaughlin, T. F., Mabee, W. S., Byram, B. J., & Reiter, S. M. (1987). Effects of academic positive practice and response cost on writing legibility of behaviorally disordered and learning-disabled junior high school students. *Journal of Child and Adolescent Psychotherapy, 4,* 216–221.

McLaughlin, T. F., Reiter, S. M., Mabee, W. S., & Byram, B. J. (1991). An analysis and of the Add-A-Word spelling program with mildly handicapped middle school students. *Journal of Behavioral Education, 1,* 413–426.

Meichenbaum, D. H., & Goodman, J. (1971). Training impulsive children to talk to themselves: A means of developing self-control. *Journal of Abnormal Psychology, 77,* 117–126.

Messick, S. (1970). The criterion problem in the evaluation of instruction: Assessing possible, not just intended, outcomes. In M. C. Wittrock & D. W. Wiley (Eds.), *The evaluation of instruction: Issues and problems* (pp. 183–201). New York: Holt, Rinehart & Winston.

Miller, G. (1986, August). *Fostering comprehension monitoring in less-skilled readers through self-instruction training.* Paper presented at the American Psychological Association, New York.

Miller, G., Giovenco, A., & Rentiers, K. A. (1987). Fostering comprehension monitoring in below average readers through self-instruction training. *Journal of Reading Behavior, 19,* 379–394.

Miltenberger, R. G. (1990). Assessment of treatment acceptability: A review of the literature. *Topics in Early Childhood Special Education, 10(3),* 24–38.

Miltenberger, R. G., & Fuqua, R. W. (1985). Evaluation of a training manual for the acquisition of behavioral assessment interviewing skills. *Journal of Applied Behavior Analysis, 18,* 323–328.

Moats, L. C. (1999). *Teaching reading is rocket science: What expert teachers of reading should know and be able to do.* Washington, DC: American Federation of Teachers.

Montague, M. (1989). Strategy instruction and mathematical problem solving. *Journal of Reading, Writing, and Learning Disabilities International, 4,* 275–290.

Montague, M., & Bos, C. S. (1986). Verbal mathematical problem solving and learning disabilities: A review. *Focus on Learning Problems in Mathematics, 8(2),* 7–21.

Mortweet, S. L., Utley, C. A., Walker, D., Dawson, H. L., Delquadri, J. C., Reddy, S. B., et al. (1999). Classwide peer tutoring: Teaching students with mild mental retardation in inclusive classrooms. *Exceptional Children, 65,* 524–536.

Myers, S. S. (1990). The management of curriculum time as it relates to student engaged time. *Educational Review, 42,* 13–23.

Naglieri, J. A., & Das, J. P. (1997). *Das-Naglieri Cognitive Assessment System (CAS).* Itasca, IL: Riverside Publishing.

Naglieri, J. A., & Johnson, D. (2000). Effectiveness of a cognitive strategy intervention in improving arithmetic computation based on the PASS theory. *Journal of Learning Disabilities, 33,* 591–597.

Naslund, R. A., Thorpe, L. P., & Lefever, D. W. (1978). *SRA Achievement Series.* Chicago: Science Research Associates.

Nastasi, B. K., & Clements, D. H. (1991). Research on cooperative learning: Implications for practice. *School Psychology Review, 20,* 110–131.

National Reading Panel. (2000). *Teaching children to read: An evidence-based assessment of the scientific research literature on reading and its implications for reading.* Available online: *http://www. nichd. nih. gov/publications/nrp/smallbook. htm.*

National Research Council. (1998). *Preventing reading difficulties in young children.* Washington, DC: National Academy Press.

Neef, N. A., Iwata, B. A., & Page, T. J. (1980). The effects of interspersal training versus high density reinforcement on spelling acquisition and retention. *Journal of Applied Behavior Analysis, 13,* 153–158.

Neill, M., & Medina, N. (1989). Standardized testing: Harmful to educational health. *Phi Delta Kappan, 70,* 688–697.

Nelson, R. O. (1977). Methodological issues in assessment via self-monitoring. In J. D. Cone & R. P. Hawkins (Eds.), *Behavioral assessment: New directions in clinical psychology* (pp. 217–240). New York: Brunner/Mazel.

Nelson, R. O. (1985). Behavioral assessment in the school setting. In T. R. Kratochwill (Ed.), *Advances in school psychology* (Vol. 4, pp. 45–88). Hillsdale, NJ: Erlbaum.

Nelson, R. O. (1988). Relationships between assessment and treatment within a behavioral perspective. *Journal of Psychopathology and Behavioral Assessment, 10,* 155–170.

Nelson, R. O., & Hayes, S. C. (1981). Theoretical explanations for reactivity in self-monitoring. *Behavior Modification, 5,* 3–14.

Nelson, R. O., & Hayes, S. C. (1986). *Conceptual foundations of behavioral assessment.* New York: Guilford Press.

Newman, B., Reinecke, D. R., & Meinberg, D. L. (2000). Self-management of varied responding in three students with autism. *Behavioral Interventions, 15,* 145–151.

Noll, M. B., Kamps, D., & Seaborn, C. F. (1993). Prereferral intervention for students with emotional or behavioral risks: Use of a behavioral consultation model. *Journal of Emotional and Behavioral Disorders, 1,* 203–214.

Northrup, J., Wacker, D. P., Berg, W. K., Kelly, L., Sasso, G., & DeRaad, A. (1994). The treatment of severe behavior problems in school settings using a technical assistance model. *Journal of Applied Behavior Analysis, 27,* 33–48.

O'Connor, R. (2000). Increasing the intensity of intervention in kindergarten and first grade. *Learning Disabilities Research and Practice, 51,* 43–54.

O'Connor, R. E., Notari-Syverson, A., & Vadasy, P. F. (1996). *Ladders to literacy: An activity book for kindergarten children.* Seattle: Washington Research Institute.

O'Donnell, P., Weber, K. P., & McLaughlin, T. F. (2003). Improving correct and error rate and reading comprehension using key words and previewing: A case report with a language minority student. *Education and Treatment of Children, 26,* 237–254.

Ollendick, T. H., & Hersen, M. (1984). *Child behavior assessment: Principles and procedures.* New York: Pergamon Press.

Ollendick, T. H., Matson, J. L., Esvelt-Dawson, K., & Shapiro, E. S., (1980). Increasing spelling achievement: An analysis of treatment procedures utilizing an alternating treatments design. *Journal of Applied Behavior Analysis, 13,* 645–654.

Ownby, R. L., Wallbrown, F., D'Atri, A., & Armstrong, B. (1985). Patterns of referrals for school psychological services: Replication of the referral problems category system. *Special Services in the School, 1*(4), 53–66.

Parker, R., Hasbrouck, J. E., & Tindal, G. (1992). Greater validity for oral reading fluency: Can miscues help? *Journal of Special Education, 25,* 492–503.

Peterson, K. M. H., & Shinn, M. R. (2002). Severe discrepancy models: Which best explains school identification practices for learning disabilities? *School Psychology Review, 31,* 459–476.

Phillips, N. B., Fuchs, L. S., & Fuchs, D. (1994). Effects of classwide curriculum-based measurement and peer tutoring: A collaborative research–practitioner interview study. *Journal of Learning Disabilities, 27,* 420–434.

Phillips, N. B., Hamlett, C. L., Fuchs, L. S., & Fuchs, D. (1993). Combining classwide curriculum-based measurement and peer tutoring to help general educators provide adaptive education. *Learning Disabilities Research and Practice, 8*(3), 148–156.

Pickens, J., & McNaughton, S. (1988). Peer tutoring of comprehension strategies. *Educational Psychology, 8*(1–2), 67–80.

Powell-Smith, K. A. (2004, February). *Individual differences in FCAT performance: A national context for our results.* Paper presented at the 12th annual Pacific Coast Research Conference, San Diego, CA.

Powell-Smith, K. A., & Bradley-Klug, K. L. (2001). Another look at the "C" in CBM: Does it really matter if curriculum-based measurement reading probes are curriculum-based? *Psychology in the Schools, 38,* 299–312.

Powell-Smith, K. A., & Stewart, L. H. (1998). The use of curriculum-based measurement in the reintegration of students with mild disabilities. In M. R. Shinn (Ed.), *Advanced applications of curriculum-based measurement* (pp. 254–298). New York: Guilford Press.

Power, T. J., & Eiraldi, R. B. (2000). Educational and psychiatric classification systems. In E. S. Shapiro & T. R. Kratochwill (Eds.), *Behavioral assessment in schools: Theory, research, and clinical foundations* (2nd ed., pp. 464–488). New York: Guilford Press.

Prater, M. A., Hogan, S., & Miller, S. R. (1992). Using self-monitoring to improve on-task behavior and academic skills of an adolescent with mild handicaps across special and regular education settings. *Education and Treatment of Children, 15,* 43–55.

Pratt-Struthers, J., Struthers, B., & Williams, R. L. (1983). The effects of the Add-a-Word spelling program on spelling accuracy during creative writing. *Education and Treatment of Children, 6,* 277–283.

Priest, J. S., McConnell, S. R., Walker, D., Carta, J. J., Kaminski, R. A., McEvoy, M. A., et al. (2001). General growth outcomes for young children: Developing a foundation for continuous progress measurement. *Journal of Early Intervention, 24,* 163–180.

Rathvon, N. (1999). *Effective school interventions: Strategies for enhancing academic achievement and social competence.* New York: Guilford Press.

Reid, R. (1996). Research in self-monitoring with students with learning disabilities: The present, the prospects, the pitfalls. *Journal of Learning Disabilities, 29,* 317–331.

Reid, R., & Harris, K. R. (1993). Self-monitoring of attention versus self-monitoring of performance: Effects on attention and academic performance. *Exceptional Children, 60,* 29–40.

Reimers, T. M., Wacker, D. P., Cooper, L. J., & deRaad, A. O. (1992). Acceptability of behavioral treatments for children: Analog and naturalistic evaluations by parents. *School Psychology Review, 21,* 628–643.

Reimers, T. M., Wacker, D. P., Derby, K. M., & Cooper, L. J. (1995). Relation between parental attributions and the acceptability of behavioral treatments for their child's behavior problems. *Behavioral Disorders, 20,* 171–178.

Reschly, D. J., & Grimes, J. P. (1991). State department and university cooperation: Evaluation of continuing education in consultation and curriculum-based assessment. *School Psychology Review, 20,* 522–529.

Resnick, L. B., & Ford, W. W. (1978). The analysis of tasks for instruction: An information-processing approach. In A. C. Cantania & T. A. Brigham (Eds.), *Handbook of applied behavior analysis: Social and instructional processes* (pp. 378–409). Englewood Cliffs, NJ: Prentice-Hall.

Reynolds, M. C. (1984). Classification of students with handicaps. In E. W. Gordon (Ed.), *Review of research in education* (pp. 63–92). Washington, DC: American Education Research Association.

Rhode, G., Morgan, D. P., & Young, K. R. (1983). Generalization and maintenance of treatment gains of behaviorally handicapped students from resource rooms to regular classrooms using self-evaluation procedures. *Journal of Applied Behavior Analysis, 16,* 171–188.

Rich, H. L., & Ross, S. M. (1989). Students' time on learning tasks in special education. *Exceptional Children, 55,* 508–515.

Roberts, A. H., & Rust, J. O. (1994). Role and function of school psychologists, 1992–93: A comparative study. *Psychology in the Schools, 31,* 113–119.

Roberts, M., & Smith, D. D. (1980). The relationship among correct and error oral reading rates and comprehension. *Learning Disability Quarterly, 3,* 54–64.

Roberts, M. L., Marshall, J., Nelson, J. R., & Albers, C. A. (2001). Curriculum-based assessment procedures embedded within functional behavioral assessments: Identifying escape-motivated behaviors in a general education classroom. *School Psychology Review, 30,* 264–277.

Roberts, M. L., & Shapiro, E. S. (1996). The effects of instructional ratios on students' reading performance in a regular education program. *Journal of School Psychology, 34,* 73–92.

Roberts, M. L., Turco, T., & Shapiro, E. S. (1991). Differential effects of fixed instructional ratios on student's progress in reading. *Journal of Psychoeducational Assessment, 9,* 308–318.

Roberts, R. N., & Dick, M. L. (1982). Self-control in the classroom: Theoretical issues and practical applications. In T. R. Kratochwill (Ed.), *Advances in school psychology* (Vol. 2, pp. 275–314). Hillsdale, NJ: Erlbaum.

Roberts, R. N., Nelson, R. O., & Olsen, T. W. (1987). Self-instruction: An analysis of the differential effects of instruction and reinforcement. *Journal of Applied Behavior Analysis, 20,* 235–242.

Robertson, S. J., Simon, S. J., Pachman, J. S., & Drabman, R. S. (1980). Self-control and generalization procedures in a classroom of disruptive retarded children. *Child Behavior Therapy, 1,* 347–362.

Rohrbeck, C. A., Ginsburg-Block, M. D., Fantuzzo, J. W., & Miller, T. R. (2003). Peer-assisted learning interventions with elementary school students: A meta-analytic review. *Journal of Educational Psychology, 95,* 240–257.

Rose, T. L., & Beattie, J. R. (1986). Relative effects of teacher-directed and taped previewing on oral reading. *Learning Disability Quarterly, 9,* 193–199.

Rosenfield, S. A. (1987). *Instructional consultation.* Hillsdale, NJ: Erlbaum.

Rosenfield, S. A. (1995). The practice of instructional consultation. *Journal of Educational and Psychological Consultation, 6,* 317–327.

Rosenfield, S. A., & Gravois, T. (1995). *Organizational consultation.* New York: Guilford Press.

Rosenfield, S., & Kuralt, S. (1990). Best practices in curriculum-based assessment. In A. Thomas & J. Grimes (Eds.), *Best practices in school psychology* (Vol. 2, pp. 275–286). Washington, DC: National Association of School Psychologists.

Rosenshine, B. V. (1979). Content, time, and direct instruction. In P. L. Peterson & H. J. Walberg (Eds.), *Research on teaching* (pp. 28–56). Berkeley, CA: McCutchan.

Rosenshine, B. V. (1981). Academic engaged time, content covered, and direct instruction. *Journal of Education, 3,* 38–66.

Rosenshine, B. V., & Berliner, D. C. (1978). Academic engaged time. *British Journal of Teacher Education, 4,* 3–16.

Rousseau, M. K., Tam, B. K., & Ramnarain, R. (1993). Increasing reading proficiency of language-minority students with speech and language impairments. *Education and Treatment of Children, 16,* 254–271.

Salvia, J. A., & Hughes, C. (1990). *Curriculum-based assessment: Testing what is taught.* New York: Macmillan.

Salvia, J. A., & Ysseldyke, J. E. (2001). *Assessment in special and remedial education* (8th ed.). Boston: Houghton Mifflin.

Santogrossi, D. A., O'Leary, K. D., Romanczyk, R. G., & Kaufman, K. F. (1973). Self-evaluation by adolescents in a psychiatric hospital school token program. *Journal of Applied Behavior Analysis, 6,* 277–287.

Saudargas, R. A. (1992). *State–Event Classroom Observation System (SECOS).* Knoxville: Department of Psychology, University of Tennessee.

Saudargas, R. A., & Creed, V. (1980). *State–Event Classroom Observation System.* Knoxville: University of Tennessee, Department of Psychology.

Saudargas, R. A., & Lentz, F. E. (1986). Estimating percent of time and rate via direct observation: A suggested observational procedure and format. *School Psychology Review, 15,* 36–48.

Sawyer, R. J., Graham, S., & Harris, K. R. (1992). Direct teaching, strategy instruction, and strategy instruction with explicit self-regulation: Effects on the composition skills and self-efficacy of students with learning disabilities. *Journal of Educational Psychology, 84,* 340–352.

Schermerhorn, P. K., & McLaughlin, T. F. (1997). Effects of the Add-a-Word spelling program on test accuracy, grades, and retention of spelling words with fifth and sixth grade regular education students. *Child and Family Behavior Therapy, 19,* 23–35.

Schumaker, J. B., Denton, P. H., & Deshler, D. D. (1984). *The paraphrasing strategy.* Lawrence: University of Kansas Press.

Schumaker, J. B., & Deshler, D. D. (2003). Can students with LD become competent writers? *Learning Disability Quarterly, 26,* 129–141.

Schumaker, J. B., Deshler, D. D., Alley, G. R., & Denton, P. H. (1982). Multipass: A learning strategy for improving reading comprehension. *Learning Disabilities Quarterly, 5,* 295–304.

Schumaker, J. B., Deshler, D. D., Alley, G. R., & Warner, M. M. (1983). Toward the development of an intervention model for learning disabled adolescents. *Exceptional Education Quarterly, 3*(4), 45–50.

Schunk, D. H., & Rice, J. M. (1992). Influence of reading-comprehension strategy information on children's achievement outcomes. *Learning Disability Quarterly, 15,* 51–64.

Schunk, D. H., & Schwartz, C. W. (1993). Goals and progress feedback: Effects on self-efficacy and writing achievement. *Contemporary Educational Psychology, 18,* 337–354.

Scruggs, T. E., & Mastropieri, M. A. (2002). On babies and bathwater: Addressing the problems of identification of learning disabilities. *Learning Disability Quarterly, 25,* 155–168.

Scruggs, T. E., Mastropieri, M., Veit, D. T., & Osguthorpe, R. T. (1986). Behaviorally disordered students as tutors: Effects on social behavior. *Behavioral Disorders, 11*(4), 36–43.

Serenty, M. L., & Kundert, D. K. (1987, August). *Curriculum-based assessment of spelling programs.* Paper presented at the American Psychological Association, New York.

Sexton, M., Harris, K. R., & Graham, S. (1998). Self-regulated strategy development and the writing process: Effects on essay writing and attributions. *Exceptional Children, 64,* 295–311.

Shapiro, E. S. (1981). Self-control procedures with the mentally retarded. In M. Hersen, R. M. Eisler, & P. M. Miller (Eds.), *Progress in behavior modification* (Vol. 12, pp. 265–297). New York: Academic Press.

Shapiro, E. S. (1984). Self-monitoring. In T. H. Ollendick & M. Hersen (Eds.), *Child behavior assessment: Principles and procedures* (pp. 148–165). New York: Pergamon Press.

Shapiro, E. S. (1987a). *Behavioral assessment in school psychology.* Hillsdale, NJ: Erlbaum.

Shapiro, E. S. (1987b). Intervention research methodology in school psychology. *School Psychology Review, 16,* 290–305.

Shapiro, E. S. (1987c). Academic problems. In M. Hersen & V. Van Hasselt (Eds.), *Behavior therapy with children and adolescents: A clinical approach* (pp. 363–384). New York: Wiley.

Shapiro, E. S. (1989). *Academic skills problems: Direct assessment and intervention.* New York: Guilford Press.

Shapiro, E. S. (1990). An integrated model for curriculum-based assessment. *School Psychology Review, 19,* 331–349.

Shapiro, E. S. (1992). Gickling's model of curriculum-based assessment to improve reading in elementary age students. *School Psychology Review, 21,* 168–176.

Shapiro, E. S. (1996a). *Academic skills problems: Direct assessment and intervention* (2nd ed.). New York: Guilford Press.

Shapiro, E. S. (1996b). *Academic skills problems workbook.* New York: Guilford Press.

Shapiro, E. S. (2003a). *Behavioral Observation of Students in Schools—BOSS* [Computer software]. San Antonio, TX: Psychological Corporation.

Shapiro, E. S. (2003b, October). *Issues in conducting curriculum-based normative data in mathematics*. Paper presented at the 37th annual Penn State School Psychology Conference, State College, PA.

Shapiro, E. S., & Ager, C. L. (1992). Assessment of special education students in regular education programs: Linking assessment to instruction. *Elementary School Journal, 92,* 283–296.

Shapiro, E. S., Angello, L. M., & Eckert, T. L. (2004). Has curriculum-based assessment become a staple of school psychology practice?: An update and extension of knowledge, use, and attitudes from 1990 to 2000. *School Psychology Review, 33,* 243–252.

Shapiro, E. S., & Bradley, K. L. (1995). Treatment of academic problems. In M. A. Reinecke, F. M. Datillio, & A. Freeman (Eds.), *Cognitive therapy with children and adolescents* (pp. 344–366). New York: Guilford Press.

Shapiro, E. S., Browder, D. M., & D'Huyvetters, K. K. (1984). Increasing academic productivity of severely multi-handicapped children with self-management: Idiosyncratic effects. *Analysis and Intervention in Developmental Disabilities, 4,* 171–188.

Shapiro, E. S., & Cole, C. L. (1994). *Behavior change in the classroom: Self-management interventions.* New York: Guilford Press.

Shapiro, E. S., & Cole, C. L. (1999). Self-monitoring in assessing children's problems. *Psychological Assessment, 11,* 448–457.

Shapiro, E. S., & Derr, T. F. (1987). An examination of overlap between reading curricula and standardized achievement tests. *Journal of Special Education, 21,* 59–67.

Shapiro, E. S., DuPaul, G. J., & Bradley-Klug, K. L. (1998). Self-management as a strategy to improve the classroom behavior of adolescents with ADHD. *Journal of Learning Disabilities, 31,* 545–555.

Shapiro, E. S., & Eckert, T. L. (1993). Curriculum-based assessment among school psychologists: Knowledge, attitudes, and use. *Journal of School Psychology, 31,* 375–384.

Shapiro, E. S., & Eckert, T. L. (1994). Acceptability of curriculum-based assessment by school psychologists. *Journal of School Psychology, 32,* 167–184.

Shapiro, E. S., Edwards, L., Lutz, J. G., & Keller, M. (2004, March). *Relationships of general outcomes measurement normative data and standardized tests in Pennsylvania.* Paper presented at the meeting of the National Association of School Psychologists, Dallas, TX.

Shapiro, E. S., Edwards, L., & Zigmond, N. (in press). Progress monitoring of mathematics among students with learning disabilities. *Assessment for Effective Intervention.*

Shapiro, E. S., & Goldberg, R. (1986). A comparison of group contingencies in increasing spelling performance across sixth grade students. *School Psychology Review, 15,* 546–559.

Shapiro, E. S., & Goldberg, R. (1990). *In vivo* rating of treatment acceptability by children: Group size effects in group contingencies to improve spelling performance. *Journal of School Psychology, 28,* 233–250.

Shapiro, E. S., & Heick, P. (2004). School psychologist assessment practices in the evaluation of students referred for social/behavioral/emotional problems. *Psychology in the Schools, 41,* 551–561.

Shapiro, E. S., & Kratochwill, T. R. (Eds.). (2000). *Behavioral assessment in schools: Theory, research, and clinical foundations* (2nd ed.). New York: Guilford Press.

Shapiro, E. S., & Lentz, F. E. (1985). Assessing academic behavior: A behavioral approach. *School Psychology Review, 14,* 325–338.

Shapiro, E. S., & Lentz, F. E. (1986). Behavioral assessment of academic behavior. In T. R. Kratochwill (Ed.), *Advances in school psychology* (Vol. 5, pp. 87–139). Hillsdale, NJ: Erlbaum.

Shapiro, E. S., & McCurdy, B. L. (1989). Direct and generalized effects of a taped-words treatment on reading proficiency. *Exceptional Children, 55,* 321–326.

Shapiro, E. S., McGonigle, J. J., & Ollendick, T. H. (1981). An analysis of self-assessment and self-reinforcement in a self-managed token economy with mentally retarded children. *Applied Research in Mental Retardation, 1,* 227–240.

Shavelson, R. J., & Towne, L. (Eds.). (2002). *Scientific research in education.* Washington, DC: National Academy Press.

Shaywitz, S. E., Escobar, M. D., Shaywitz, B. A., Fletcher, J. M., & Makuch, R. (1992). Distribution and temporal stability of dyslexia in an epidemiological sample of 414 children followed longitudinally. *New England Journal of Medicine, 326,* 145–150.

Shimabukuro, S. M., Prater, M. A., Jenkins, A., & Edelen-Smith, P. (1999). The effects of self-monitoring of academic performance on students with learning disabilities and ADD/ADHD. *Education and Treatment of Children, 22,* 397–414.

Shinn, M. R. (1988). Development of curriculum-based local norms for use in special education decision-making. *School Psychology Review, 17,* 61–80.

Shinn, M. R. (Ed.). (1989a). *Curriculum-based measurement: Assessing special children.* New York: Guilford Press.

Shinn, M. R. (1989b). Identifying and defining academic problems: CBM screening and eligibility. In M. R. Shinn (Ed.), *Curriculum-based measurement: Assessing special children* (pp. 90–129). New York: Guilford Press.

Shinn, M. R. (Ed.). (1998). *Advanced applications of curriculum-based measurement.* New York: Guilford Press.

Shinn, M. R., Good, R. H., III, & Stein, S. (1989). Summarizing trend in student achievement: A comparison of models. *School Psychology Review, 18,* 356–370.

Shinn, M. R., Habedank, L., Rodden-Nord, L., & Knutson, N. (1993). Using curriculum-based measurement to identify potential candidates for reintegration into general education. *Journal of Special Education, 27,* 202–221.

Shinn, M. R., Powell-Smith, K. A., & Good, R. H. (1996). Evaluating the effects of responsible reintegration into general education for students with mild disabilities on a case-by-case basis. *School Psychology Review, 25,* 519–539.

Shinn, M. R., Tindal, G., & Stein, S. (1988). Curriculum-based assessment and the identification of mildly handicapped students: A research review. *Professional School Psychology, 3,* 69–86.

Shinn, M. R., Walker, H. M., & Stoner, G. (Eds.). (2002). *Interventions for academic and behavior problems: II. Preventive and remedial approaches.* Washington, DC: National Association of School Psychologists.

Shriner, J., & Salvia, J. (1988). Chronic noncorrespondence between elementary math curricula and arithmetic tests. *Exceptional Children, 55,* 240–248.

Sideridis, G. D., Utley, C., Greenwood, C. H., Delquadri, J., Dawson, H., Palmer, P., et al. (1997). Classwide peer tutoring: Effects on the spelling performance and social interactions of students with mild disabilities and their typical peers in an integrated instructional setting. *Journal of Behavioral Education, 7,* 435–462.

Simmons, D., & Kame'enui, E. (1999). *Optimize.* Eugene: College of Education, Institute for Development of Educational Achievement, University of Oregon.

Skinner, C. H. (2002). An empirical analysis of interspersal research evidence, implications, and applications of the discrete task completion hypothesis. *Journal of School Psychology, 40,* 347–368.

Skinner, C. H., Bamberg, H. W., Smith, E. S., & Powell, S. S. (1993). Cognitive cover, copy, and compare: Subvocal responding to increase rates of accurate division responding. *RASE: Remedial and Special Education, 14*(1), 49–56.

Skinner, C. H., Cooper, L., & Cole, C. L. (1997). The effects of oral presentation previewing rates on reading performance. *Journal of Applied Behavior Analysis, 30,* 331–333.

Skinner, C. H., Dittmer, K. I., & Howell, L. A. (2000). Direct observation in school settings: Theoretical issues. In E. S. Shapiro & T. R. Kratochwill (Eds.), *Behavioral assessment in schools: Theory, research, and clinical foundations* (2nd ed., pp. 19–45). New York: Guilford Press.

Skinner, C. H., Fletcher, P. A., Wildmon, M., & Belifore, P. J. (1996). Improving assignment preference through interspersing additional problems: Brief versus easy problems. *Journal of Behavioral Education, 6,* 427–436.

Skinner, C. H., Ford, J. M., & Yunker, B. D. (1991). A comparison of instructional response requirements on the multiplication performance of behaviorally disordered students. *Behavioral Disorders, 17,* 56–65.

Skinner, C. H., Hall-Johnson, K., Skinner, A. L., Cates, G., Weber, J., & Johns, G. A. (1999). Enhancing perceptions of mathematics assignments by increasing relative problem completion rates through the interspersal technique. *Journal of Experimental Education, 68,* 43–59.

Skinner, C. H., Hurst, K. L., Teeple, D. F., & Meadows, S. O. (2002). Increasing on-task behavior during mathematics independent seat-work in students with emotional disturbance by interspersing additional brief problems. *Psychology in the Schools, 39,* 647–659.

Skinner, C. H., McLaughlin, T. F., & Logan, P. (1997). Cover, copy, and compare: A self-managed academic intervention effective across skills, students, and settings. *Journal of Behavioral Education, 7,* 295–306.

Skinner, C. H., & Shapiro, E. S. (1987). A comparison of a taped-words and drill interventions on reading fluency in adolescents with behavior disorders. *Education and Treatment of Children, 12,* 123–133.

Skinner, C. H., Shapiro, E. S., Turco, T. L., Cole, C. L., & Brown, D. K. (1992). A comparison of self- and peer-delivered immediate corrective feedback on multiplication performance. *Journal of School Psychology, 30,* 101–116.

Skinner, C. H., & Smith, E. S. (1992). Issues surrounding the use of self-management interventions for increasing academic performance. *School Psychology Review, 21,* 202–210.

Skinner, C. H., Turco, T. L., Beatty, K. L., & Rasavage, C. (1989). Cover, copy, and compare: A method for increasing multiplication performance. *School Psychology Review, 18,* 412–420.

Skinner, C. H., Wallace, M. A., & Neddenriep, C. E. (2002). Academic remediation: Educational applications of research on assignment preference and choice. *Child and Family Behavior Therapy, 24,* 51–65.

Slate, J. R., & Saudargas, R. A. (1986). Differences in learning disabled and average students classroom behaviors. *Learning Disability Quarterly, 9,* 61–67.

Slavin, R. E. (1977). Classroom reward structure: An analytic and practical review. *Review of Educational Research 47,* 633–650.

Slavin, R. E. (1980). Cooperative learning. *Review of Educational Research, 50,* 315–342.

Slavin, R. E. (1983a). *Cooperative learning.* New York: Longman.

Slavin, R. E. (1983b). Team assisted individualization: A cooperative learning solution for adaptive instruction in mathematics. *Center for Organization of Schools Report No. 340.* Baltimore: Johns Hopkins University.

Slavin, R. E. (1991). Cooperative learning and group contingencies. *Journal of Behavioral Education, 1,* 105–115.

Slavin, R. E., Madden, N. A., & Leavey, M. (1984). Effects of team-assisted individuation on the mathematics achievement of academically handicapped and non-handicapped students. *Journal of Educational Psychology, 76,* 813–819.

Smith, A. M., & Van Biervliet, A. (1986). Enhancing reading comprehension through the use of a self-instructional package. *Education and Treatment of Children, 9,* 40–55.

Smith, C., & Arnold, V. (1986). *Macmillan-R series.* New York: Macmillan.

Smith, D. J., Young, K. R., Nelson, J. R., & West, R. P. (1992). The effect of a self-management procedure on the classroom academic behavior of students with mild handicaps. *School Psychology Review, 21,* 59–72.

Smith, D. J., Young, K. R., West, R. P., Morgan, D. P., & Rhode, G. (1988). Reducing the disruptive behavior of junior high school students: A classroom self-management procedure. *Behavioral Disorders, 13,* 231–239.

Smith, S. B., Simmons, D. C., & Kame'enui, E. J. (1998). Phonological awareness: Instructional and curricular basics and implications. In D. C. Simmons & E. J. Kame'enui (Eds.), *What reading research tells us about children with diverse learning needs: Bases and basics.* Mahwah, NJ: Erlbaum.

Speece, D. L., & Case, L. P. (2001). Classification in context: An alternative approach to identifying early reading disability. *Journal of Educational Psychology, 93,* 735–749.

Speltz, L. L., Shimamura, J. W., & McReynolds, W. T. (1982). Procedural variations in group contingencies: Effects on children's academic and social behaviors. *Journal of Applied Behavior Analysis, 15,* 533–544.

Staats, A. W., Minke, K. A., Finley, J. R., Wolf, M. M., & Brooks, L. O. A. (1964). Reinforcer system and experimental procedure for the laboratory study of reading acquisition. *Child Development, 36,* 925–942.

Stage, S. A., & Jacobsen, M. D. (2001). Predicting student success on a state-mandated performance-based assessment using oral reading fluency. *School Psychology Review, 30,* 407–419.

Stanley, S. D., & Greenwood, C. R. (1981). *CISSAR: Code for Instructional Structure and Student Academic Response: Observer's manual.* Kansas City: Juniper Gardens Children's Project, Bureau of Child Research, University of Kansas.

Stanley, S. D., & Greenwood, C. R. (1983). Assessing opportunity to respond in classroom environments through direct observation: How much opportunity to respond does the minority, disadvantaged student receive in school? *Exceptional Children, 49,* 370–373.

Stecker, P. M., & Fuchs, L. S. (2000). Effecting superior achievement using curriculum-based measurement: The importance of individual progress monitoring. *Learning Disabilities Research and Practice, 15,* 128–134.

Stein, C. L., & Goldman, J. (1980). Beginning reading instruction for children with minimal brain dysfunction. *Journal of Learning Disabilities, 13,* 219–222.

Sternberg, R. J., & Grigorenko, E. L. (2002). Difference scores in the identification of children with learning disabilities: It's time to use a different method. *Journal of School Psychology, 40,* 65–83.

Stevenson H. C., & Fantuzzo, J. W. (1984). Application of the "generalization map" to a self-control intervention with school-aged children. *Journal of Applied Behavior Analysis, 17,* 203–212.

Stewart, C. A., & Singh, N. N. (1986). Overcorrection of spelling deficits in moderately mentally retarded children. *Behavior Modification, 10,* 355–365.

Stinnett, T. A., Havey, J. M., & Oehler-Stinnett, J. (1994). Current test usage by practicing school psychologists: A national survey. *Journal of Psychoeducational Assessment, 12,* 351–350.

Stoddard, B., & MacArthur, C. A. (1993). A peer editor strategy: Guiding learning-disabled students in response and revision. *Research in the Teaching of English, 27*(1), 76–103.

Stoddard, K., Valcante, G., Sindelar, P., & O'Shea, L. (1993). Increasing rate and comprehension: The effects of repeated readings, sentence segmentation, and intonation training. *Reading Research and Instruction, 32,* 53–65.

Stoner, G., Carey, S. P., Ikeda, M. J., & Shinn, M. R. (1994). The utility of curriculum-based measurement for evaluating the effects of methylphenidate on academic performance. *Journal of Applied Behavior Analysis, 27,* 101–113.

Stowitschek, C. E., Hecimovic, A., Stowitschek, J. J., & Shores, R. E. (1982). Behaviorally disordered adolescents as peer tutors: Immediate and generative effects on instructional performance and spelling achievement. *Behavior Disorders, 7,* 136–147.

Stromer, R. (1975). Modifying letter and number reversals in elementary school children. *Journal of Applied Behavior Analysis, 8,* 211.

Struthers, J. P., Bartlamay, H., Bell, S., & McLaughlin, T. F. (1994). An analysis of the Add-a-Word spelling program and public posting across three categories of children with special needs. *Reading Improvement, 31*(1), 28–36.

Struthers, J. P., Bartlamay, H., Williams, R. L. O., & McLaughlin, T. F. (1989). Effects of the Add-a-Word spelling program on spelling accuracy during creative writing: A replication across two classrooms. *British Columbia Journal of Special Education, 13*(2), 151–158.

Stuebing, K. K., Fletcher, J. M., LeDoux, J. M., Lyon, G. R., Shaywitz, S. E., & Shaywitz, B. A. (2002). Validity of IQ-discrepancy classification of reading disabilities: A meta-analysis. *American Educational Research Journal, 39,* 469–518.

Sulzer-Azaroff, B., & Mayer, G. R. (1986). *Achieving educational excellence: Using behavioral strategies.* New York: Holt, Rinehart, & Winston.

Swanson, H. L. (1981). Modification of comprehension deficits in learning disabled children. *Learning Disability Quarterly, 4,* 189–202.

Swanson, H. L., Harris, K. R., & Graham, S. (Eds.). (2003). *Handbook of learning disabilities.* New York: Guilford Press.

Swanson, H. L., & Hoskyn, M., & Lee, C. (1999). *Interventions for students with learning disabilities: A meta-analysis of treatment outcomes.* New York: Guilford Press.

Swanson, H. L., & Scarpati, S. (1984). Self-instruction training to increase academic performance of educationally handicapped children. *Child and Family Behavior Therapy, 6*(4), 23–39.

Szykula, S., Saudargas, R. A., & Wahler, R. G. (1981). The generality of self-control procedures following a change in the classroom teacher. *Education and Treatment of Children, 4,* 253–264.

Tabacek, D. A., McLaughlin, T. F., & Howard, V. F. (1994). Teaching preschool children with disabilities tutoring skills: Effects on preacademic behaviors. *Child and Family Behavior Therapy, 16*(2), 43–63.

Tarver, S. G., & Dawson, M. M. (1978). Modality preference and the teaching of reading: A review. *Journal of Learning Disabilities, 11,* 5–7.

Talor, L. K., Alber, S. R., & Walker, D. W. (2002). The comparative effects of a modified self-questioning strategy and story mapping on the reading comprehension of elementary students with learning disabilities. *Journal of Behavioral Education, 11,* 69–87.

Taylor, N. E., & Conner, U. (1982). Silent vs. oral reading: The rational instructional use of both processes. *Reading Teacher, 35,* 440–443.

Terry, M. N., Deck, D., Huelecki, M. B., & Santogrossi, D. A. (1978). Increasing arithmetic output of a fourth-grade student. *Behavior Disorders, 7,* 136–147.

Texas Center for Reading and Language Arts. (1998). *Professional Development Guide.* Austin: Texas Center for Reading and Language Arts, University of Texas at Austin.

Thomas, A., & Grimes, J. (2002). *Best practices in school psychology.* Silver Spring, MD: National Association of School Psychologists.

Thurber, R. S., Shinn, M. R., & Smolkowski, K. (2002). What is measured in mathematics tests?: Construct validity of curriculum-based mathematics measures. *School Psychology Review, 31,* 498–513.

Thurlow, M. L., Graden, J., Greener, J. W., & Ysseldyke, J. E. (1983). LD and non-LD student's opportunities to learn. *Learning Disability Quarterly, 6,* 172–183.

Thurlow, M. L., & Ysseldyke, J. E. (1982). Instructional planning: Information collected by school psychologists vs. information considered useful by teachers. *Journal of School Psychology, 20,* 3–10.

Thurlow, M. L., Ysseldyke, J. E., Graden, J. L., & Algozzine, B. (1983). What's "special" about the special education resource room for learning disabled students? *Learning Disability Quarterly, 6,* 283–288.

Thurlow, M. L., Ysseldyke, J. E., Graden, J., & Algozzine, B. (1984). Opportunity to learn for LD students receiving different levels of special education services. *Learning Disabilities Quarterly, 7,* 55–67.

Thurlow, M. L., Ysseldyke, J. E., Wotruba, J. W., & Algozzine, B. (1993). Instruction in special education classrooms under varying student–teacher ratios. *Elementary School Journal, 93,* 305–320.

Tiegs, E. W., & Clarke, W. W. (1970). *California Achievement Test.* Monterey, CA: CTB/McGraw-Hill.

Tindal, G., Fuchs, L. S., Fuchs, D., Shinn, M. R., Deno, S. L., & Germann, G. (1985). Empirical validation of criterion-referenced tests. *Journal of Educational Research, 78,* 203–209.

Tindal, G., & Parker, R. (1989). Development of written retell as a curriculum-based measurement in secondary programs. *School Psychology Review, 18,* 328–343.

Tindal, G., Wesson, C., Deno, S. L., Germann, G., & Mirkin, P. K. (1985). The Pine County model for special education delivery: A data-based system. In T. R. Kratochwill (Ed.), *Advances in school psychology* (Vol. 4, pp. 223–250). Hillsdale, NJ: Erlbaum.

Tingstrom, D. H., Edwards, R. P., & Olmi, D. J. (1995). Listening previewing in reading to read: Relative effects on oral reading fluency. *Psychology in the Schools, 32,* 318–327.

Todd, A. W., Horner, R. H., & Sugai, G. (1999). Self-monitoring and self-recruited praise: Effects on problem behavior, academic engagement, and work completion in a typical classroom. *Journal of Positive Behavior Interventions, 1,* 66–76.

Topping, K., & Ehly, S. (Eds.). (1998). *Peer-assisted learning.* Mahwah, NJ: Erlbaum.

Topping, K., & Whiteley, M. (1993). Sex differences in the effectiveness of peer tutoring. *School Psychology International, 14,* 57–67.

Torgesen, J. K., & Bryant, B. T. (1994). *Phonological awareness training for reading.* Austin, TX: Pro-Ed.

Tralli, R., Colombo, B., Deshler, D. D., & Schumaker, J. B. (1996). The Strategies Intervention Model: A model for supported inclusion at the secondary level. *Remedial and Special Education, 17,* 204–216.

Trammel, D. L., Schloss, P. J., & Alper, S. (1994). Using self-recording, evaluation, and graphing to increase completion of homework assignments. *Journal of Learning Disabilities, 27,* 75–81.

Trice, A. D., Parker, F. C., & Furrow, F. (1981). Written conversations and contingent free time to increase reading and writing in a non-reading adolescent. *Education and Treatment of Children, 1,* 25–29.

Trout, A. L., Epstein, M. H., Mickelson, W. T., Nelson, J. R., & Lewis, L. M. (2003). Effects of a reading intervention for kindergarten students at risk for emotional disturbance and reading deficits. *Behavioral Disorders, 28,* 313–326.

Trovato, J., & Bucher, B. (1980). Peer tutoring with or without home-based reinforcement for reading remediation. *Journal of Applied Behavior Analysis, 13,* 129–141.

Tucker, J. A. (1985). Curriculum-based assessment: An introduction. *Exceptional Children, 52,* 199–204.

Tucker, J. A. (1989). *Basic flashcard technique when vocabulary is the goal.* Unpublished teaching materials, Berrien Springs, MI.

Truchlicka, M., McLaughlin, T. F., & Swain, J. C. (1998). Effects of token reinforcement and response cost on the accuracy of spelling performance with middle-school special education students with behavior disorders. *Behavioral Interventions, 13*(1), 1–10.

Turco, T. L., & Elliott, S. N. (1990). Acceptability and effectiveness of group contingencies for improving spelling achievement. *Journal of School Psychology, 28,* 27–37.

U.S. Department of Education. (2001). *Twenty-third annual report to Congress on the implementation of the Individuals with Disabilities Education Act.* Washington, DC: Author.

Utley, C. A., Reddy, S. S., Delquadri, J. C., Greenwood, C. R., Mortweet, S. L., & Bowman, V. (2001). Classwide peer tutoring: An effective teaching procedure for facilitating the acquisition of health education and safety facts with students with developmental disabilities. *Education and Treatment of Children, 24,* 1–27.

Vaac, N. N., & Cannon, S. J. (1991). Cross-age tutoring in mathematics: Sixth graders helping students who are moderately handicapped. *Education and Training in Mental Retardation, 26,* 89–97.

Vallecorsa, A. L., & deBettencourt, L. U. (1997). Using a mapping procedure to teach reading and writing skills to middle grade students with learning disabilities. *Education and Treatment of Children, 20,* 173–188.

Van Houten, R., Hill, S., & Parsons, M. (1975). An analysis of a performance feedback system: The effects of timing and feedback, public posting, and praise upon academic performance and peer interaction. *Journal of Applied Behavior Analysis, 8,* 449–457.

Van Houten, R., & Lai Fatt, D. (1981). The effects of public posting on high school biology test performance. *Education and Treatment of Children, 4,* 217–226.

Van Houten, R., & Thompson, C. (1976). The effect of public posting on high school biology test performance. *Journal of Applied Behavior Analysis, 9,* 227–230.

Van Houten, R., & Van Houten, J. (1977). The performance feedback system in a special education classroom: An analysis of public posting and peer comments. *Behavior Therapy, 8,* 366–376.

Van Luit, J. E. H., & Naglieri, J. A. (1999). Effectiveness of the MASTER program for teaching special children multiplication and division. *Journal of Learning Disabilities, 32,* 98–107.

Vellutino, F. R., Scanlon, D. M., & Lyon, G. R. (2000). Differentiating between difficult-to-remediate and readily remediated poor readers: More evidence against the IQ-achievement discrepancy definition of reading disability. *Journal of Learning Disabilities, 33,* 233–238.

Ward, L., & Traweek, D. (1993). Application of a metacognitive strategy to assessment, intervention, and consultation: A think-aloud technique. *Journal of School Psychology, 31,* 469–485.

Wechsler, D. (2001). *Wechsler Individual Achievement Test—II.* San Antonio, TX: Psychological Corporation/Harcourt Brace Jovanovich.

Wechsler, D. (2003). *Wechsler Intelligence Scale for Children—IV.* San Antonio, TX: Psychological Corporation/Harcourt Brace Jovanovich.

Wepman, J. (1967). The perceptual basis for learning. In E. C. Frierson & W. B. Barbe (Eds.), *Educating children with learning disabilities: Selected readings* (pp. 353–362). New York: Appleton–Century–Crofts.

Whinnery, K. W., & Fuchs, L. S. (1993). Effects of goal and test-taking strategies on the computation performance of students with learning disabilities. *Learning Disabilities Research and Practice, 8,* 204–214.

White, O. R., & Haring, N. G. (1980). *Exceptional teaching* (2nd ed.). Columbus, OH: Merrill.

White, W. A. T. (1988). A meta-analysis of the effects of direct instruction in special education. *Education and Treatment of Children, 11,* 364–374.

Whitman, T., & Johnston, M. B. (1983). Teaching addition and subtraction with regrouping to educable mentally retarded children: A group self-instructional training program. *Behavior Therapy, 14,* 127–143.

Wiggins, G. (1989). A true test: Toward a more authentic and equitable assessment. *Phi Delta Kappan, 70,* 703–713.

Wildmon, M. E., Skinner, C. H., McCurdy, M., & Sims, S. (1999). Improving secondary students' perception of the "dreaded mathematics word problem assignment" by giving them more word problems. *Psychology in the Schools, 36,* 319–325.

Wilkenson, G. S. (1993). *Wide Range Achievement Test* (3rd ed.). Wilmington, DE: Wide Range.

Wilson, M. S., & Reschly, D. J. (1996). Assessment in school psychology training and practice. *School Psychology Review, 25,* 9–23.

Winterling, V. (1990). The effects of constant time delay, practice in writing or spelling, and reinforcement on sight word recognition in a small group. *Journal of Special Education, 24,* 101–116.

Witt, J. C. (1990). Complaining, precopernican thought, and the univariate linear mind: Questions for school-based behavioral consultation research. *School Psychology Review, 19,* 367–377.

Witt, J. C., & Elliott, S. N. (1983). Assessment in behavioral consultation: The initial interview. *School Psychology Review, 12,* 42–49.

Witt, J. C., & Elliott, S. N. (1985). Acceptability of classroom intervention strategies. In T. R. Kratochwill (Ed.), *Advances in school psychology* (Vol. IV, pp. 251–288). Hillsdale, NJ: Erlbaum.

Witt, J. C., Erchul, W. P., McKee, W. T., Pardue, M., & Wickstrom, K. F. (1991). Conversational control in school-based consultation: The relationship between consultant and consultee topic determination and consultation outcome. *Journal of Educational and Psychological Consultation, 2,* 101–116.

Witt, J. C., & Martens, B. K. (1983). Assessing the acceptability of behavioral interventions used in classrooms. *Psychology in the Schools, 20,* 510–517.

Wood, D. A., Rosenberg, M. S., & Carran, D. T. (1993). The effects of tape-recorded self-instruction cues on the mathematics performance of students with learning disabilities. *Journal of Learning Disabilities, 26,* 250–258, 269.

Wood, S. J., Murdock, J. Y., & Cronin, M. E. (2002). Self-monitoring and at-risk middle school students: Academic performance improves, maintains, and generalizes. *Behavior Modification, 26,* 605–626.

Woodcock, R. E., McGrew, K., & Mather, N. (2001). *Woodcock–Johnson III (WJ III) Tests of Achievement.* Allen, TX: Riverside.

Woodcock, R. W. (1987). *Woodcock Reading Mastery Tests—Revised.* Circle Pines, MN: American Guidance Service.

Woodcock, R. W. (1998). *Woodcock Reading Mastery Tests—Revised/Normative Update.* Circle Pines, MN: American Guidance Service.

Woodcock, R. W., & Muñoz-Sandoval, A. F. (1996). *Woodcock–Muñoz Language Survey/Normative Update.* Allen, TX: Riverside.

Xin, Y. P., Jitendra, A., Deatline-Buchman, A., Hickman, W., & Bertram, D. (2002). *A comparison of two instructional approaches on mathematical word problem solv-*

ing by students with learning problems (Eric Document Reproduction Service No. ED473061). Lafayette, IN: Purdue University.

Yopp, H. K. (1992). Developing phonemic awareness in young children. *Reading Teacher, 45,* 696–703.

Young, C., Hecimovic, A., & Salzberg, C. L. (1983). Tutor-tutee behavior of disadvantaged kindergarten children during peer tutoring. *Education and Treatment of Children, 6,* 123–135.

Young, K. R., West, R. P., Smith, D. J., & Morgan, D. P. (1991). *Teaching self-management strategies to adolescents.* Longmont, CO: Sopris West.

Ysseldyke, J. E., & Christenson, S. (1987). *The Instructional Environment Scale.* Austin, TX: Pro-Ed.

Ysseldyke, J. E., & Christenson, S. (1993). *TIES-II, the Instructional Environment System II.* Longmont, CO: Sopris West.

Ysseldyke, J. E., & Mirkin, P. E. (1982). The use of assessment information to plan instructional interventions: A review of the research. In C. R. Reynolds & T. B. Gutkin (Eds.), *The handbook of school psychology* (pp. 395–409). New York: Wiley.

Ysseldyke, J. E., Spicuzza, R., Kosciolek, S., & Boys, C. (2003). Effects of a learning information system on mathematics achievement and classroom structure. *Journal of Educational Research, 96,* 163–173.

Ysseldyke, J. E., Thurlow, M. L., Christenson, S. L., & McVicar, R. (1988). Instructional grouping arrangements used with mentally retarded, learning disabled, emotionally disturbed, and nonhandicapped elementary students. *Journal of Educational Research, 81,* 305–311.

Ysseldyke, J. E., Thurlow, M. L., Mecklenberg, C., Graden, J., & Algozzine, B. (1984). Changes in academic engaged time as a function of assessment and special education intervention. *Special Services in the Schools, 1*(2), 31–44.

Zigmond, N., & Miller, S. E. (1986). Assessment for instructional planning. *Exceptional Children, 52,* 501–509.

Zipprich, M. A. (1995). Teaching web making as a guided planning tool to improve student narrative writing. *Remedial and Special Education, 16,* 3–15.

Index

♦

"f" following a page number indicates a figure;
"t" following a table number indicates a table.